Medicinal Plants in Folk Tradition

AN ETHNOBOTANY OF BRITAIN & IRELAND

T0345365

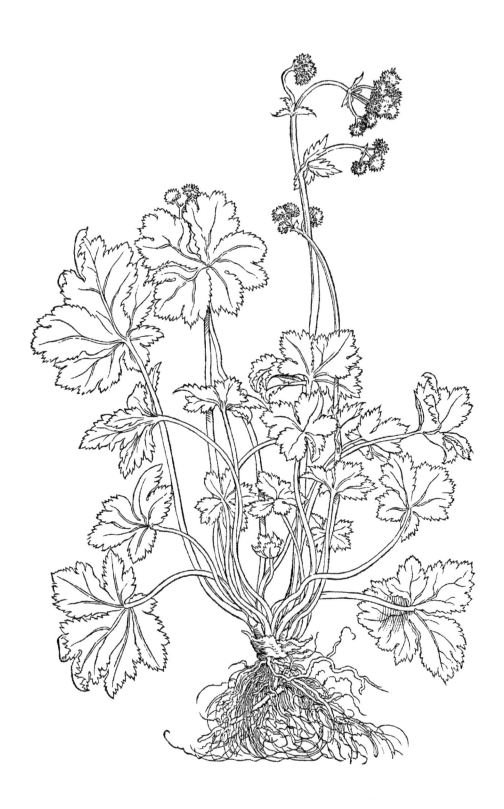

MEDICINAL PLANTS
in Folk Tradition

AN ETHNOBOTANY OF
BRITAIN & IRELAND

David E. Allen
&
Gabrielle Hatfield

Timber Press
Portland • London

The authors and publisher cannot accept any responsibility for any situation or problems which could arise from experimentation with any of the remedies mentioned in this book.

Page 2, *Sanicula europaea*, sanicle (Brunfels 1530, fig. 80).
Map, page 33, by Jamie Quinn and Elanor McBay, The Drawing Office, Department of Geography, University College London.

Published in 2004 by Timber Press, Inc.

The Haseltine Building
133 S.W. Second Avenue, Suite 450
Portland, Oregon 97204-3527, U.S.A.
timberpress.com

2 The Quadrant
135 Salusbury Road
London NW6 6RJ
timberpress.co.uk

Printed in the United States of America
ISBN 978-1-60469-429-1

The Library of Congress has previously cataloged the hardcover edition as follows:

Allen, David E.
    Medicinal plants in folk tradition : an ethnobotany of Britain & Ireland / David E. Allen and Gabrielle Hatfield.
        p.   cm.
    ISBN 0-88192-638-8 (hardcover)
    1. Ethnobotany—Great Britain. 2. Ethnobotany—Ireland. 3. Medicinal plants—Great Britain. 4. Medicinal plants—Ireland. 5. Traditional medicine—Great Britain. 6. Traditional medicine—Ireland. I. Hatfield, Gabrielle. II. Title.
GN585.G7 A45 2004
581.6'34'0941—dc22

                                                                2003019706

A catalog record for this book is also available from the British Library.

To Clare and John,
with love

Contents

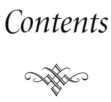

Preface

*S*o many people for so many years have been collecting and reporting the herbal remedies used by country folk that it must seem surprising that the resulting mass of data has not been brought together long since and surveyed overall. Certainly, it seemed surprising to the two of us, as interlopers from the world of botany. For more than a century and a half, records of where in Britain and Ireland each species of wild plant is known to occur (or have occurred) have been sedulously logged and published. So well established is this tradition that the regular disciplined effort that sustains it has come to be taken for granted. Unfortunately, the study of folklore failed to attract individuals with the necessary time and inclination to perform a similar service for records of plant use, and the magnitude of that task has increased with the passage of time.

The problem is not so much the quantity of the information that exists as its scattered nature. Much of it is in rare, privately published, often ephemeral printed sources, many of them concerned only peripherally with folk medicine. There are hardly any libraries that combine the necessary open access to their shelves with a sufficiently representative collection of seemingly relevant titles to allow research to be concentrated in just a single place. Worse, though, there is even more material remaining unpublished than has found its way into print, and extracting that in repositories that happen to be distant can be costly in time and money, especially when repeated visits are required. Doubtful plant identifications and obscure or vaguely described ailments, to say nothing of the Celtic languages, are further difficulties that may have to be wrestled with even after a productive source has been located.

Fortunately, the full arduousness of the undertaking that has culminated

11

in *Medicinal Plants in Folk Tradition: An Ethnobotany of Britain & Ireland* was not apparent at the outset, or it might well not have been attempted at all. Nor was it apparent at that time, now more than sixteen years ago, that other research and administrative commitments would shortly intervene and reduce it to a part-time activity and one with a far longer timescale than originally envisaged. To those who have assisted with the project in one way or another and have had so long to wait to see the fruits of that assistance in print, we can but apologise and thank them for their patience.

Among those to whom we are indebted more particularly, Sylvia Reynolds must be mentioned first and foremost. One of Ireland's leading field botanists, she could not have been a more appropriate choice for the lengthy and onerous task of sifting for herbal remedies the many volumes constituting the Schools' Manuscript Collection of the Department of Irish Folklore, University College Dublin. The key importance to the project of that source, without compare in its size and comprehensive geographical coverage, is abundantly clear in the following pages, and we are indebted to the head of department for his kind permission to publish data from it. Several past students of the department have similarly granted us permission to cite records drawn from their undergraduate essays and postgraduate theses. Both those and the Schools' Manuscript Collection proved to contain numerous problematical names in Irish, and we are further indebted to Mrs Reynolds and to Dr Nicolas Williams of Trinity College, University of Dublin, for the trouble they went to in seeking to identify the plants and ailments in question.

For generously giving us access to two other major manuscript collections, and granting permission to cite records contained in them, we also wish to thank Roy Vickery and Dr Anne E. Williams most warmly. The latter's data rectified what would have otherwise been a serious dearth of Welsh information. The survey from which those data come, 'Folk Medicine in Living Memory in Wales, 1977–89', was carried out under the auspices of the then Welsh Folk Museum (now the Museum of Welsh Life), one of the sections of the National Museums and Galleries of Wales, whose permission to publish these records is also gratefully acknowledged. Vickery's personal files of data on folklore, obtained in large part from correspondents, yielded many useful extra records, some of which have appeared in the periodical he founded and edits, *Plant-lore Notes and News*.

Professor J. D. A. Widdowson, Director of the Centre for English Cultural Tradition and Language (now the National Centre for English Cultural Tradition) of the University of Sheffield, similarly welcomed scrutiny of that institution's extensive files and kindly granted permission for data to be taken and published from some of the undergraduate theses they contain. Three individual items of special importance came to our notice in the archives of the Folklore Society in London, the Manx National Heritage Library in Douglas and the National Botanic Gardens in Dublin. We would like to thank Dr Larch Garrad and Miss Maura Scannell for their help in the last two connections, respectively, as well as in correspondence on Manx and Irish herbal use more generally. We are also grateful to the three institutions for permission to cite records from the manuscripts in question.

Four authorities on different groups of cryptogamic plants were kind enough to remedy our defective knowledge in those areas: Dr Francis Rose and Professor Mark Seaward provided useful leads on the herbal uses of lichens; Francis Rose and Professor Roy Watling identified the likeliest species concerned in particular cases, and Roy Watling and Jenny Moore were primarily instrumental in supplying the world distributions of the fungi and seaweeds, respectively. And we thank Dr Barrie Juniper for guidance on the taxonomy and distribution of apple species. D.E.A.'s colleagues in the then Academic Unit of the Wellcome Institute for the History of Medicine (now the Wellcome Trust Centre for the History of Medicine at University College London), in particular Professor Vivian Nutton and Dr Andrew Wear, were similarly helpful in identifying some of the obscurer ailments.

We both owe a deep debt to the Wellcome Trust for grant support of this work at different periods. Its *imperium in imperio,* the Wellcome Institute for the History of Medicine (as it was known until more recently), provided an ideal base and academic environment for D.E.A. throughout the years that the book has been in preparation, for which he is no less grateful. The University of East Anglia's Centre for East Anglian Studies similarly provided not only a base for G.H. for the duration of the research on the country remedies of that region, one of the foundation stones of this book, but also a supportive environment for what would otherwise have been a solitary endeavour.

The library of the Folklore Society has proved of the greatest assistance to D.E.A. during the years it has been housed in the D. M. S. Watson Library of University College London, so conveniently close to the Wellcome Building. Similarly, G.H. would like to pay tribute to the rich resources of the Norfolk Record Office and (until its untimely destruction by fire in 1994) the Local Studies Collection of Norwich Central Library.

For the illustrations we have the specialist skill of the photographers of the Wellcome Trust's Medical Photographic Library to thank, including Chris

Carter for the photographs of the authors. Those from medieval German herbals are reproduced from volumes in the magnificent collection of those in the Wellcome Library for the History and Public Understanding of Medicine. Hans Weiditz was the illustrator of the Brunfels (1530) herbal; Albrecht Meyer, the Fuchs (1543) herbal; and Emily Margaret Wood, the Green (1902) flora, whose drawings are reproduced here. We warmly thank Deni Bown for generously providing the colour photographs. The locating of information for the map of British and Irish county boundaries prior to the 1974 U.K. local government reorganisation came at the end of a very long search, for it turned out that libraries have thoughtlessly disposed of their atlases with maps of counties as they were before that period. The one that appears here is based on one produced for *A Reader's Guide to the Place-names of the United Kingdom,* edited by Jeffrey Spittal and John Field (1990), and we are grateful to the first-named editor and Shaun Tyas of Paul Watkins Publishing for permission to adapt it for our use.

Finally, Sylvia Reynolds and Roy Vickery placed us still further in their debt by reading the text in draft and making numerous helpful comments. We are no less grateful to Elizabeth Platts for also undertaking that major task.

We cannot close without thanking in the warmest terms the staff of Timber Press for unfailing helpfulness throughout the period of our association. It has been a great comfort to have a botanist for an editor and to know that our queries would receive answers from a background of publishing expertise combined with a wide knowledge of the two subjects that come together in ethnobotany. We also thank our spouses for their understanding and patience during the very long period the compiling and writing of the book has occupied our attention—and Clare more particularly for the key part she has played in the chain of communications.

G.H. would like to take this opportunity to thank D.E.A. publicly for his generosity in sharing with her what was originally his own project, and for allowing her to co-author this book, of which the lion's share of work was his.

CHAPTER 1

Herbs Without the Herbals:
Retracing a Lost Tradition

Medicinal Plants in Folk Tradition: An Ethnobotany of Britain & Ireland arose out of a conviction, arrived at by each of the authors independently, that the history of Western medicine as usually recounted suffers from a serious distortion as far as the use of herbal remedies is concerned. Written on the assumption that it is only through the study of surviving texts that the medical practices of the past can be reconstructed, that history has been conceived in terms of tracing the gradual diffusion of written knowledge from the ancient civilisations around the shores of the Mediterranean. Because the texts were originally written in Greek or Latin (though many had been preserved in Arabic), it was the practices of the Classical world, seen through these texts, on which historians concentrated. The story of the rise of Western medicine has been carried forward through the herbals of the Dark Ages to the eventual selective filtering of that received body of learning and its culmination, after various false turnings, in the professional practices of today.

That version has two major flaws. The first is that it overlooks the fact that the herbal expertise of the Classical world was based primarily on the flora of the Mediterranean basin and its vicinity. The Greeks and Romans had little or no knowledge of what grew in the colder and wetter parts of Europe and probably saw few if any of the plants restricted to those different climates. Away from the Mediterranean, their herbals consequently had at best only a limited relevance, a fact which their successors were for many centuries in no position to realise.

The second major flaw in that standard version of the history of Western medicine is that it ignores the traditional use of local plant remedies on which the main mass of people depended for everyday first aid. Mostly illiterate and with a herbal repertory built up over the generations by trial and error, they neither knew nor cared about the Classical authorities. As their knowledge was transmitted by word of mouth, it is almost unrepresented in the written record until the nineteenth century.

Although it can be assumed that Greek and Roman colonists took their herbal knowledge wherever they went, the extent to which it became incorporated into the ordinary domestic practices of those among whom they settled is very hard to determine. In the colder parts of Europe many Mediterranean plants would have been difficult or impossible to cultivate. The raw material for those remedies would therefore have had to be imported in dried form if it was to be available at all. Imports, however, by reason of the distance they had to be brought and the risks they had to survive, would have been costly and available only to the relatively well-off. On the outer reaches of the Empire the proportion of their herbal heritage that the Romans would have had access to was small, their pharmacopoeia bearing little resemblance to its native Mediterranean richness in that respect. To make up for this deficiency, borrowing from the locals is likely to have taken place. Unfortunately, archaeological excavation throws little light on the extent of this. One purely medicinal plant of presumptively Roman introduction, the greater celandine, *Chelidonium majus,* has been detected in settlement remains of that period in two places in the south of England and Wales; of the many other species that have been identified from Romano-British levels, though, there is none whose presence can be attributed unequivocally to therapeutic use.

After the Romans left Britain, the medical practices they had introduced were perpetuated by the early Christian Church. A reminder of how much further within the British Isles that alien Romanised culture was later diffused is provided by the lingering presence down to this day of elecampane, *Inula helenium,* around early monastic sites in Ireland and on islets off the Irish and Manx coasts.[1] This plant is probably a native of central Asia, and had the dual attraction of being a subsistence food as well as a source of medicine. It owed its spread across Europe entirely to human favour, and once planted, it could indefinitely survive the competition of natural vegetation and grazing by animals.

A second influx of alien herbs, or at least novel uses of herbs already present, is perhaps attributable to the waves of Germanic immigrants who settled in Britain, especially in England, in the post-Roman era. The one Anglo-Saxon medical text written in the vernacular that survives, known to scholars as *Leechbook III*,[2] provides evidence of a northern European herbal tradition substantially distinct from that of the Romans and presumably independent in its origins. But how far did that tradition retain a discrete identity once transported to a country with its own well-rooted body of herbal knowledge? That solitary text could have been an attempt to set down 'best practice' in the eyes of just a conservative minority, and its prescriptions may not be representative of the behaviour of Anglo-Saxon society more generally. It may even be a treasured relic of a time before that immigrant tradition had begun to lose its coherence—or conceivably before that immigration had even taken place. If plant remains unearthed in Denmark[3] are anything to go by, at least by the Viking Age herbal cultures on both sides of the North Sea had much in common, and species of known Roman origin such as greater celandine had been to all appearances assimilated.

However great or small that northern influence may have been, it was essentially southwards, to the legacy of Rome, that the monasteries looked in the following centuries. Classical texts copied and recopied and copied yet again, frequently undergoing corruption in the process, increasingly filled their libraries. The herbs were crudely depicted and all too briefly described— if described at all—and were hopefully matched as far as possible with plants growing locally. Literacy, a near-monopoly of the monks, had become largely identified with the ability to translate and imbibe the writings of Classical authors, that body of ancient wisdom and experience deemed superior to any contemporary equivalent. Literacy at the same time conferred upon its possessors a privileged apartness, an apartness which could be placed at risk by giving credence to practices and beliefs unsanctioned by Classical authority. Among these were the remedies that the unlettered peasantry derived from plants that grew around them in the wild.

The eventual advent of herbals with illustrations painted or etched direct from nature improved matters only slightly. They were still accessible only to the few, as rare as they were expensive and with texts normally in Latin. John Gerard's much-celebrated *Herball* of 1597 was exceptional in this latter respect. It seems to have been intended by its barber-surgeon author to serve also as a practical guide for those fellow members of the lowlier ranks of the medical fraternity who were not above going into the fields and woods in search of their own raw material. From his personal knowledge, Gerard gave directions to particular places in England where some of the scarcer herbs could be found. What he did not make clear, though, and possibly did not realise, was that almost exactly half the plants covered in his work cannot be found in the wild in Britain—and many were probably not even available in the best-stocked of the country's physic gardens at that period. Either Gerard or his publisher could not resist trying to appeal to an international readership, for by re-using a set of woodcuts made for a previous Dutch herbal the work was given a spuriously pan-European appearance that was at odds with its England-oriented text. Gerard's own contributions to field botany are overlaid by the customary farrago of Classical lore topped up with the assertions of a miscellany of later learned authors. Consequently, the work emerges as an awkward hybrid between a pioneer field manual and a run-of-the-mill encyclopaedia for fellow practitioners. For all its promise of opening up herbal expertise to a now much-enlarged literate lay public, Gerard's volume was still emphatically a work by a member of the medical profession, addressed to fellow professionals. Only rarely are there patronizing mentions of 'the common people' or 'the country people' and of certain remedies used by them. And that attitude was shared by leading non-medical authors even of the stature of John Ray. Science was still struggling to free itself from folk beliefs, and those who wished to be seen as serious students had to distance themselves from anything redolent of older ways of thinking.

The herbals indeed were trebly misleading. They reflected the general conspiracy of silence among the learned about the extent and efficacy of folk medicine; they gave indiscriminate endorsement to just about every alleged plant virtue that had ever appeared in print; and they were written largely in obliviousness of the differences imposed by geography which make the flora of one region dissimilar from that of another. Until the seventeenth century, at the earliest, the natural distributions of Europe's indigenous plants were little known. The same was true of the range in climate and soil types that each plant could tolerate. It was natural, as well as very convenient, to assume that most of Europe had inherited the same broad legacy of natural herbal wealth.

The Columbian rediscovery of the New World and the opening up of trade with the Indies were to alter the picture profoundly, though not wholly for the better. The great influx of new drugs that resulted from this trade further widened the gulf between learned practitioners and the majority of the people—three-fifths as far as England was concerned—who continued to live in rural isolation, away from even the smallest settlement worthy of being called a town. The very fact that these remedies were novel and came from far away allowed premium prices to be charged, leaving them way out of general reach. As John Parkinson tartly observed in his 1640 *Theatrum Botanicum*, 'Men more willingly spend their cost on strange things fetch from farre, than upon their owne hombred and country plants.'[4] Most people did not have this choice; they had to use their own home-bred remedies or nothing.

By the seventeenth century a few were questioning the advisability of taking such profoundly alien remedies. The poet George Herbert warned the country parson and his wife to steer clear of the 'outlandish gums' of the city and seek their remedies in their gardens and fields, 'for home-bred medicines are both more easy for the parsons purse, and more familiar for all mens bodyes.'[5] In such protests an element of national pride is detectable as well. William Coles in *The Art of Simpling* held the maidenhair of Britain, *Adiantum capillus-veneris?*, 'never a whit inferior to the Assyrian', just as 'our Gentian is as good as that which is brought from beyond sea' and 'our Angelica . . . as that of Norway and Ireland [Iceland?]'.[6] Some believed that the rearrangement of nature caused by importing plants was going against Divine intention. This point was well made in an 'advertisement' inserted by Thomas Johnson (1636) by way of a postscript to his edition of Gerard's *Herball*:

> I verily believe that the divine Providence had a care in bestowing
> plants in each part of the earth, fitting and convenient to the fore-
> knowne necessities of the future inhabitants; and if wee throughly
> knew the vertues of these, we needed no Indian nor American drugges.[7]

Johnson could be accused of self-interest in advancing this view since his uniquely extensive first-hand knowledge of Britain's native flora was now in danger of being rendered obsolete. However, his opinion was probably honestly held.

Ironically, the discovery of such an unsuspected diversity of valuable plant-based drugs in distant parts of the world eventually led to the notion that Britain's own little-known hinterland might have something of the same kind to offer as well. To this extent the alien influx had a beneficial side effect. Folk medicine was at last to be taken seriously in progressive learned quarters.

The first sign of this major change of heart was the dispatching in 1695 of Martin Martin on a general research inspection of Scotland's Western Isles. A resident of that region as factor to the laird of Macleod, Martin owed this commission to some leading figures in the then-burgeoning Scottish Enlightenment in Edinburgh, one of whom, Archibald Pitcairne, ensured that enquiring about remedies in use was included in the brief. Martin's conscientious, refreshingly non-judgemental coverage of that aspect in his subsequent report is outstanding in its value today, not just on account of its early date but also because most of the remedies he came across appear to have fallen into disuse during the following century. In 1772 the Rev. John Light-foot, who accompanied the non-botanical Thomas Pennant on his tour of much the same region, came back with a much more slender haul, confirming Martin's information in only one or two respects (though admittedly, medicine was not his primary interest). Though there were to be no comparably ambitious expeditions in which the noting of folk remedies was a significant feature, the precedent had been set for making at least some mention of these in the many accounts of gentlemen's tours to various parts of Britain that thereafter became a publishing vogue.

Meanwhile on the international scene it was becoming increasingly fashionable in medical circles to investigate some of the long-disdained herbs of the backwoods, in the hope that there might after all be at least a kernel of truth in their claims to cure. Advances in chemical knowledge provided a spur to this. In 1746, bemoaning that so few of his fellow practitioners 'now know the common virtues of our own herbs', a Sheffield physician, Thomas Short, published a treatise expressly for their benefit on those herbal species 'generally to be found in the fields or gardens in Great-Britain'.[8] Yet it was not a member of that profession at all but a country parson, the Rev. Thomas Stone, who ten years later brought to medical attention the properties of a species of willow, *Salix alba*, and opened up the path that would eventually lead to the multi-purpose aspirin. It is ironic, too, that this discovery and the even more epoch-making one by William Withering that followed twenty years later were both made in the English Midlands, virtually on the back-doorstep of the College of Physicians. Withering's confirming of the folk reputation long enjoyed by the foxglove, *Digitalis purpurea*, as a remedy for heart trouble was an historic addition to the armoury of orthodox medicine. And it could not have been achieved had Withering not been alert to the possibility already and possessed the necessary training and insight for the lengthy series of experiments that transformed a hunch into proof. He might not have made the discovery in the first place had he not taken up botany as a leisure pursuit some five or six years earlier. Just as important in this context is the fact that the three-volume, widely bought manual on Britain's flowering plants that he went on to produce had observations on their medical potential as one of its notable features.

Thanks particularly to Withering, and to the fashionable interest in botany among the cultivated classes at that period, at least some mention of the folk usage of appropriate species became *de rigueur* in published catalogues of the wild flora. Several of those had doctors for their authors—and not always for reasons that one might suppose. *Flora Sarisburiensis,* for instance, was produced by the head of the Salisbury Infirmary, Henry Smith, from a notion that was unashamedly economic: 'Every saving of expensive medicines in hospital practice is in these days important, and particularly so when an equally efficacious and much cheaper [one] can be introduced.'[9] There were substitutes to be had for free in the countryside round about, and the primary purpose of his book was to stimulate their collection by enabling some of the more useful ones to be identified.

That favourable trend was massively reinforced by the Apothecaries' Act of 1815, which required all medical students wishing to be licenced to practise in England or Wales—and thus comprising many graduates of Scottish medical schools as well—to pass an exam that included a test of herbal knowledge. The act established botany firmly within the medical curriculum and for at least a generation afterwards produced a good many practitioners who retained that subject as a hobby, especially if they went to live in a country area. Some of these naturally made a note of the rustic remedies they encountered, resulting in local lists of exceptional value because of their above-average botanical precision. The publications of Dr George Johnston on Berwickshire are doubly valuable in view of the shortage of herbal information for the whole of lowland Scotland. Several of his counterparts in rural Ireland, where folk cures were particularly prominent, also made noteworthy contributions—as indeed country doctors have continued to do, in Britain as well, long after the disappearance of botany from the medical curricula.

The second half of the nineteenth century saw a complementary surge of lay interest in what till then had passed under the name of 'popular antiquities', part of a wider antiquarianism that had led up to the Romantic Movement and been boosted by that. By 1846 that interest was sufficiently widespread and distinctive to have 'folk-lore' coined for it.[10] The field collecting of the folklorists in the decades that followed was unsystematic and rarely informed by much botanical knowledge, but it served to show that the number of remedies still surviving, if only in the memories of the aged, was very much greater than generally supposed. Unfortunately, though, there were no moves to collate all the data for Britain and Ireland, as Hewett Cottrell Watson and his imitators were doing so impressively in several branches of natural history. Thus the mass of information collected was deprived of effect by remaining fragmentary and, too often, by being published obscurely. It was not until the 1930s, and then only in Ireland, that the first large-scale systematic survey at a national level was carried out.

Long after that nineteenth-century ample harvest of herbal data had been gathered, historians continued to dismiss folk medicine as having little or no relevance to the rise of the Western medical tradition. Many were reluctant to accept that in a highly developed country like Britain it consisted of anything other than cultural detritus. As late as the 1960s, Charles Singer, a much-respected authority, dismissed it as 'usually medieval or renaissance medicine misunderstood'.[11] A more general reason why historians largely ignored it was that, being an oral tradition, it has left next to nothing in the way of documentary evidence for scholars to study. Until the advent of oral history, following the spread of tape recorders, the belief that the past could be safely reconstructed only from written records had the force of gospel. Till then, historians were happy to leave cross-questioning of the illiterate to folklorists and anthropologists. For the same reasons, glimpses of folk medicine available in such sources as folk tales, ballads and proverbs received little serious attention from them either.

Yet even among folklorists, interest in herbal remedies has been marginalised. Compared with the tales, rituals and superstitions that form the staple of their study, herbs and their uses are a discordantly down-to-earth matter, a kind of primitive science, more akin perhaps to folk *life*—that separate study of such practical matters as farming methods and the layout of cottages. Lack of botanical knowledge among folklorists has been a further reason for their neglecting this area, for it is awkward to make enquiries about herbal remedies unless one can recognise by name the plants concerned.

Until all the scraps of folk medical information collected in the ways described have been collated and presented as a whole, it will be impossible to convince historians or other scholars of their worth and importance. The main aim of this book is to provide such a corpus. The body of information that has resulted is so substantial, and involves such a high proportion of our native flora, that it is hard to avoid the conclusion that it represents a full-scale tradition of its own. In order for so much to have survived, this tradition must have retained its own identity, existing alongside the learned medical tradition of the literate population but keeping its basic essence.

It is highly likely that some form of medicine existed in this part of Europe from the time of its first inhabitants. All known primitive peoples possess a mixture of rituals and natural therapies to cope with injury and pain, those pressing realities on a par with hunger and death. Even apes have been observed eating particular leaves for their apparent therapeutic effect. By the time the Romans settled in Britain, one or more medical systems of considerable sophistication and stability were probably already established and would have been highly resistant to alien traditions. The more remote parts of Britain and Ireland have remained out of contact with towns and cities until the eighteenth or nineteenth century at the earliest and would have proved largely impenetrable by new ideas. Such was the degree of isolation of many smaller islands in particular that few had any resident medical practitioner even in the mid-Victorian period. In such areas, where the inhabitants had to be medically self-reliant, ancestral practices had an especially good chance of surviving, particularly if, like the herbal ones, they met compelling needs and seemed to have a basis in more than superstition.

To present a picture of a solid mass of herbal lore coming down unaltered from prehistoric times would, however, be unrealistic. Unquestionably, over the years much modification must have taken place. Irrespective of the infiltration of alien remedies from outside sources, particularly through the influence of the Church, there would have been processes at work internally that continually brought about change. Many folk cures remain the treasured property of individual families, or of individual 'wise men' and 'wise women'. They are passed on by word and deed from one generation to the next, but when a supply of suitable successors dies out, that line of knowledge is lost. There may in addition have been elements of secrecy involved. This was particularly the case where an individual set him or herself up as a local healer and made a living from dispensing cures. Even where no material rewards were involved, there may have been a strong motivation for women in particular to keep very quiet about their knowledge or risk being branded as witches. A less important factor inducing secrecy was the conviction that the power to cure certain ailments would be lost if communicated to someone else. In the sphere of wart-charming this belief persists to this day. However, it is probable that within a community much herbal knowledge was shared despite not being written down.

Even though innately conservative, folk medicine would have changed and evolved over the years, replacing older remedies with newly discovered ones or remedies borrowed from other sources. As learned medicine extended its sway, interchange between the two traditions must surely have increased. By the thirteenth century, for instance, it had been received into the depths of Carmarthenshire by the physicians of Myddvai[12] and taken to Scotland's Western Isles by the no less renowned Beaton dynasty in the sixteenth.[13] This interchange must have accelerated as populations grew, mobility increased and there was less reluctance to try the unfamiliar. Nicholas Culpeper's *Lon-*

don Dispensatory of 1649, William Buchan's *Domestic Medicine* of 1769 and other books that sought to break the secrecy cultivated by the physicians and make the best-available medical guidance accessible to the populace in general may well have furthered the process. Information probably moved in both directions, from country to city and *vice versa*. Robert Boyle produced his *Medicinal Experiments* of 1692 'chiefly for the use of those that live in the Country, in Places where Physicians are scarce, if at all to be had, especially by Poor People'; John Wesley's more famous *Primitive Physic* of 1747 was written expressly from that motive, too. By the eighteenth century the itinerant chapman with his stock of books that so often included a herbal had become a familiar figure in rural areas. The long-established trade of gathering herbs from the wild for sale in city markets or to apothecaries and druggists also began to expand to such proportions that it constituted a major threat to the local survival of some plant species as well as a serious nuisance to the owners of the land on which they grew.

The influences for change within folk medicine were gathering pace. As land enclosure led to increased rural poverty and migration to cities and towns, communities and their traditions were fragmented. Massive emigrations to North America increased this fragmentation, especially of the rural traditions of Scotland and Ireland. For the Irish, the physical severance from country ways that resulted was so abrupt and wholesale that their traditional herbal lore must inevitably have been largely forgotten. The Scots, on the other hand, had some chance of preserving their traditional herbal remedies in rural eastern Canada, where the native flora was fairly similar to the one they had left behind. The early colonists in North America had taken a selection of herbs along with them, but because many of them came from urban Britain, that selection could have been drawn only in part at best from the folk medical tradition.

Even before the nineteenth century, British folk medicine had lost much of its diversity. The folk uses of many plants recorded by sixteenth- and seventeenth-century writers were not heard of again. If so much had been lost so early, then what was lost subsequently must have been great indeed.

Yet the story has not been entirely one of loss. Uses of the more versatile herbs have proliferated, though on what scale it is hard to tell with such incomplete records. Additional herbs were also brought into service. Two that were demonstrably recruited since 1860 feature in the following pages: pineapple-weed, *Matricaria discoidea,* and Hottentot-fig, *Carpobrotus edulis* and *C. acinaciformis,* natives respectively of north-eastern Asia and South

Africa which are known to have joined the wild flora of these islands some-time after.

Such gains apart, however, the period since 1800 can hardly have been kind to the folk tradition as far as Britain has been concerned (with Ireland it has been a different matter). The eighteenth-century wave of new respect for folk medicine as a repository of potential extra weapons in the armoury of learned medicine failed to last. So many alternatives of proven value poured in from all around the globe that searching so close to home no longer seemed worth the effort. Though professional herbalism was sent under-ground by legislation secured by the orthodox medical community, it soon enjoyed a resurgence in the guise of physiomedicalism, a re-import from North America (along with some North American plant usage). That was too alien a development, however, to affect folk tradition significantly. Rus-tic remedies consequently disappeared once again into obscurity, becoming survivals from the past to be appreciated by the learned merely for their quaintness. The national health services, providing free treatments of appar-ent reliability and potency, finally brought to a rapid end what remained of a living tradition.

The main purpose of *Medicinal Plants in Folk Tradition: An Ethnobotany of Britain & Ireland* is to demonstrate that a large enough body of evidence has survived to show that the folk medical tradition was impressively wide in its botanical reach and equally impressive in the range of ailments it treated. Many of the plants recorded within this tradition, even some of them that were used over wide areas, do not appear in the herbals. This lends strong support to the idea that the rural tradition retained much of its autonomy through the centuries and was substantially self-sufficient.

Folk medicine had, of course, its limitations. The complaints treated on the whole were necessarily relatively minor: coughs, colds, burns, skin com-plaints, aches and pains, the staple of today's doctor's consulting room. Some of its exponents could heal broken limbs, some would even treat tumours, but few went as far as surgery. For all its limitations, however, folk medicine does not deserve all the contempt heaped upon it by followers of learned medicine. It probably did less harm overall, and may even have been more effective, than all their bleeding and purging.

However, the effectiveness or otherwise of folk medicine is not a prof-itable area for discussion. Hardly any of its remedies have yet been subjected to randomised double-blind trials, the only testing method recognised by the medical profession today as conclusive. Most of the claims made for them will remain unproven until more work is done or new approaches formulated. On the whole, those claims are in any case hardly extravagant ones. At a common-sense level, who will want to disbelieve that members of the mint family, the Lamiaceae, contain substances that ease coughing, for example? Or how can anyone reasonably question that such a readily observable effect as an increased flow of urine resulting from eating the leaves of dandelions (*Taraxacum officinale*) or the young tops of broom (*Cytisus scoparius*)? But as the detailed practical instructions for gathering and preparing the remedies have in many cases been lost, misinterpretations can and do arise. Herbs boiled for too long or stored in the wrong conditions can lose their potency. Individual plants within a species may vary in their chemical constituents with the type of environment, the season and even the time of day. Most species have genetically distinct populations as well, another source of chemical variation.

Patients, too, have their individual reactions: where some are hypersensitive, others may be immune. Some medicines, particularly herbal ones, work too subtly and slowly to convince the impatient of their effectiveness and are discontinued prematurely. Many minor illnesses are self-limiting, and the results of any treatment may in these cases be irrelevant. Symptoms can come and go regardless of any cures claimed for them; warts, for example, may eventually disappear with or without any intervention. Above all, there is the placebo effect: faith in the treatment itself may help effect a cure, especially if it includes a prescribed element of ritual, such as reciting a familiar prayer backwards or wearing some substance in a bag about one's person.

Because of all these uncertainties, deliberately little is said about this aspect in these pages. That a remedy is mentioned should not be taken as endorsement of its effectiveness. Similarly, the mention of a particular ailment does not imply any judgement as to the accuracy of the diagnosis; it is merely what the person relating or recording it supposed it to be. Given the looseness of folk terminology, attempting to bring that into line with modern medical usage is too full of pitfalls to be a sensible procedure in most cases. An exception has been made for obsolete terms that have unambiguous modern equivalents: 'chincough' has been translated into whooping cough (pertussis), for instance, and 'St Anthony's fire' into erysipelas.

Plant identifications are a further major source of uncertainties. Users of country remedies do not make such fine distinctions as botanists, so related species that look broadly similar—most of the St John's-worts (*Hypericum*), for instance—tend to pass as all one and the same. That is unlikely to matter unless beneath the outward similarity there are substantial differences in chemical potency, as could well be the case with willows (*Salix*) or mints of the genus *Mentha,* for example; information on that score, however, is at present mainly lacking. More seriously, in the lowlier and more obscure sections of the plant world, separation of species is by and large not attempted and nothing more enlightening than 'grass' or 'moss' too often features in the folk medicine records. But this last may be just as much the fault of the collectors of folk remedies themselves, unskilled as so many of them are in field botany. That also helps to explain why there is so much tedious repetition in the records of remedies so common that they must surely be well known already (such as the use of dock leaves for stings). It is far easier to note down those than probe for ones involving plants unfamiliar to the collector.

It is vernacular names, though, that cause most problems. These can bear little or no relation to the ones used in books for the plants in question, and they may be peculiar just to a single area or even a single household. The same name can be shared by several plants that are unrelated. Conversely, one species may have accumulated a large number of country names down the centuries; for the red campion (*Silene dioica*) more than sixty English-language ones have been recorded from Britain and Ireland, and the Celtic languages could produce still more.

A problem special to a primarily oral study is the mishearing of names, especially if they are ones unfamiliar to the enquirer. This may account for the existence of some that have defeated all attempts to identify the plant referred to—they are perhaps just ghosts, without any substance in the first place. Mishearings are all the more likely to occur when enquirers are unfamiliar not only with the name but with the local accent or even the language in which it is told to them. Many of the names borne by plants in Ireland or the Scottish Highlands are Gaelic ones that have been garbled in the process of being written down, like so many of the place-names there. Gaelic speakers, equipped to recognise sounds that may have occasioned misunderstandings in transmission, have fortunately proved able to supply identifications in the case of many records which would otherwise have had to be omitted from this work.

Inherent in this field of study there is also an altogether more fundamental difficulty. The more developed a country becomes, the ever less obvious the distinction that remains between its folk medicine in the sense of the aboriginal, underlying layer of folk medicine practices and beliefs and the increasingly hybrid entity superimposed on that, the product of multiple intrusive influences. The difficulty is exactly comparable with that faced by botanists in trying to distinguish pristine vegetation from that altered by humans, often unintentionally and in some cases so subtly that only an expert eye can detect the manipulation that has occurred. Just as there is the greatest likelihood of pristine vegetation surviving in remote places, so one looks to similar areas to find folk culture at its least contaminated. Collectors of folk medicine have naturally concentrated on such areas, and they have indeed proved rich in herbal lore. In the nineteenth century much collecting was done in the Shetlands and the Isle of Man, while Hebridean lore is well represented in the records from a range of periods. In addition, large-scale primary surveys of Wales and the greater part of Ireland within living memory have made outstandingly valuable contributions to our knowledge of folk herbal medicine. Between them, these provide a good comparative basis for reconstructing the salient features of the plant-based therapies that formerly reigned more or less unchallenged in the north and west of the British Isles. In turn, these data provide a means of disentangling what is putatively indigenous from what is seemingly intrusive from other cultures and sectors of society.

Outside that belt of presumptively minimal contact, the disentangling becomes much more difficult. The problems arise not only from the length of time over which different traditions have mingled but also from the ambiguity of the very term folk. For some this is synonymous with the practices of the least-educated layer of the rural population, practices which have been passed down largely or wholly by word of mouth. For others it embraces the equivalent social layer in the towns and cities as well. Still others seem to equate the term with any system outside the bounds of orthodox, official medicine, sweeping into that capacious category commercial herbalism of every kind and every degree of sophistication, including imports like Thomsonianism and, ultimately, even homoeopathy. Michael Moloney's *Irish Ethno-botany* of 1919 is an example of the third kind. Despite its title, the temptingly long list of remedies turns out on close examination to be an only partly differentiated *mélange* drawn from herb-based systems of a variety of kinds, for which reason it needs to be approached with great caution (the more so as it includes some obviously erroneous plant identifications as well). Unfortunately, many other published lists conceal their suspected hybrid character more successfully. Much information derived from learned medicine, in however an indirect and attenuated form, has been unwittingly incorporated as a result into published accounts of ostensibly folk usage. That process has been so widespread that the two traditions are now inextricably and irremediably mixed in the literature. All that it is possible to do is to indicate instances where, on the balance of probability, a particular record appears to belong to one tradition rather than the other. This has accordingly been done in the pages that follow. In cases where the folk credentials of a species as a whole seem doubtful, this has been indicated by introducing the text of the entry with '(Folk credentials questionable)' or '(Folk credentials lacking)'. In other instances, reservations are expressed in the body of the text. The same course has been followed wherever a plant identification is judged either wrong or at least open to question, and if a species as a whole is judged to have been misidentified, the text of its entry is introduced with '(Identification dubious)', '(Name ambiguity suspected)' or something similar.

Because so much that has appeared on paper about the use of plants for medicine has been written in ignorance of these different ways in which 'folk' has been understood and the composite character of the term as a result, very little of the printed literature is safe to draw upon for reconstruction of the folk tradition. The herbals have to be firmly disregarded except in so far as they explicitly identify a few uses as those of the rustic or unlettered. For the same reason, the remarkable number of household books of remedies that survive in the countries' archives have regretfully had to be set aside, too. A high proportion of the remedies these contain are probably folk ones, and it may eventually be possible to identify which those are; attaining the level of expertise necessary for that still lies in the future, though.

Besides steering clear of so much of the published literature, it has also seemed advisable to treat very circumspectly information relating to herbs grown in gardens, even if they are cottage gardens. In many cases the herbs may have been transplanted from the wild, so their use is little different from going out into the countryside to collect them as required. In many more cases, though, such plants will have originated exclusively from cultivated stocks and probably owe their presence to recommendations in the herbals. Some of the best-known garden herbs do not feature in these pages in view of this.

Finally, deliberately little or nothing has been said about the marked revival of interest in the therapeutic potential of wild plants that has taken place in the West from World War II onwards. It is difficult to open a newspaper these days without being reminded that roughly half the world's pharmaceutical products in use today are plant-derived. Yet most of this recent wave of research has focused on the floras of the tropics. The herbal potential of Europe and other temperate regions has been relatively neglected, perhaps in the belief that it can have little more to offer after so many centuries of empirical use. But if we assume that over the millennia the users of country remedies have experimented with all the wild plants around them, we would probably be wrong. There is a notable lack of folk remedies drawn from some groups of common plants, such as the legumes (the Fabaceae). Perhaps a plant needed some tangible scent or taste to encourage experimentation. Those groups omitted from the folk record may have been rejected as inactive or may simply not have been tried at all. There is still much to be learned from native plant medicines of Britain and Ireland, and it is hoped that this book may provide some leads to further remedies worthy of closer investigation.

Notes

1. Praeger, 155; Webb & Scannell, 110; L. S. Garrad, in litt.
2. Cockayne 1864–6; Grattan & Singer 1952
3. Robinson 1994
4. Parkinson, 947
5. Herbert, 82
6. Coles 1656, 52
7. Johnson 1636, unnumbered last page
8. Short 1746, ix
9. Smith, 8 verso
10. Dorson, 1
11. Singer, i, xlvii
12. Williams ab Ithel; Turner & Turner 1983
13. Anon. 1906; MacFarlane; Comrie, i, 23–4

CHAPTER 2

Introduction to the Compendium of Uses

The compendium in the following chapters lists all the folk medical uses traced for plants growing wild in Britain, Ireland or the Isle of Man. Some domestic uses, such as in pest control and cosmetics, are also included. Veterinary uses are the subject of a more concise list in the Appendix. Though fungi have been shown to be more animal than vegetable, and lichens as part-fungi share that character in some measure, they have traditionally been regarded as plants, for which reason it seemed appropriate to include them.

Excluded from coverage are (i) the Channel Islands, which though part of the British Isles in the strict geographical sense have inherited very different, essentially French folk traditions, (ii) all uses identified with Romany or other more recent immigrant peoples with folk herbal traditions based on floras substantially or wholly different from those of Britain and Ireland, and (iii) all uses of plants not accepted as indigenous to those two islands or not established in them in the wild in sufficient enduring quantity to have been capable of serving as genuinely folk herbs (which thus excludes a high proportion of plants that feature in medieval and early modern herbals).

Geographical Areas

As far as the evidence permits, records are cited in terms of counties, the smallest administrative unit to which the greatest number of records can be tied. As far as Britain is concerned, though, the counties for the purposes of *Medicinal Plants in Folk Tradition: An Ethnobotany of Britain & Ireland* are the ones that preceded the radical changes that accompanied the local government reorganisation of 1974, as they were the ones obtaining (with only minor boundary adjustments) throughout all but a tiny part of the period to which the records in the following pages relate. Note that the -shire ending was at one time borne by some English counties, such as Devon and Dorset, but latterly fell into disuse. Though the Irish county boundaries also underwent numerous adjustments in 1898, none of those was sizeable enough to have affected the assignment of the records in this book. An exception has had to be allowed for certain records from the Lake District and its environs that have failed to distinguish between the different components of Cumberland, Westmorland and the isolated part of Lancashire sometimes distinguished as Furness; for these, the post-1974 'Cumbria' has had to do duty instead. Exceptions have also been made for (i) island groups, such as Scilly, that enjoy a distinctiveness even though formally part of a county and (ii) individual islands of the far-extending Hebrides in view of the great differences in size and location of these.

'The border' in Irish contexts refers to the political line separating the six counties constituting the U.K. portion of the province of Ulster from the Irish Republic. 'The Borders' is a vague term for the physical borderland between England and Scotland. East Anglia is a collective term for the counties of Norfolk and Suffolk only, an area broadly coterminous with the one-time Anglo-Saxon kingdom of this name, strictly speaking, but commonly used in a vaguer and broader sense. Eastern Counties is East Anglia in the strict sense plus the several counties immediately to the west and south of those. Galloway is a collective term for Wigtownshire and Kirkcudbrightshire. South Wales refers to the southernmost Welsh counties of Monmouthshire (now Gwent), Glamorganshire and Carmarthenshire. For records regarded as lacking that specificity, the vaguer 'southern Wales' has been used.

Some records exist just for a city or for a well-marked topographical region, such as the Fens of East Anglia, that cannot be identified with one county alone, and there is no alternative but to repeat those designations. Particularly regrettable is the use of an undifferentiated 'Highlands' for a large proportion of the records from the vast northern half of Scotland, a term which may or may not embrace the Inner and Outer Hebrides (*alias* the Western Isles) as well. More vaguely still, 'the north [of Britain]' may be all that one is told; but that is thankfully rare.

To save space, the 'Co.' conventionally employed before the names of many Irish counties has been omitted, except in the case of Co. Dublin, in order to avoid confusion with Dublin city.

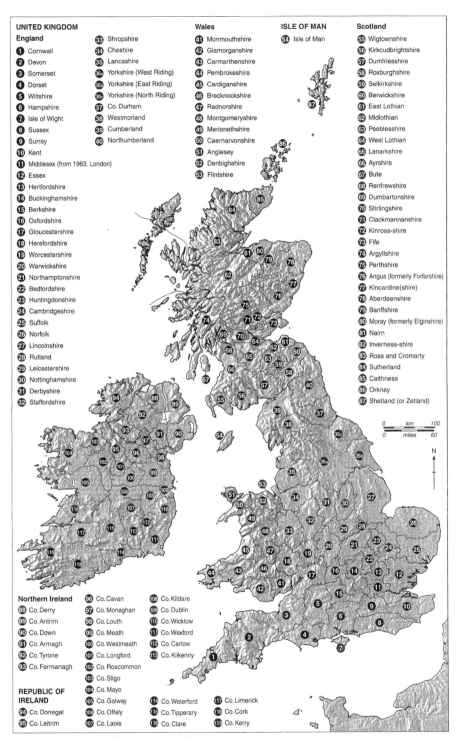

UNITED KINGDOM

England

1. Cornwall
2. Devon
3. Somerset
4. Dorset
5. Wiltshire
6. Hampshire
7. Isle of Wight
8. Sussex
9. Surrey
10. Kent
11. Middlesex (from 1963, London)
12. Essex
13. Hertfordshire
14. Buckinghamshire
15. Berkshire
16. Oxfordshire
17. Gloucestershire
18. Herefordshire
19. Worcestershire
20. Warwickshire
21. Northamptonshire
22. Bedfordshire
23. Huntingdonshire
24. Cambridgeshire
25. Suffolk
26. Norfolk
27. Lincolnshire
28. Rutland
29. Leicestershire
30. Nottinghamshire
31. Derbyshire
32. Staffordshire
33. Shropshire
34. Cheshire
35. Lancashire
36a. Yorkshire (West Riding)
36b. Yorkshire (East Riding)
36c. Yorkshire (North Riding)
37. Co. Durham
38. Westmorland
39. Cumberland
40. Northumberland

Wales

41. Monmouthshire
42. Glamorganshire
43. Carmarthenshire
44. Pembrokeshire
45. Cardiganshire
46. Brecknockshire
47. Radnorshire
48. Montgomeryshire
49. Merionethshire
50. Caernarvonshire
51. Anglesey
52. Denbighshire
53. Flintshire

ISLE OF MAN

54. Isle of Man

Scotland

55. Wigtownshire
56. Kirkcudbrightshire
57. Dumfriesshire
58. Roxburghshire
59. Selkirkshire
60. Berwickshire
61. East Lothian
62. Midlothian
63. Peeblesshire
64. West Lothian
65. Lanarkshire
66. Ayrshire
67. Bute
68. Renfrewshire
69. Dumbartonshire
70. Stirlingshire
71. Clackmannanshire
72. Kinross-shire
73. Fife
74. Argyllshire
75. Perthshire
76. Angus (formerly Forfarshire)
77. Kincardine(shire)
78. Aberdeenshire
79. Banffshire
80. Moray (formerly Elginshire)
81. Nairn
82. Inverness-shire
83. Ross and Cromarty
84. Sutherland
85. Caithness
86. Orkney
87. Shetland (or Zetland)

Northern Ireland

88. Co. Derry
89. Co. Antrim
90. Co. Down
91. Co. Armagh
92. Co. Tyrone
93. Co. Fermanagh

REPUBLIC OF IRELAND

94. Co. Donegal
95. Co. Leitrim
96. Co. Cavan
97. Co. Monaghan
98. Co. Louth
99. Co. Meath
100. Co. Westmeath
101. Co. Longford
102. Co. Roscommon
103. Co. Sligo
104. Co. Mayo
105. Co. Galway
106. Co. Offaly
107. Co. Laois
108. Co. Kildare
109. Co. Dublin
110. Co. Wicklow
111. Co. Wexford
112. Co. Carlow
113. Co. Kilkenny
114. Co. Waterford
115. Co. Tipperary
116. Co. Clare
117. Co. Limerick
118. Co. Cork
119. Co. Kerry

Pre-1974 counties of Britain and Ireland

'Ulster' has been used in the records loosely and variously. All or just a part or parts of that Irish province may be meant, or it may be shorthand for just the six counties that constitute the U.K. portion. For this reason, unless the province is clearly intended, that word is placed in quotation marks throughout the book.

GEOGRAPHICAL ORDER OF RECORDS

In the case of that majority of plants with entries containing records from both Britain and Ireland, normally the British records are cited *en bloc* first and approximately from south to north in turn. The Irish ones are normally grouped together in a separate paragraph and are cited in reverse order, from north to south, to reflect that island's greater proximity to Scotland and the marked cultural affinities between the two. Overall, the order is thus spirally anticlockwise.

The separation of the Irish records makes it possible to tell at a glance which of the two islands has yielded the greater range of recorded uses traced (though not necessarily the greater *volume* of use, an aspect on which, as on all quantitative ones, little information exists or can safely be deduced). The separation also serves as a reminder of the limited comparability of the Irish and the British records by reason of the much greater completeness of the Irish ones geographically. A further justification is the substantial degree of autonomy that Irish folk medicine seems to have enjoyed, a matter discussed in more detail in Chapter 17.

Records

Any statement, published or unpublished, regarding a use for one of the purposes with which *Medicinal Plants in Folk Tradition: An Ethnobotany of Britain & Ireland* is concerned is treated as 'a record'. A reference is given for the source of each, individually cited in the text as a number referring to the Notes at the end of that chapter, and to a particular page in cases where the statement could otherwise be found only with difficulty. There is much unacknowledged repetition of records in the literature and in such cases only the *original* source is given in so far as that has proved traceable; in surprisingly few instances seemingly independent records have been found for a particular use in a particular area, in which case references to clearly different sources appear against the same number.

Records differ greatly in their degree of precision. Very few, and those mostly in works of a general character, are entirely unspecific either geographically or about the use or uses to which the plant in question has been put (though even if a medicinal use is mentioned, that may be in unhelpfully vague terms). Records collected in more recent years by those versed in 'best practice' as folklorists represent the opposite extreme in normally identifying the informant, his or her location down to the level of a village or parish, and the date when the information was gathered Most records, however, probably even including a majority of these latter ones, rest on oral statements unchecked by first-hand observation by whoever noted them down, who in any case may not have had sufficient botanical knowledge for that purpose or not have sought it from someone who had. A plant familiar to the informant may be known to him or her by a name that rightly belongs to some other one, or by a name peculiar to just the one family or community. Mishearing of names, too, can easily occur. Anomalous records must often have arisen from such causes, but they seldom betray their untrustworthy character and there is no alternative but to take them at face value.

A further weakness special to a study of the present kind is that a use mentioned by an informant may have been learned of in some quite different area, perhaps even a different country, from where he or she was living at the time the information was communicated, but without that being made clear. This must be a particular risk with records from towns and cities, where people are liable to call on their memory of an earlier rural period in their life. Though the great majority of folk records come from those living in country areas, fortunately, many even of them may have lived in other counties or regions for periods. Usually, though, such an experience is likely to have been within the same region, so the attribution of a record to just the one county may be relatively unimportant in such cases.

ABBREVIATIONS USED IN NOTES

The following abbreviations for frequently cited sources of records are used in the Notes at the end of each chapter:

CECTL   Centre for English Cultural Tradition and Language,
        University of Sheffield
IFC S   Irish Folklore Commission, Schools' Survey
PLNN   *Plant-lore Notes and News*

Plant Names

The scientific names of flowering plants and ferns are those of the list by Kent (1992) and its supplements or, in the case of plants not in that, those of the *New Flora of the British Isles* (Stace 1997). Similarly for those of the lower plants, the most authoritative publications have been followed.

For vernacular names, the nearest to a standard list of the English ones of British and Irish flowering plants and ferns is that sponsored by the Botanical Society of the British Isles (Dony et al. 1986), which has been adhered to, and extended to many species not included in that work, by Stace (1997). This is now in general use, at least for scientific publications. It has been thought advisable to make it the basis for the purposes of *Medicinal Plants in Folk Tradition: An Ethnobotany of Britain & Ireland*, too, for the number of vernacular names on record is bewilderingly large (cf. Grigson 1955) and different ones enjoy currency in different circles and different areas. Where names other than those of the standard list as extended by Stace have been used particularly widely, however, they have been added for ease of reference, as also have some in the Celtic languages that are encountered especially frequently in the folklore records. In these instances the name in the standard list is the one that appears first. For other than flowering plants and ferns, the vernacular name most in use in the latest handbooks has been followed.

SEQUENCE OF FAMILIES AND SPECIES

For the flowering plants, the Cronquist classification as used in the publications by Kent and Stace has been followed. The hierarchy of superorders (-iflorae) and orders (-ales) under which families (-aceae) are grouped in the modified version of the Cronquist classification of Stace (1997, xxv–xxvii) has provided a means of avoiding an otherwise unacceptably unwieldy referencing system. The need to provide a source reference for each individual record requires so many superscript numbers that, if these were to be in a single sequential series, they would run to more digits than would be practicable. The systematic list of plants has accordingly been divided into chapters, each with its separate, self-contained sequence of numbered references to the Notes at the end of each one. Conveniently, the Cronquist classification groups the flowering plant families recognised into a series of affinity clusters and subclusters. As many families are not represented among the plants with folk uses recorded in this book, those that are can be grouped in such a way that twelve subdivisions not too dissimilar in size emerge. The rest of the plants covered can be grouped in two further ones to produce fourteen sections (Chapters 3–16) in all:

Nonvascular plants
    Chapter 3 bryophytes, lichens, algae and fungi
Vascular plants
    Chapter 4 pteridophytes and conifers
  Flowering plants: dicotyledons
    Chapter 5 Magnoliiflorae: Nymphaeales to Papaverales (water-lilies, buttercups and poppies)
    Chapter 6 Hamameliflorae and Caryophylliflorae: Urticales to Plumbaginales (elms to docks)
    Chapter 7 Dilleniiflorae: Theales to Primulales (St John's-worts to primulas)
    Chapter 8 Rosiflorae: Rosales (currants, succulents and roses)
    Chapter 9 Rosiflorae: Fabales to Geraniales (legumes, spurges and geraniums)
    Chapter 10 Rosiflorae: Apiales (ivy and umbellifers)
    Chapter 11 Asteriflorae: Gentianales and Solanales (gentians and nightshades)
    Chapter 12 Asteriflorae: Lamiales (comfrey, vervain and mints)
    Chapter 13 Asteriflorae: Callitrichales to Scrophulariales (plantains, figworts, foxglove and speedwells)
    Chapter 14 Asteriflorae: Rubiales and Dipsacales (bedstraws, valerian and scabious)
    Chapter 15 Asteriflorae: Asterales (daisies)
  Flowering plants: monocotyledons
    Chapter 16 Alismatiflorae to Liliiflorae: Alismatales to Orchidales (pondweeds, grasses, lilies and orchids)

Names of Ailments

The restriction of folk medicine mainly to surface complaints is reflected in a comparatively limited set of terms, non-technical in character but doubtless commonly deceptive in an unreal broadness. Most, however, refer to everyday complaints that are reasonably unambiguous. The only sensible course has seemed to be to repeat the terms as they appear in the records themselves, confining attempts at translation to those that are archaic and have a recognised modern synonym.

All too often, unfortunately, folk records have been mediated through practitioners of official medicine or pharmacy, who have placed their own sophisticated interpretations on the ailments in question when reporting them. This may well have led to an element of distortion. Allegedly folk records of complaints such as diabetes sound particularly suspicious, though it is always possible that a genuinely folk remedy has been used before or after diagnosis by a physician.

MODE OF USE

Many records extend to details, sometimes quite elaborate, of how a particular remedy is or has been prepared and applied. For reasons of space it has only been possible to include these in the following pages in a few cases. Readers seeking information on this aspect may find following up the reference to the source of the record is well rewarded.

CHAPTER 3

Bryophytes, Lichens, Algae and Fungi

The non-vascular plants include the bryophytes (liverworts and mosses) and organisms that are not truly plants but that have traditionally been treated as plants: lichens (associations of fungi and algae), algae and fungi.

Bryophytes

LIVERWORTS

Marchantia polymorpha Linnaeus
  liverwort
  cosmopolitan
'Liverwort' or, in some areas, 'liver-grass', commonly assumed to refer to *Marchantia polymorpha,* has, as the name indicates, enjoyed an age-old reputation, propagated in herbals, as a remedy for liver complaints. The only allegedly folk record of that use traced, however, is from Lincolnshire.[1] In Berwickshire these plants were valued instead as a cure for colds and consumption, for 'a binding at the heart' and as a diuretic for dropsy.[2]

In Shetland a plant known as 'dead man's liver' and popularly supposed to be a lichen—though in fact a liverwort, according to a local botanist—served at one time as a remedy for asthma.[3]

MOSSES

Sphagnum Linnaeus
  bog-moss
  arctic to subtropical zones of the northern and southern hemispheres

Fontinalis antipyretica Hedwig
willow moss
disjunct circumpolar

Apart from a record of 'river moss' (presumably the aquatic species *Fontinalis antipyretica,* which can grow in dense bunches) from Limerick, used there to staunch bleeding,[4] *Sphagnum* is the only kind of moss which seems to have been separately distinguished in folk medicine. The abundant remains of *S. palustre* Linnaeus accompanying a skeleton in a Bronze Age grave in Fife have been interpreted as packing for a wound,[5] but that may be fanciful; certainly, though, the absorbency of bog-moss has been widely valued in the Highlands for such purposes as menstrual bleeding and as a forerunner of the disposable nappy.[6] Fomentations of warm water in which this moss has been simmered have also been popular there as a rub for sore feet, while in Somerset a treatment for sore eyes has been to bathe them with seawater and dry them with it.[7]

In Ireland the mildly antiseptic property of *Sphagnum* has been well appreciated: the moss has either been simply left on wounds or sores after first being washed, as in Westmeath,[8] or clay has been plastered over it as an added protection, as in Devon.[9] In Offaly[10] and at least one other part of Ireland[11] a treatment for a sprain has been to pack this plant tightly round the limb affected, in Limerick[12] a dressing with it is one accepted answer to a rash, and in that county[13] and Louth[14] it has also been applied to burns.

In one or two other cases a habitat detail with a record of 'moss' in the collective sense may allow the species most probably involved to be surmised. Thus in Norfolk a kind used for insect bites and stings has been taken from the tiles on roofs,[15] and a popular home remedy for a nosebleed in parts of Ireland has been to sniff up moss (or lichen?) collected off tree-trunks and dried.[16] But it is anyone's guess which kind has been used for staunching bleeding in records from a wide spread of Irish counties (most, if not all, *Sphagnum* again?), or for easing a pain in the leg in Limerick,[17] or for the decoction applied to boils that fail to respond to other treatment, which at least one Londoner has found successful on following the advice of 'an old man'.[18]

Lichens

CLADONIACEAE

Cladonia chlorophaea (Floerke ex Sommerfeldt) Sprengel,
in the broad sense
chalice-moss, cup-moss, Our Lady's chalice
northern and southern temperate, alpine and polar regions

An old whooping-cough remedy, recommended in some of the herbals and still in John Quincy's day 'mightily in vogue among the good wives' though largely ignored by official medicine,[19] *Cladonia chlorophaea* has continued into more or less contemporary folk medicine in Britain in two Welsh counties (Merionethshire and Denbighshire) under the name *cwpanau pas*.[20]

In Ireland, this lichen, boiled in new milk, has had the same role in Waterford.[21]

PARMELIACEAE

Parmelia Acharius
crotal
northern and southern temperate zones

Parmelia omphalodes (Linnaeus) Acharius, abundant in the upland and rockier regions of the British Isles, is the species most commonly used for the brown dyes colloquially known by their English spelling as 'crottle'. Familiar though that use is, lichens of this genus have also attracted some applications in folk medicine as well. In the Highlands they were traditionally sprinkled on stockings at the start of a journey to prevent the feet becoming inflamed.[22] The *fiasgag nan creag*, a name translating as 'rock lichen' but not further identified, was probably one of these; it was used for healing sores.[23]

In Ireland it was as a cure for a bad sore under the chin that *crotal* found one of its uses in Donegal,[24] where it has also been valued for burns and cuts.[25] In Kerry, on the other hand, *crotal* has been one of several herbs put into a *carragheen*-like (referring to *Chondrus crispus* or *Mastocarpus stellatus*) soup given to invalids to drink.[26]

Usnea Dillenius ex Adanson
beard lichen
northern and southern temperate zones

Usnea has traditionally had a reputation for curing diseases of the scalp, allegedly for no better reason than that its appearance recalls a head of long hair (and it is still sold in the best chemist shops as an ingredient in anti-dandruff shampoos). The only unambiguously folk record traced, however, is a treatment in Ireland for sore eyes: in Leitrim the 'greyish mossy substance' growing on the blackthorn trunks is presumably *U. subfloridana* Stirton, which commonly grows on the twigs of that tree. It was mixed with tobacco and butter, boiled and then cooled before being applied as a lotion.[27]

Perhaps an *Usnea* species was also the mysterious 'brighten', a lichen known by that name in the New Forest in Hampshire and recommended there for use on weak eyes at one time.[28]

PELTIGERACEAE

Peltigera aphthosa (Linnaeus) Willdenow
sea-green lichen
northern and southern temperate and alpine zones

As its specific name indicates, the widespread and formerly more common *Peltigera aphthosa* was regarded as specific for that fungus infection of the mouth and tongue, especially found in children, known to learned medicine as aphthae and colloquially as 'the thrush'. The sole evidence traced of this lichen's use in folk medicine is provided by Withering, according to whom 'the common people' in his day made an infusion of it in milk and gave it to children afflicted with that complaint. He added that in large doses it caused purging and vomiting and was effective against intestinal worms.[29]

Peltigera canina (Linnaeus) Willdenow, in the broad sense
dog lichen, liverwort lichen, ash-coloured liverwort
cosmopolitan

With fruit-bodies resembling dogs' teeth, *Peltigera canina* was long regarded as a supposedly certain specific antidote to the bite of a rabid dog or of resulting hydrophobia. The lichen is said to have been still in widespread use for that in the early nineteenth century in the Snowdonia area of Caernarvonshire, where it was dried, reduced to a black powder and mixed with black pepper.[30]

LOBARIACEAE

Lobaria pulmonaria (Linnaeus) Hoffman
tree lungwort, lungs of oak, lung lichen
nearly circumboreal in northern hemisphere, south to Korea, Mexico
and Canaries; South Africa

A frequent species on old oaks, *Lobaria pulmonaria* was recommended in the herbals from the fifteenth century onwards for lung complaints, allegedly because it has an irregular pitted surface superficially resembling that human organ (but that explanation could well be fanciful). Whether or not from that source, it became highly rated as a remedy for consumption. In the New Forest in Hampshire in the mid-nineteenth century it was still being collected and an infusion of it extensively drunk for that ailment.[31] The plant similarly persisted in use in the Highlands.[32] Sold today by herbalists primarily for asthma and bladder complaints and as a bitter tonic to promote appetite, its mucilaginous character has also made it attractive as a soothing syrup.

According to one Irish source,[33] a very common lichen in Sligo variously known there as 'tree lungwort', 'hazel rag' or 'crottles' has been used locally as a cure for piles. That sounds like a conflation of more than one kind and perhaps refers more particularly to *Parmelia* species, which have been put to related purposes.

Xanthoria parietina (Linnaeus) Th. Fries
cosmopolitan

As in the case of the mosses, there has predictably been a measure of vagueness in folk medicine about the kinds of lichens used, and sometimes people can get no further than 'a leaf called lichen which grows in mossy fields', in the words of one Kilkenny informant.[34] In that particular one, as it happens, the plant in question was mentioned as boiled in milk and drunk for yellow jaundice, which suggests *Xanthoria parietina*, a species common throughout the British Isles which, allegedly on account of its bright yellow colour, is known to have had a reputation for curing that ailment. In the case of *dub-cosac*, on the other hand, a lichen considered good for heart trouble in the Clare-Galway borderland,[35] there is no such clue to its identity.

Algae

Algae comprise a variety of quite distantly related organisms that have been recognised as belonging to a number of separate divisions. The algae included here are *Nostoc*, a blue-green alga that is more closely related to bacteria, and red, green and brown algae of the divisions Rhodophycota, Chlorophycota and Chromophycota, respectively.

Nostoc commune Vaucher
cosmopolitan

(Folk credentials questionable) There has been a widespread European folk belief that jelly-like masses that appear on the ground after rain are the remains of shooting stars fallen to earth and, as such, possess special medicinal potency. Known as 'star-shot', 'star-jelly' or 'star-fall'n', these were apparently most often either *Nostoc commune,* a member of the blue-green algae (or cyanobacteria) fairly common in bare dry places, or a gelatinous fungus of the genus *Tremella*[36] (q.v.). While there is reliable evidence that the latter has featured in British Isles folk medicine, records attributable to *Nostoc* are less certain. The most probable comes from Skye: 'a jelly-like shiny stuff . . . a kind of lichen or mould which grew on the rocks at the burn mouth' and, in accordance with a recipe passed down in one family from a 'wise woman' ancestor, was brewed (but not boiled) and given for puerperal fever.[37]

In Ireland the 'green slime' from the top of stagnant water which has been applied to burns in Meath[38] is presumably some other member of the blue-green algae.

RED ALGAE

Chondrus crispus Stackhouse
   colder northern Atlantic

Mastocarpus stellatus (Stackhouse) Guiry
   Gigartina stellata (Stackhouse) Batten
   Irish moss, *carragheen*
   colder northern Atlantic

Chondrus crispus and *Mastocarpus stellatus,* both generally distributed around the British Isles, are very similar in appearance, often grow together and are not distinguished by present-day harvesters of Irish moss. Extensively collected for eating and the source of a former teetotal beverage ('Sobriety'), they have been popular in the coastal counties of Ireland as folk cures for colds, coughs, sore throats and chest and lung ailments (including tuberculosis). The plants were boiled in milk or water, strained and drunk hot. They have also been used for burns in Leitrim[39] and for kidney trouble in Cavan.[40]

British folk uses of Irish moss have been recorded much more scantily, for different purposes and apparently only from the Hebrides: for poulticing a sore stomach in South Uist[41] and as a rub for tired feet in Skye.[42]

Palmaria palmata (Linnaeus) Kuntze
   Rhodymenia palmata (Linnaeus) Greville
   dulse, dillisk, *duileasc, crannach, creathnach*
   colder northern Atlantic, Arctic

Eaten raw, fresh or dried, or cooked like spinach, *Palmaria palmata* has long held a place in Scottish and Irish folk medicine as a protection against ill-health in general. In Orkney there was once a saying, 'he who eats the dulse [of a local rocky creek] . . . will escape all maladies except Black Death'.[43] A soup of it, taken at least three times a week, was popular in the Highlands as a means of purifying the blood.[44] It was eaten in Berwickshire[45] and Skye[46] for the same purpose. In the Highlands and Western Isles it has also been regarded as one of the best cures for indigestion and stomach disorders.[47]

Indeed, few other plants were recorded by early observers as used for such a range of ailments. From Ireland a physician in Kilkenny reported to John Ray in 1696 that it was esteemed effective against both worms and scurvy[48] and was eaten to sweeten the breath, while his contemporary Martin Martin learned of its use in Skye for constipation, scurvy, poor vision, migraine, colic, the stone, worms and stomach pain. Martin also found that the people of Skye shared with those of Edinburgh the belief that, when fresh, it removes the afterbirth safely and easily.[49] Two later visitors to Skye confirmed and added to Martin's information: James Robertson in 1768 noted that the inhabitants dissolved a bladder stone by drinking a dilute solution of the ashes of a seaweed[50] (which he left unidentified but which was doubtless this), and Lightfoot in 1772 learned that it was sometimes employed to pro-mote a sweat in cases of fever.[51]

In Ireland in more recent times, dulse has been used in the Aran Islands for worming children,[52] while in Mayo it has been chewed and its juice drunk to ease a sore throat.[53]

Porphyra umbilicalis (Linnaeus) Kützing
purple laver, slake, sloke, slouk, *sloucan*
Arctic, northern Atlantic south to Canaries, Mediterranean,
   northern Pacific

Species of the genus *Porphyra*, perhaps more particularly *P. umbilicalis*, have been eaten extensively in Ireland, Scotland and Wales but records of their use in folk medicine are rare, surprisingly. In eighteenth-century Cornwall, William Borlase was informed that three spoonfuls of the juice, taken every morning, fasting, for three weeks had proved very effective against cancers. One cure of breast cancer was claimed to be due to that alone, but it is unclear which medical tradition, the folk or the learned one, was being referred to.[54] We can be sure, however, that it is as a folk cure that *sleabhcán* has won a fol-lowing in the Aran Islands for easing indigestion.[55] Similarly, Martin Martin found it being boiled and given to the cows on Skye to clear up their spring-time costiveness.[56]

GREEN ALGAE

Ulva lactuca Linnaeus
  sea lettuce, green laver
  northern and southern Atlantic, northern Pacific

Enteromorpha Link
  northern Atlantic, Arctic, northern Pacific

Cladophora Kützing
  cosmopolitan

(Identification dubious) A kind of seaweed known as *linarich* and described as 'a very thin small green plant, about 8–12 inches long', growing on stones, shells or bare sand, was noted by Martin Martin in 1695 in use on the Hebridean islands of Skye and Lingay for healing the wounds made by a blistering plaster, for 'drawing up' the tonsils and for poulticing the temples and forehead, to dry up a runny nose, ease migraine or induce sleep in cases of fever.[57] A few years later Lightfoot attributed to *Ulva lactuca* a poulticing function in the 'Western Isles' in the words used by Martin of *linarich*, strongly suggestive of an unacknowledged repeat of the latter's information.[58] It is possible that Lightfoot did personally see *U. lactuca* being applied in this manner and thus solved the identity of *linarich;* other authors, however, have thought some species of *Enteromorpha* or *Cladophora* best fits Martin's description.

'Sea lettuce' described by the informant as variously green, brown and dark red in colour—which could apply only in part to *Ulva lactuca,* even if the name were correctly applied—has been stewed in sea-water on the Essex coast and the resulting liquid used to ease the pain of bunions and arthritis in the feet.[59]

BROWN ALGAE

Fucus vesiculosus Linnaeus
  bladder wrack, lady wrack, button seaweed, sea-wrack,
    bubbling wrack
  northern Atlantic, Arctic

The jelly-like mucilage contained in the swollen vesicles (or pneumatocysts) of *Fucus vesiculosus* is an age-old embrocation in coastal areas for rheumatism, bruised limbs and sprains. In Britain it has been recorded from Cornwall,[60] Somerset,[61] Essex,[62] Cumbria[63] and Angus.[64] It was boiled into an oily lotion and rubbed in or simply placed hot against the skin or, more simply still, put in a bath of hot sea-water. The relaxing effect has been valued in Yorkshire fishing villages especially as a cure for bow legs in small children; the fresh fronds and sliced vesicles together with equal parts of water and gin or rum were placed in a corked bottle for a week and then applied as a rub.[65] Another unusual use for the plant was encountered by Martin Martin in 1695 in Jura in the Inner Hebrides: steam from the boiled plant was inhaled to cure a stitch after a fever.[66]

Irish records of the standard use as an embrocation are known from as many and as scattered coastal counties as in Britain. As it was this kind of seaweed specifically that was valued in Londonderry[67] for 'weak feet' and in Leitrim[68] for sore or sweaty ones, it was presumably the unnamed one too that has been prized for easing swollen legs in Galway.[69] A less orthodox practice recorded from Donegal has been to suck the mucilage out of the vesicles and swallow it to cure a sore throat.[70] In official medicine the mucilage was also applied to throats—but externally, as a poultice for glandular swellings.

Pelvetia canaliculata (Linnaeus) Decaisne & Thuret
channelled wrack
Atlantic coasts of Europe
Carefully distinguished in Gaelic as *feamain chìrein*, *Pelvetia canaliculata* was held to contain more potash than any other local seaweed and consequently was much used in the Highlands and Western Isles for poulticing and other medical purposes.[71] Boiled in sea-water and bandaged on hot, it was particularly used for easing rheumaticky knees.[72]

In Ireland's Aran Islands, besides being employed as a general prophylactic, this species also served to worm children.[73]

Laminaria digitata (Hudson) Lamouroux

Laminaria hyperborea (Gunnerus) Foslei
tangle
colder northern Atlantic, Arctic
Laminaria digitata and *L. hyperborea* are very similar and unlikely to have been distinguished for folk medicine purposes. The records traced are exclusively from the Scottish Western Isles. Martin Martin in 1695 found tangle valued there as a cure for loss of appetite, boiled with butter[74]; in South Uist

it has been shredded, chewed and swallowed for constipation[75] and in Skye it has been eaten to purify the blood.[76]

Four unidentified seaweeds are

'Seafog', a cure for paralysis in Leitrim, used as a wash three times a day either on its own or in combination with bladder wrack.[77]

'Red-fog', found by Martin Martin in 1695 being boiled on Jura with bladder wrack and then inhaled to cure a stitch after a fever.[78]

Luireach, a 'filmy, skin-like form of seaweed', baked strips of which bound over the swelling were an ancient cure for goitre in the Highlands.[79]

'Sleek', a long, thin hairy seaweed common on the coast of Fife and employed there to poultice sprains, rheumatism, etc.[80] This is not a recorded use of sloke (*Porphyra* spp.) and the name could belong to some other alga.

Fungi

Fungi include a wide variety of organisms actually more closely related to animals than to true plants. The fungi included here belong to the classes Hymenomycetes (mushrooms), Gasteromycetes (puffballs) and Pyrenomycetes (powdery mildews and related fungi).

HYMENOMYCETES

Agaricus campestris Linnaeus ex Fries
field mushroom
northern and southern temperate zones and Caribbean; possibly introduced into many parts of southern hemisphere

Though the word mushroom has doubtless always been applied loosely, for most people it more particularly refers to *Agaricus campestris,* the one traditionally most sought after and collected for cooking. Unexpectedly, though, only a single instance has been traced of what is fairly unambiguously this being employed in the British Isles as a folk medicine—in Norfolk, where it has been stewed in milk to soothe cancer of the throat.[81]

Fomes fomentarius (Fries) Kickx
tinder fungus
circumboreal on birch, extending south to North Africa on beech

Phellinus igniarius (Fries) Quélet
willow fomes
circumpolar and northern temperate zone

Of the two related species that have shared the names 'touchwood' or 'funk' down the centuries, *Fomes fomentarius* is the more likely to have been the one used in Suffolk 'since time immemorial' to staunch bleeding and cure slight wounds,[82] as it is said to have grown on oaks, which this species favours, whereas *Phellinus igniarius* tends to occur on other deciduous trees, especially willows. On the other hand, the former is rare in England, and the latter common. The hard outer part was cut off and the soft inner substance hammered to soften it further.[83]

Phellinus pomaceus (Fries) Maire
northern temperate zone and where *Prunus* is cultivated

The very hard fruit-bodies of *Phellinus pomaceus*, a fungus of fruit trees of the rose family, formerly enjoyed a reputation in West Sussex villages for poulticing facial swelling. Before being applied, they first had to be ground down on a nutmeg grater and then heated in the oven.[84]

Piptoporus betulinus (Bulliard ex Fries) P. Karsten
birch bracket
circumboreal

In Sussex, pieces of *Piptoporus betulinus*, a common fungus of birches, were slowly steamed in tins to produce a charcoal valued as an antiseptic and disinfectant.[85] Regular strips of the thick, elastic flesh were also cut and kept there whenever required for staunching bleeding (in the same way as puffballs); with a hole punched in the middle, they were found to make very comfortable corn pads.[86] Perhaps these are the 'mushroom slices' reputed to cure corns in Galway when applied to them on three successive nights.[87]

Fistulina hepatica Schaeffer ex Fries
poor man's beefsteak
northern temperate zone, Caribbean, mountains of subtropical
    India; introduced (?) into Australia

The botanist William Sherard, during his brief residence in north-eastern Ireland in 1690–4, found the local peasants searching out a certain fungus from the clefts of rotten oaks and using it to heal old ulcers, laying a portion on the sore. In his edition of Ray's *Synopsis*, Dillenius was able to provide a sufficiently good description of it, under the pre-Linnaean name *Fungus cariaceus quercinus haematodes*,[88] to leave little doubt that this was the species in question.[89]

Tremella mesenterica Retzius ex Hooker
jelly fungus, yellow brain-fungus
Arctic and northern temperate region, Caribbean, North Africa,
    Australasia, Falkland Islands

The early Anglesey botanist Hugh Davies insisted that the gelatinous mass known in those parts under the name 'star-shot', which he had found very effective when rubbed on chilblains, was a species of *Tremella* and not, as then usually assumed, the blue-green alga *Nostoc commune*[90] (q.v.).

Auricularia auricula-judae (Bulliard ex Fries) Wettstein
ear fungus
northern temperate zone, Caribbean

The very common *Auricularia auricula-judae,* a fungus of dead or moribund trees, almost wholly on elder in Europe (though on a wider range in North America), once enjoyed a reputation for easing sore throats, coughs and hoarseness when boiled in water to a jelly-like consistency. It was warmly recommended by Gerard and other authors of herbals. The only allegedly folk records of its use, however, are from the Highlands, as a gargle for sore throats,[91] and from the north-western part of central Ireland, where it has been boiled in milk as a cure for jaundice.[92]

GASTEROMYCETES

Bovista nigrescens (Persoon) Persoon; and other Lycoperdaceae
puffball, bolfer, fuzzball, blind man's buff, devil's snuffbox
Europe, Middle East, East Africa

The spores and the absorbent inner tissue of various members of the family Lycoperdaceae share a well-founded reputation for effectiveness in staunching all but the most profuse forms of bleeding. This reputation is not only common to much of Europe, but on the evidence of an archaeological find is also probably very ancient. At Skara Brae in Orkney, the best-preserved pre-historic village in northern Europe, in undisturbed layers of a midden which yielded a calibrated radiocarbon date of 1750–2130 B.P., ten mature fruit-bodies of one of these species, *Bovista nigrescens,* were excavated from a single trench in 1972–3. So many in one spot strongly pointed to collection for a purpose, and as they are inedible when mature, it is most unlikely that it had been for food.[93] According to John Parkinson, country surgeons in seventeenth-century England were often in the practice of stringing up skeins of puffballs to use, when required, for stopping up a wound[94]; and till only very recently many farmers and cottagers in, for example, Norfolk[95] and Sussex[96] anticipated accidents by doing the same.

Apart from their deployment against bleeding, records of which can be found from most parts of the British Isles, puffballs have been valued in Britain for burns in East Anglia,[97] for warts in Cumbria,[98] for piles in the Highlands[99] and for carbuncles in Suffolk.[100] To that list Parkinson could have added chapped heels and any chafing of the skin.[101] In Norfolk the spores have even been held to prevent tetanus.[102]

In comparison, Ireland has yielded far fewer records of such lesser uses. The one for burns is known from Fermanagh.[103] One for chilblains in Wicklow[104] has apparently no British counterpart.

PYRENOMYCETES

Claviceps purpurea (Fries ex Fries) Tulasne & C. Tulasne, in the
   broad sense
   ergot
   northern temperate zone, wherever rye is cultivated
More than fifty compounds have been isolated from the microfungus *Claviceps purpurea*, which attacks the inflorescences of numerous grass genera the world over, besides those of the cereals on which its poisonous action is most notorious. One or more have long been known to have the effect of bringing on uterine contractions in pregnant women of a sufficient severity to expel the foetus. Ergot derivatives have consequently long been is use officially for inducing or speeding labour and inhibiting postpartum bleeding as well as unofficially for procuring abortions. Though only a solitary folk record of the latter (in Norfolk[105]) has been traced, it may well have been a widespread practice down the centuries.

Daldinia concentrica (Bolton ex Fries) Cesati & De Notaris
   cramp balls, King Alfred's cakes
   the least common member of a cosmopolitan species complex
The hard, hemispherical, black or dark brown fruit-bodies produced by the common fungus *Daldinia concentrica* on the dead parts of ash trees were at one time in use on the Surrey-Sussex border to ward off cramp by being carried about the person.[106] That sounds more like a superstition than a genuinely medical practice, however.

Notes

1. Woodruffe-Peacock
2. Johnston 1853, 263–4
3. Tait
4. IFC S 485: 53
5. Darwin, 11; Dickson & Dickson, 79, 226
6. Beith
7. Tongue
8. IFC S 736: 22
9. St Clair
10. IFC S 811: 64
11. Logan, 124
12. IFC S 506: 229
13. IFC S 483: 89
14. IFC S 658: 275
15. Hatfield MS
16. Wilson
17. IFC S 484: 30
18. *PLNN*, no. 7 (1989), 32
19. Quincy, 227
20. Williams MS
21. IFC S 654: 245; 655: 150, 267
22. Cameron; MacFarlane
23. Carmichael, vi, 72
24. McGlinchey, 85
25. IFC S 1112: 54
26. IFC S 476: 217
27. IFC S 226: 569
28. Wise, 176
29. Withering 1787–92, 718
30. Trevelyan, 314
31. Wise, 176; de Crespigny & Hutchinson, 106
32. Cameron
33. Wood-Martin
34. IFC S 862: 376
35. Gregory, 7–8
36. Belcher & Swale
37. Swire, 63
38. IFC S 690: 40
39. Vickery 1995, 60
40. Maloney
41. Shaw, 48
42. Martin, 237
43. Neill, 25
44. Beith
45. Johnston 1829–31, ii, 228
46. *Folk-lore,* 34 (1923), 91
47. Beith; Shaw, 48
48. Lankester, 305
49. Martin, 223, 226, 229, 230
50. Henderson & Dickson, 93
51. Lightfoot, ii, 935
52. Ó hEithir
53. IFC S 93: 233
54. Borlase 1758, 236
55. Ó hEithir
56. Martin, 229
57. Martin, 145, 203, 225
58. Lightfoot, ii, 972
59. Hatfield, 46 and MS
60. Macpherson MS
61. Gifford, xxxix
62. Hatfield MS
63. Freethy, 82
64. Hatfield MS
65. Quelch, 38
66. Martin, 267
67. Moore MS
68. IFC S 190: 171
69. IFC S 5: 163
70. IFC S 1090: 439
71. Carmichael, ii, 276: McDonald
72. Beith
73. Ó Síocháin
74. Martin
75. Shaw, 48
76. *Folk-lore,* 34 (1923), 91
77. IFC S 190: 170, 172
78. Martin, 267
79. Macdonald
80. Simpkins
81. Hatfield, 26
82. Warner

83. Withering 1787–92, 767
84. Swanton
85. Swanton
86. Swanton; *Sussex County Magazine,*
    no. 6 (1932), 709
87. IFC S 22: 119
88. Dillenius, 25
89. R. Watling, in litt.
90. Davies 1813, 117
91. Beith
92. Logan, 47
93. Watling; Watling & Seaward
94. Parkinson, 1324

95. Hatfield, 32
96. Swanton
97. Evans 1966, 90
98. Newman & Wilson
99. Beith
100. Hatfield MS
101. Parkinson, 1324
102. Wigby, 67
103. Glassie, 308
104. McClafferty
105. Hatfield, 20
106. Swanton

CHAPTER 4

Pteridophytes and Conifers

Pteridophytes

Pteridophytes consist of a number of not very closely related plants sometimes referred to as 'fern allies', comprising clubmosses and horsetails, of the families Lycopodiaceae and Equisetaceae, respectively; adder's-tongue and moonworts, of the unusual fern family Ophioglossaceae; as well as true ferns of which members of the following families are included here: Osmundaceae, Adiantaceae, Polypodiaceae, Dennstaedtiaceae, Aspleniaceae, Woodsiaceae, Dryopteridaceae and Blechnaceae.

LYCOPODIACEAE

Huperzia selago (Linnaeus) Bernhardi ex Schrank & C. Martius
 Lycopodium selago Linnaeus
 fir clubmoss
 northern temperate zone
Huperzia selago and *Lycopodium clavatum* are the only two of the seven species in the family Lycopodiaceae native to the British Isles to have been credibly distinguished in the folk medicine records. Not only is *H. selago* the most widely distributed, but a related *Huperzia* species long used in Chinese medicine has been found to produce a substance, huperzine A, with the power to block a brain enzyme. *Huperzia selago,* known in both the Scottish Highlands and Western Isles as *garbhag an t'slèibhe* and valued there, as in Scandinavia, as a powerful emetic, was well known to be dangerous if taken in anything but a small dose, being said to induce giddiness and convulsions[1] or (as reported in Skye in 1768) causing a pregnant woman to abort.[2]

At the same time, as its specific name indicates, *Huperzia selago* was widely identified with a herb recorded by Pliny the Elder in his *Natural History* (Book 24, Section 62) as valued by the druids of Gaul for its 'smoke', which they held to be efficacious for eye ailments. Although some authors[3] have held that Pliny's *selago* was much more probably a kind of juniper, there are records from the Highlands[4] and Cornwall[5] of the use of 'club-moss' as an allegedly folk medicine for treating the eyes. In both those areas, though, this use was either as a fomentation or in an ointment rubbed on the eyelids: 'smoke', i.e. the spores, does not feature. Certain ritual prescribed for collecting and preparing clubmoss for this particular purpose could be evidence that this is a genuine survival in folk tradition; equally, though, the use could have been taken over, maybe in the distant past, from Classical medicine via the herbals.

Strengthening the likelihood that use for the eyes is an import from the learned tradition is the fact that other uses traced in the folk records are for quite unrelated ailments: as an emetic, an emmenagogue and a skin tonic in the Highlands,[6] and for 'any sickness' in the Outer Hebrides.[7]

Lycopodium clavatum Linnaeus
stag's-horn clubmoss
temperate zones, tropical mountains
A herb featuring in two Cardiganshire uses, for 'the back' (which sometimes refers to a kidney complaint) and for a cold or sore throat respectively, has been botanically identified as *Lycopodium clavatum*.[8]

EQUISETACEAE

Equisetum Linnaeus
horsetail
cosmopolitan except Australasia
As the recommendation of *Equisetum* as a vulnerary goes back to Galen in Classical medicine, its status in the folk records would look more suspicious were it not for the impressive concentration of those in parts of Britain that were heavily settled from Scandinavia. Only in the Highlands and/or Western Isles,[9] and the Isle of Man,[10] moreover, do one or more species of this genus feature for staunching the flow of blood (apparently because the minutely rough surface of these plants stimulates clotting). In Yorkshire, equisetums have served as a wash to a bad back,[11] in the Shetlands as an indigestion remedy[12] and in the Isle of Man also as a diuretic.[13]

OPHIOGLOSSACEAE

Ophioglossum vulgatum Linnaeus
adder's-tongue
northern temperate zone, North Africa

Perhaps because of a fancied resemblance of *Ophioglossum vulgatum* to a hooded snake preparing to strike, it has had a reputation for curing adder bites. Large quantities were gathered in the mid-nineteenth century in Sussex and the counties round London[14, 15] and also in Devon[16] for inclusion with various other herbs in a then very popular potion, 'Adder's-spear Ointment', employed for that purpose. However, that geographical distribution and the large scale of the gathering suggest a commercial impetus behind this, and even if it had genuinely a folk origin, the potion may have been a late import and not indigenous to Britain at all. Similarly, because so many of the herbals long recommended the fronds for healing wounds and cuts, it is hard to feel confident that the plant's use for that purpose in Lincolnshire[17] (other records[18–20] are unlocalised as well as vague or ambiguous) was other than a borrowing from that source. However, in Oxfordshire[21] and perhaps some other areas[22] a tea made from the fronds has been drunk as a spring tonic and that may well have a purer pedigree.

Botrychium lunaria (Linnaeus) Swartz
moonwort
Arctic and northern temperate zone, Australasia

Despite the magical powers widely credited to *Botrychium lunaria,* there appears to be only a solitary record of its use in British folk medicine—and that an early one. John Ray in his *Catalogus Angliae* cites his medical friend Walter Needham as the source of the information that the Welsh considered an ointment of this, when well rubbed into the region of the kidneys, an infallible cure for dysentery.[23] Needham had practised in Shrewsbury and may have learned of this from friends or patients from across the Welsh border (he also told Ray of a herbal use of rowan, *Sorbus aucuparia*).

OSMUNDACEAE

Osmunda regalis Linnaeus
royal fern, bog-onion
all continents except Australasia

The most striking and distinctive of the ferns native to the British Isles, *Osmunda regalis* seems to have substituted as the standard cure for sprains, dislocations and bruises in those boggier parts of the north and west from which *Symphytum officinale* (comfrey), elsewhere used for those, is largely or wholly absent. Its rhizomes, like those of comfrey, contain an astringent mucilage with an apparently similar soothing and relaxing effect. These were collected from young plants, chopped up, steeped in water and the resulting liquid bathed on the injured joint or other part. This use is on record in Britain from Cumberland,[24] Westmoreland and Furness,[25] the Scottish Highlands[26] and Colonsay in the Inner Hebrides.[27]

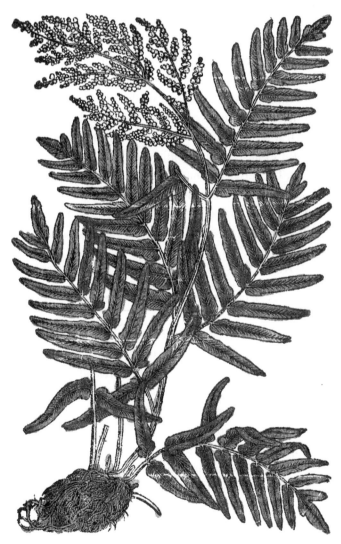

Osmunda regalis, royal fern (Bock 1556, p. 206)

Ireland has experience of that use, too, in the neighbouring counties of Limerick[28] and Clare,[29] but the plant has been further valued there in (unidentified) parts as a cure for rickets[30] (presumably because of its reputation for healing bone troubles) and in Galway for easing rheumatism and sciatica.[31]

But despite an assertion by the leading mid-Victorian authority on ferns that it 'is much used as a rustic vulnerary',[32] no localised folk records of its application to bleeding have been uncovered.

ADIANTACEAE

Adiantum capillus-veneris Linnaeus
maidenhair fern
almost worldwide in tropical and temperate zones

The only convincing evidence that *Adiantum capillus-veneris* has truly been a folk herb in Britain or Ireland comes from the latter's remote Aran Islands, where it is sufficiently frequent in the wild for its dried fronds to have been used to make a tea.[33] Elsewhere, though, this fern is surely too scarce for wild populations of it to have been credibly drawn on medicinally, at least in recent centuries. The vernacular name is shared by several other, more common plants, especially the somewhat similar spleenwort *Asplenium trichomanes,* which those enthused by the praise heaped on 'maidenhair' by the herbals and by physicians presumably used instead.

POLYPODIACEAE

Polypodium vulgare Linnaeus, in the broad sense
polypody
northern temperate zone, South Africa

Polypodium vulgare is one of a number of herbs whose uses have magico-religious overtones. In early eighteenth-century Ireland a careful distinction was made between the epiphytic 'polypody of the oak' and the supposedly different kind to be found so commonly there on walls, the former rated so much the more effective that, given the scarcity of Irish woodland by then, it was having to be imported.[34] More than a century later the belief still lingered there in the Aran Islands that the rhizomes had to be pulled at the time of the new moon and buried in porridge overnight before being potent medicinally.[35]

It is from Ireland that most of the few folk records come, doubtless in reflection of the plant's greater profusion there overall. Those records, as also in Britain, are for very diverse uses, and the ailments treated seem largely determined by whether the rhizomes or the fronds were utilised. An infusion of the rhizomes was valued as a mild laxative in Classical medicine, and it was perhaps from that source that it persisted in use into the last century in Donegal,[36] just as in adjacent Londonderry[37] a decoction of the fronds, much favoured in official herbalism for coughs and colds, lingered on as a mixture with liquorice for remedying the severer kinds of those and asthma. Both parts of the plant, however, feature in a marked cluster of records from Cavan,[38] spilling across into Leitrim,[39] for application to burns or scalds.

In Britain the rhizomes are said to have persisted in use for an unspecified

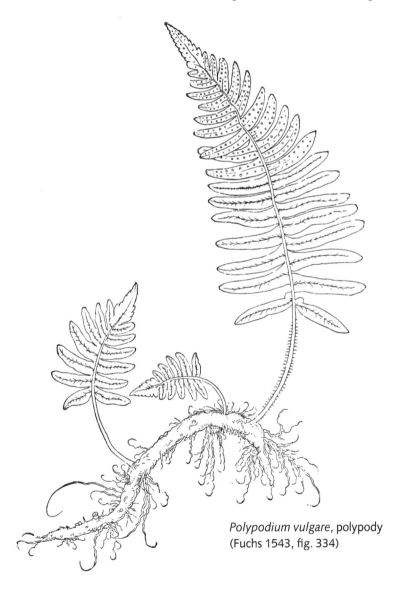

Polypodium vulgare, polypody
(Fuchs 1543, fig. 334)

ailment in 'some parts of England'.[40] In the Highlands they have served as
the source of a snuff taken to alleviate catarrh.[41] The only record traced of the
use of the fronds is from Herefordshire, where they had to be bearing spores
if they were to be effective for whooping cough.[42]

DENNSTAEDTIACEAE

Pteridium aquilinum (Linnaeus) Kuhn
   bracken
   cosmopolitan except temperate South America
(Identity as a folk herb questionable) Though 'fern' more often than not
means *Pteridium aquilinum* when used by non-botanists, when that word is
met with in folk medicine it apparently refers to other species in most if not
all cases. Even John Lightfoot's eighteenth-century report, cited by many later
authors, that the country people in Scotland reckoned a bed of 'bracken' a
sovereign remedy for rickets in children[43] has to be treated with reserve, for
it is suspicious in that the ability to cure rickets was attributed to *Osmunda
regalis* (royal fern) in Ireland. Though allegedly used in Classical medicine
and recommended in herbals,[44] *P. aquilinum* is poisonous to humans as well
as farm animals, often containing cyanide and also now known to be car-
cinogenic.

ASPLENIACEAE

Phyllitis scolopendrium (Linnaeus) Newman
   Asplenium scolopendrium Linnaeus
   hart's-tongue; fox-tongue, cow's-tongue (Ireland)
   Europe, Macaronesia, west-central Asia, Japan, North America
As with *Polypodium vulgare* and *Osmunda regalis*, the greater prevalence of
Phyllitis scolopendrium in the west of the British Isles explains why the records
of its use are predominantly from there. In those from England and Scotland, ailments treated by it have been diverse: in Devon[45] and the Hebrides[46]
colds and pulmonary congestion, in Wiltshire warts[47] and in the Isle of Wight
to cool erysipetaloid eruptions on the legs.[48] The last may perhaps have
involved the same plaster as James Robertson found being applied in Ross-
shire in 1767 'to extract an animalcule which nestling in their legs or other
places produces exquisite pain'.[49]

   In Ireland, in sharp contrast, the plant has enjoyed a very wide use for one
quite different purpose: as an ointment made from the boiled fronds for

soothing burns and scalds. The only records of that traced for certain from Britain are from south-eastern Wales.[50] In those two regions it would appear to have shared the role of *Umbilicus rupestris* (navelwort) in standing in for *Sempervivum tectorum* (house-leek, sengreen) as the pre-eminent salve for burns. Its use in Donegal[51] for soothing insect stings, in Wexford[52] for dog bites and in Limerick[53] for ringworm are doubtless variations on that, but the same can hardly be true of its application to warts[54] in Meath, where it has also been the main ingredient in a remedy for jaundice,[55] or asthma in Wexford.[56]

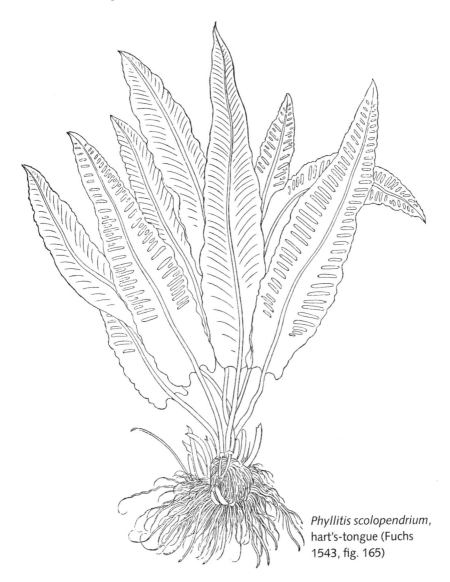

Phyllitis scolopendrium, hart's-tongue (Fuchs 1543, fig. 165)

Asplenium trichomanes Linnaeus
maidenhair spleenwort
temperate zones, tropical mountains

Long and widely promoted by learned authors, *Asplenium trichomanes* must be regarded as doubtfully an age-old member of the folk medicine repertory. Its principal use, for severe coughs and chest complaints, certainly goes back at least to the seventeenth century in certain of the Inner Hebrides,[57] but a lack of evidence to justify its Gaelic name of *lus na seilg*[58] suggests that prescribing it for that supposed malfunctioning of the spleen was a borrowing from the herbals or learned medicine, while use of it in Cumbria as a hair tonic[59] may be late and idiosyncratic.

In Ireland a cough cure known as 'maidenhair' once popular among country people in Londonderry[60] was presumably this, as also an ingredient under that name boiled with honeysuckle and oatmeal into a concoction taken for dysentery in Cavan.[61]

Asplenium ruta-muraria Linnaeus
wall-rue
Eurasia, eastern North America

Like *Asplenium trichomanes,* and for the same reason, the membership of *A. ruta-muraria* in the folk tradition is problematical. Moreover, a plant so widespread could be expected to have left more evidence of its use had it been much prized, yet only a solitary record has been traced for Britain and that not a certain one: a plant abundant on walls in Skye and believed to be this from the verbal description was held to be effective there in drawing the 'fire' from the skin in cases of erysipelas.[62]

In Ireland it has been identified as a 'herb of the seven gifts', valued in Tipperary for its ability to cure seven diseases,[63] and possibly it was also the 'wall fern' employed in Kilkenny for kidney trouble.[64] That it was boiled in milk and taken for epilepsy in Cavan,[65] however, is seemingly more certain.

WOODSIACEAE

Athyrium filix-femina (Linnaeus) Roth
lady-fern
northern temperate zone, southern Asian mountains, tropical America

(Identification dubious) 'Female fern', a remedy for burns and scalds in Wicklow,[66] has been taken to be *Athyrium filix-femina,*[67] but the propensity of folk taxonomy for he-and-she herb pairs lacking in any modern scientific rationale renders such an assumption unsafe.

DRYOPTERIDACEAE

Dryopteris filix-mas (Linnaeus) Schott, in the broad sense
male-fern
Europe, temperate Asia, North America

Because male-fern (in the old aggregate sense) was recommended as a vermifuge by all the leading Classical writers, it is hard to be sure of the genuineness of its place in the folk repertory as the cure for tapeworm *par excellence*. It is

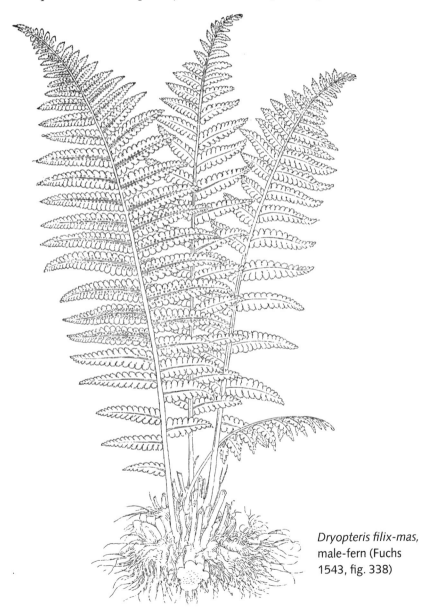

Dryopteris filix-mas,
male-fern (Fuchs
1543, fig. 338)

nevertheless suggestive that the numerous records for that are all from the 'Celtic fringe' and that it has been used in Ireland for other ailments as well: for burns in Waterford,[68] shingles in Tipperary[69] and erysipelas in Limerick.[70] Greatly confusing the picture, however, was the extensive publicity for its use produced by two papers in the *Edinburgh Monthly Medical Journal* in 1852–3 ('On the treatment of Tape-worm by the Male Shield Fern'), which brought to notice a more reliable method of exploiting the plant—by soaking the fresh rhizomes in ether—and thereafter gave it respectability in official medical circles.[71] The powerful anthelminthic properties attributed to the rhizomes certainly have a well-attested clinical basis but their use is regarded today as dangerous.

BLECHNACEAE

Blechnum spicant (Linnaeus) Roth
hard-fern
Europe, Japan, western North America

Despite the distinctiveness of its fronds, *Blechnum spicant* has been encountered only once in the folk use records—and that as merely one of eight ingredients in a juice drunk for a cough after a fever in Mayo.[72] Though employed by midwives in the Faeroe Islands in the eighteenth century to staunch bleeding in childbirth,[73] it would appear not to have found favour in the British Isles, at least in more recent times, as a specific.

Conifers

Conifers are seed plants but, unlike in the true flowering plants, the seeds are borne on cones rather than in fruits. Conifers included here are pines, junipers and yews, of the families Pinaceae, Cupressaceae and Taxaceae, respectively.

PINACEAE

Pinus sylvestris Linnaeus
Scots pine
Europe, temperate Asia; introduced into North America and
New Zealand

Reduced now to a few fragments from its one-time prevalence in the Scottish Highlands, the native populations of the tree *Pinus sylvestris* cannot have helped but decline in use proportionately as a source of folk remedies. Relics of that use that have been recorded there are the consumption of the astringent bark as a remedy for fevers[74] and, in the Badenoch district of Inverness-shire, the making of a plaster for boils and sores from the resin mixed with beeswax and hog's lard.[75] Extensive pinewoods of considerably long standing, even though probably all planted originally, are to be found in East Anglia, and within living memory a child suffering from a polio-like illness was taken to those in Norfolk to breathe in the fragrance, which was believed to have a therapeutic effect.[76] A child is likewise on record as having been taken to the coast in Wales in order to sniff 'the pines' there for an hour or two daily.[77] *Pinus* species have enjoyed a reputation as bronchial cleansants since Classical times, and these cases are presumably a distant echo of that—as has been the use of the young shoots for a cough medicine, recorded from Essex.[78]

Ireland shares only with Essex[79] evidence of the resin's having been employed also as a vulnerary: to stop a cut finger bleeding in Wicklow[80] and, though with the introduced larch (*Larix decidua* Miller) apparently standing in for a pine, in Limerick[81] too. Some part of the tree is known to have been applied also in Galway for the mysterious *fanmadh*.[82]

CUPRESSACEAE

Juniperus communis Linnaeus   PLATE 1
juniper, savin
Arctic and northern temperate zone

In the guise of the drink distilled from the berries (though an infusion made from the whole plant is an alternative that has had its followers), members of the genus *Juniperus* have long enjoyed a reputation as abortifacients. This use has been dubiously ascribed to the Doctrine of Signatures, on the argument that a plant so often conspicuously sterile itself must have been placed on this earth for human beings to have the benefit of the special property that that implied. Widely known as savin, a name which strictly speaking belongs to a related species native to other parts of Europe, *J. sabina* Linnaeus (which is more potent and toxic), the use of *J. communis* for this particular purpose is doubtless as ancient as it has been widespread—though much under-reported by folklorists. In Somerset[83] and Lincolnshire,[84] indeed, it is only from suggestive vernacular names that have been employed for it that it can be inferred that it has had some popularity there. In Norfolk[85] and Galloway,[86] on the other hand, the evidence for that is more direct. Though drinking an infusion was normally deemed sufficient, the Pitt Rivers Museum in Oxford has in its collections sprigs of the plant which a local woman was found in 1914 wearing in her boots for nine days, in the belief that as the feet became hot the 'savin' soaks through the stockings into the feet and thence into the bloodstream[87]—a practice analogous to the wearing of *Urtica dioica* (nettle) in socks as a male contraceptive.[88] Giving birth 'under the savin tree' was once a euphemism in Lothian for an abortion or a miscarriage,[89] and there are similar allusions in a number of both English and Scottish ballads. That the records are all from England and Lowland Scotland may or may not reflect reality; it seems probable, however, that use for this purpose in Ireland has always been rare or over wide areas even non-existent.

That juniper has had acknowledged value in folk medicine in other directions may have served to cloak its use for 'improper purposes'. The berries, for example, had a reputation as diuretic and caused the herb to be resorted to for dropsy and kidney ailments, a use reported from Hampshire[90] and the Highlands.[91] A liniment made from the berries or two or three drops of the oil taken on a lump of sugar also served to ease rheumatism and backache in Devon,[92] Somerset[93] and Norfolk,[94] its use for teething infants in the Highlands[95] being perhaps of similar origin.

Another, certainly ancient use of juniper (for this was recommended by Hippocrates) was as a fumigant. The green branches, and in some cases the berries, too, were burnt to purify the air in sick-rooms or to prevent an infection from spreading, a practice recorded from as far apart as Devon[96] and Colonsay in the Inner Hebrides.[97] In Devon, people in contact with a contagious disease are known to have chewed the berries as an extra precaution.[98]

In common with other herbs held in especially high esteem, the plant has also attracted a miscellany of apparently more restricted uses: for indigestion in Somerset,[99] for skin disorders such as psoriasis in the Westmoreland Pennines[100] and for epilepsy[101] and snakebites[102] in the Highlands.

In Ireland the juice of the berries has been a traditional diuretic,[103] brought to bear specifically on dropsy in Cavan.[104] In Donegal a concoction of them has also been favoured as a stimulant or cleanser of the system.[105] And the gathering of them in their white unripe state (*caora aitinn*), for bottling in whiskey and keeping on hand for 'ailments', is even the subject of a special tradition, reserved for the last Sunday in July, among children on Achill Island and the neighbouring Corraun Peninsula, on the coast of Mayo.[106]

TAXACEAE

Taxus baccata Linnaeus

yew

Europe, mountains of central Asia and North Africa, close allies elsewhere in northern temperate zone; introduced into New Zealand

Various explanations have been put forward to explain the custom of planting *Taxus baccata* in churchyards, some more convincing than others, but it appears to have been generally overlooked that there might be some natural property of the species itself which caused it to be valued more directly in connection with death. In 'some parts of England' there was a practice in the early nineteenth century of sponging corpses immediately after decease with an infusion of fresh yew leaves, which was claimed to preserve the body from putrefaction for many weeks.[107]

In Britain the only other recorded uses of this tree appear to have been in Lincolnshire, where its twigs were steeped in tea and the resulting liquid drunk to remedy trouble with the kidneys,[108] and in unstated areas an infusion was given as an abortifacient by midwives—with at least one death to its discredit.[109]

Ireland, too, has supplied only a solitary localised record: an application to ringworm in Kildare.[110]

Notes

1. Lightfoot, ii, 689
2. Henderson & Dickson, 93
3. e.g. Anon., *Phytologist,* n.s. 3 (1859), 202–12
4. Carmichael ii, 298; Pratt 1859, 128
5. Hunt, 415, who identifies the species used there as *Lycopodiella inundata* (Linnaeus) Holub, but that may be merely a guess. Though now rare in Cornwall, this was probably the commonest clubmoss there formerly.
6. Beith
7. McDonald, 136
8. Williams MS
9. Beith
10. Quayle, 70
11. Vickery MSS
12. Jamieson
13. Quayle, 70
14. *Phytologist,* 4 (1853), 976
15. Pratt 1859, 122; Britten 1881b, 182
16. *Phytologist,* 4 (1853), 976
17. Gutch & Peacock
18. Pratt 1859, 122
19. Folkard, 207
20. Lightfoot, 652
21. 'E.C.'
22. Hole, 14
23. Ray 1670, 199
24. Hodgson, 371
25. *Phytologist,* 5 (1854), 30
26. Macdonald
27. McNeill

28. IFC S 506: 229
29. Logan, 124; IFC S 593: 43
30. Page, 22
31. IFC S 50: 458
32. Moore 1855, 35
33. Ó hEithir
34. Threlkeld
35. *Journal of Botany,* 11 (1873), 339
36. Hart 1898, 380
37. Moore MS
38. Maloney; IFC S 968: 183, 223; 969: 24
39. IFC S 266: 481
40. Johnson 1862
41. Beith
42. Newman 1844, 112
43. Lightfoot, 661
44. Rymer
45. Collyns
46. Martin, 228; McNeill
47. Whitlock 1976, 164
48. Broomfield, 634
49. Henderson & Dickson, 56
50. *Phytologist,* 1 (1843), 521, 583, 589
51. IFC S 1090: 275
52. IFC S 897: 82
53. IFC S 499: 201
54. IFC S 689: 100
55. IFC S 710: 43
56. IFC S 876: 239
57. Martin, 228; McNeill
58. Cameron
59. Freethy, 91
60. Moore MS
61. Maloney
62. *Folk-lore,* 34 (1923), 90
63. IFC S 572: 91, 297
64. IFC S 861: 212
65. Maloney
66. IFC S 914: 322
67. McClafferty
68. IFC S 637: 21
69. IFC S 572: 70
70. IFC S 512: 523
71. Lindsay
72. IFC S 132: 97
73. Svabo
74. Beith
75. McCutcheon
76. Hatfield MS
77. Vickery 1995
78. Hatfield MS
79. Hatfield MS
80. IFC S 921: 26
81. IFC S 505: 148
82. IFC S 21: 12
83. Grigson
84. Woodruffe-Peacock
85. Taylor 1929, 118
86. Mactaggart, 418
87. *PLNN,* no. 36 (1994), 172
88. Macpherson MS
89. Mabey, 27
90. Hatfield MS
91. Beith
92. Lafont
93. Palmer 1976, 115
94. Taylor MS (Hatfield, 45); Wigby, 67
95. Polson, 33
96. Lafont
97. McNeill
98. Lafont
99. Tongue
100. Duncan & Robson, 71
101. Carmichael, iv, 268
102. Beith
103. Logan, 38
104. Maloney
105. McGlinchey, 83
106. MacNeill, 191–2
107. Rootsey
108. Hatfield MS
109. Taylor 1848, 790
110. IFC S 780: 129

CHAPTER 5

Water-lilies, Buttercups and Poppies

Dicotyledonous flowering plants in the orders (and families) Nymphaeales (Nymphaeaceae, water-lilies), Ranunculales (Ranunculaceae, buttercups; Berberidaceae, barberries) and Papaverales (Papaveraceae, poppies; Fumariaceae, fumitories) are included in this chapter.

NYMPHAEACEAE

Nymphaea alba Linnaeus
  white water-lily
  Europe; introduced into Australasia

Nuphar luteum (Linnaeus) Smith
  yellow water-lily
  Europe, northern Asia, North Africa, subspecies or allied species in
    North America; introduced into New Zealand
The Scots Gaelic name *duilleaga-bhàite*, 'drowned leaf', is ascribed in dictionaries[1] to water-lilies, but the healing herb bearing that name on the Inner Hebridean island of Colonsay, when sent to a botanist for identification, was found to be bog pondweed, *Potamogeton polygonifolius*.[2] Although the similar name in Irish Gaelic, applied to plants used for a cure in Waterford,[3] has also been assumed to refer to water-lilies, such familiar plants would surely not have had to be described to informants in Limerick as a 'green leaf that grows on the top of water in the bog',[4] a description that fits bog pondweed better than anything else, even though the 'green leaf' in question was a corn

cure—a use for water-lily roots according to a recipe written on the back of an early eighteenth-century account at Inverary Castle in Argyllshire.[5] A further complication is that bog pondweed in its turn may have been confused in part with marsh pennywort, *Hydrocotyle vulgaris,* for that seems the likeliest possessor of the 'penny leaves that are got in the bog' mentioned by two other Limerick informants[6]; they used them, however, for putting on burns, which, suspiciously, was the principal application of the pondweed on Colonsay[7] (as it has also been in parts of Wales[8]). What have also been recorded as water-lily roots were more recently used in Cavan to staunch bleeding or applied as a poultice for 'drawing' a boil.[9] The roots of yellow water-lily, *Nuphar luteum,* evidently possess some chemical potency, for William Withering[10] claimed that, when rubbed with milk, they are effective against cockroaches and crickets. The likeliest inference would seem to be that both pondweeds and water-lilies were utilised herbally, perhaps in different regions and for on the whole different purposes, but failure to draw a clear distinction has led to some confusion.

RANUNCULACEAE

Caltha palustris Linnaeus   PLATE 2
marsh-marigold, kingcup; mayflower (northern half of Ireland)
arctic and temperate Eurasia, North America

Although John Parkinson in his comprehensive seventeenth-century herbal could find no evidence of the use of *Caltha palustris* medicinally, its flowers are reputed to have been much valued for such purposes in Ireland formerly.[11] In Meath they are known to have been boiled into a posset or a soup and the contents drunk for heart ailments—perhaps on 'sympathetic' grounds, as the heart-shape of the leaves was stressed to the informant.[12] The fleshiness of these, as one might expect, was also an attraction: in Roscommon, three were plucked and one at a time stewed and then tied hot on a bandage to a boil.[13]

Helleborus foetidus Linnaeus
stinking hellebore, setterwort
western and southern Europe

Though mainly used for cattle and horses, *Helleborus foetidus* was widely grown in cottage gardens or (as Gilbert White observed at Selborne in Hampshire) gathered in the wild and the powdered leaves administered to children troubled with worms. But it was so violent a purge that Parkinson[14] considered only country folk had bodies robust enough to stand its strength. Fatal-ities are even recorded. In one such case, in Wiltshire, it had been mistaken for the less toxic green hellebore, *H. viridis*.[15]

Helleborus viridis Linnaeus
green hellebore, bear's-foot
western and central Europe
(Folk credentials questionable) If the very few records of *Helleborus viridis* in folk use rest on correct identi-fications, it was even more exclusively a veterinary herb than setterwort, *H. foetidus*. Thomas Johnson, in his 1633 edition of Gerard's *Herball*, mentions that an infusion of the leaves was believed to be prophylactic against smallpox and other contagions, but whether that extended into the folk repertory is not clear.

Anemone nemorosa Linnaeus
wood anemone
northern temperate zone of Europe and western Asia;
   introduced into eastern Canada, New Zealand
Too many misadventures with the toxic *Anemone nemorosa* in village medicine[16] appear to have largely eliminated it from the folk repertory. The only British record traced is an eighteenth-century one of its use as a blis-tering plaster in Ross-shire.[17]

Irish records are almost as rare: there is an unlocalised one of its application to wounds as a plaster,[18] and in the Clare-Galway border district the leaves were laid on the head to ameliorate a headache.[19]

All these uses echo those of buttercups (*Ran-unculus* spp.), reflecting the shared properties of anemonin.

Ranunculus acris Linnaeus
meadow buttercup (buttercups in general:
   crowfoot, eagle's-foot, *fearbán*)
arctic and temperate Eurasia, Greenland,
   Aleutian Islands; introduced into other
   temperate regions

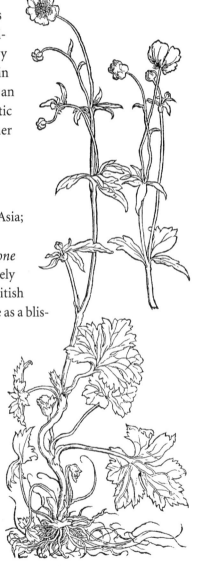

Ranunculus acris,
meadow buttercup
(Brunfels 1530, p. 123)

Ranunculus bulbosus Linnaeus
bulbous buttercup

Europe, Middle East, North Africa; introduced into North America,
New Zealand

The acrid properties of the two common grassland species *Ranunculus acris*
and *R. bulbosus* (which are unlikely to have been distinguished from one
another) are shared by most other British Isles members of the genus, with
the result that they featured in folk use almost as widely as lesser spearwort,
R. flammula Linnaeus, for their power to raise blisters and to act as a counter-
irritant for all rheumatic afflictions in the same way as nettles. Records of
that use are specially frequent in the Highlands and Western Isles in the eighteenth century, but that doubtless only reflects the fact that it persisted there
longest—later ones occur scattered across the English and Irish lowlands. All
three species similarly acted as a remedy for toothache and for headaches,
though more rarely and the latter records are wholly Irish.[20] Again, chewing
the leaf, or rubbing the affected portion with one, acted as a strong counter-
irritant.

One or both of the acrid grassland species have also attracted an impressive diversity of other uses. Marginally the most widespread of these has been
as a wart cure but, surprisingly, the British records for that are all from the far
south of England only: Devon[21] Somerset,[22] Sussex[23] and Middlesex.[24] This
cure, however, is a 'regular' in herbals back to Pliny, and that distribution
possibly betrays an inheritance solely from the medicines of the books.
Related to that use was presumably the Highland one of applying a buttercup
poultice to a swelling on the sole of the foot.[25] Other ailments for which these
plants have been valued are skin troubles in England (Cornwall,[26] Dorset[27])
and bleeding from cuts and wounds in Scotland (Berwickshire,[28] the Highlands[29]).

In common with that other yellow-flowered herb with an age-old reputation for curing eye troubles, greater celandine (*Chelidonium majus*), the
creeping buttercup, *Ranunculus repens* Linnaeus, has been identified as the
species widely renowned in parts of Cornwall as the 'kenning herb', from its
use as an ointment for healing the eye ulcers known as 'kennings'.[30] No doubt
it was carefully picked out because it was known to be non-caustic, unlike its
similar-looking relatives. Surprisingly, though, it was apparently not that but
the species known to its user(s) as 'meadow crowfoot' that has been favoured
for inflamed eyes in Norfolk.[31]

Irish uses seem to have been largely different. Apart from a repeat of the southern English cure for warts in Louth,[32] those recorded include for heartburn (Clare,[33] Limerick[34]), kidney trouble (Meath[35]), hydrophobia (the north-western Midlands),[36] mumps or swollen glands (the Aran Islands[37])—but in this case only after boiling the juice to allay the possibility of blistering—and consumption or suppurating tuberculosis (the western border counties,[38] Galway[39]). The acrid species have also shared with the non-acrid *Ranunculus repens* popularity only there as a jaundice cure (Antrim,[40] Carlow[41]).

Ranunculus aquatilis Linnaeus, in the broad sense
water-crowfoot
Eurasia, North Africa, North America; introduced into Australasia,
South America

(Identification questionable) A herb known in Manx as *lus y vuc awin*, 'the river pig wort', and used for scalds was identified as *Ranunculus aquatilis* by a local collector competent in botany,[42] but the species found in the Isle of Man to which the name in a collective sense would have been applied occur there almost exclusively in ponds, which puts the identification in doubt; the floating pondweed *Potamogeton natans,* a known scald herb, seems more likely.

Thomas Pennant reported that in the Highlands, 'the water ranunculus is used instead of cantharides to raise blisters'.[43] Although at least one later author[44] has assumed he intended by that the standard blister herb, lesser spearwort, *Ranunculus flammula,* possibly he was referring to the 'crowfoot of the moor' which his predecessor Martin Martin had been told in Skye was found the more effective there for that purpose (and used as well to alleviate sciatica).[45] Perhaps that was *R. hederaceus,* though it is one of Skye's rarer plants.

Ranunculus hederaceus Linnaeus
ivy-leaved crowfoot
western Europe
Ranunculus hederaceus was identified botanically as (at least in part) the '*peabar uisgi*', which, pounded between stones, formed a main ingredient in poultices applied to scrofula on Colonsay in the Inner Hebrides.[46] As mentioned above, one or other of the caustic species of buttercup is on record as having been in wide use in part of northern Ireland for suppurating tuberculosis; possibly this less common relative had been found in the Hebrides to be more efficacious.

Ranunculus ficaria Linnaeus

Ficaria verna Hudson

lesser celandine, pilewort, pileweed

Europe, western Asia; introduced into North America, Australasia

Though the corms of *Ranunculus bulbosus* are also on record as cures for piles, in Cornwall[47] and Antrim[48] that has been pre-eminently the role in European folk medicine of the roots and axillary bulbils of lesser celandine, *R. ficaria*, a use recorded from many and widely separate parts of the British Isles. Extensions of this have been their application to small lumps in women's breasts in the Highlands[49] (for which purpose the roots were usually placed under the arms), to corns on Colonsay[50] and to warts in Herefordshire.[51] Less expected is the use of the petals (in Cumbria)[52] or the leaves (in

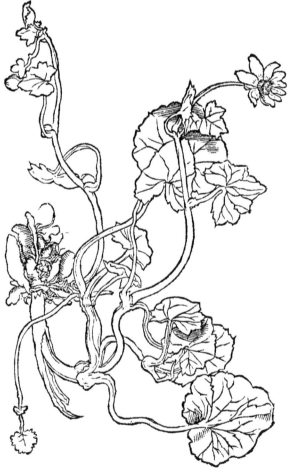

Ranunculus ficaria, lesser celandine (Brunfels 1530, p. 215)

Kent)[53] for cleaning teeth. In Norfolk an infusion of the flowers has even been used for treating sore eyes accompanying measles,[54] possibly out of mistake for the greater celandine at some time in the past.

A herb with parts used for suggestively similar-looking afflictions has inevitably acquired a reputation as one of the classic examples of the Doctrine of Signatures. As in other cases, however, that may well be merely a *post-hoc* rationalisation, for a decoction of the roots, applied with very hot compresses or as a mild ointment, has earned medical respect as an excellent remedy for haemorrhoids in its own right.

Myosurus minimus Linnaeus
mousetail
southern half of Europe, North Africa, south-western Asia, North
America, Australasia

There is a solitary, seventeenth-century record of the use of *Myosurus minimus*, a further acrid member of the buttercup family: 'the country people in some [unspecified] places of this land applied it not only to nose-bleeds, by bruising the leaves and putting them up the nose, but also to staunch heavy-bleeding wounds and heal them.'[55] The identification is borne out by a woodcut of the plant, which was formerly frequent on field margins subject to winter flooding. It is on record north to Yorkshire in England.

Aquilegia vulgaris Linnaeus
columbine
southern and central Europe, North Africa, temperate Asia;
introduced into North America, Australasia

(Folk credentials questionable) Though *Aquilegia vulgaris* has plausibly been claimed as indigenous in limestone thickets in Donegal,[56] it must surely have been too rare in that county to have served as a wild source for the use of the leaves there to poultice swellings, at least at the time of the one record for that.[57] The plant has long been grown in cottage gardens and, once introduced, reproduces very freely.

Thalictrum flavum Linnaeus
common meadow-rue
Europe, temperate Asia

The roots of all species of the genus *Thalictrum*, especially *T. flavum*, are known to be powerful laxatives, earning the collective name 'false rhubarb'. It is the 'tops', however, which feature in the sole record of its use for this purpose which has been encountered: in Buckinghamshire, boiled in ale.[58]

Thalictrum minus Linnaeus
lesser meadow-rue
Eurasia, Alaska; introduced into New Zealand

Widespread round the coast of Scotland, especially in the calcareous coastal grassland of its north and west known as machair, and on sand dunes, *Thalictrum minus* evidently substituted there for the more southerly *T. flavum*. Known as *rú beag*, it was valued in the Highlands primarily as a purge,[59] sometimes taken expressly to kill parasitic worms.[60] James Robertson on his 1768 tour found a decoction in use by women in Skye and Mull for obstruction of the menses.[61] On Colonsay, on the other hand, it was said to have been a remedy for rheumatism.[62]

BERBERIDACEAE

Berberis vulgaris Linnaeus
barberry
Europe; introduced into eastern North America, New Zealand

The use of parts of the shrub *Berberis vulgaris*, usually a decoction of the yellow inner bark, as a cure for jaundice, of which there are records from all over Britain and Ireland, has been so deeply and widely entrenched in medicine both learned and unlearned that it is impossible to be sure how far, if at all, it held a place in the folk tradition independent of herbals and their readers. Though it often grows far from habitations, even sometimes in the hedges of ancient drove roads, the best botanical opinion now is that it is doubtfully native anywhere in the British Isles, but presumptively bird-sown in all cases from planted stock, perhaps over a very long period. In Cornwall, where, as in some other parts of England, it is or was well known and widespread enough to have acquired the name 'jaundice tree', it used to be frequently planted in gardens and shrubberies expressly for herbal use.[63] Nevertheless, it seems likely that in lowland areas, particularly in England, it was grown and escaping from cultivation well back into the monastic period.

One of the very few members of the flora of the British Isles to have been drawn on emphatically for one ailment above all others, barberry has even so been utilised here and there for other purposes as well: in Devon as an ingredient in a herbal mixture given to consumptives,[64] in Lincolnshire for gall stones[65] and in the Highlands for a form of indigestion accompanied by bilious vomiting known as 'the boil'.[66]

PAPAVERACEAE

Papaver Linnaeus

poppy

northern temperate zone; introduced into Australasia

Not only was no distinction apparently drawn in folk medicine between the various red-flowered *Papaver* species of cornfields, but the name is also used as shorthand for opium poppy, *P. somniferum* Linnaeus, as well as for the product extracted from that. All have soporific and painkilling properties, but opium is not present in significant amounts in the European cornfield species. Though there is archaeological evidence that *P. somniferum* was in Britain at least by the Bronze Age (though under what circumstances is not clear), it does not appear to have been grown extensively here as a commercial crop until the nineteenth century and even then it was latterly widely abandoned as unprofitable, as Asian imports rendered opium so cheap that it could be bought over the counter for as little as twopence.

In the fen country of Cambridgeshire and Lincolnshire, where 'ague' (in part malaria) was historically endemic and still prevalent well into the Victorian era, a presumably age-old dependence there on the local cornfield species as the source of 'poppy tea', the standard treatment for both 'ague' and rheumatism, at some point mutated into a general adoption of *Papaver somniferum* instead. A patch of the favoured white-flowered form of that became a feature of cottage gardens throughout the region, enabling consumption to be raised so much that for several months of the year the Fenland people were largely drugged with opium, a fact to which their stunted physique was commonly attributed.[67] The capsules, gathered green, might be boiled in beer as an alternative to the tea.[68]

Though the cornfield species are only mildly narcotic, it can probably be safely assumed that the recorded folk uses of 'poppies' were mostly if not wholly shared by them as well, either before the advent of *Papaver somniferum* or as an inferior stand-in for that or for opium itself. Any or all, but latterly the cultivated plant in particular, appear to have been drawn on as a means of calming babies, during teething or when fevered or otherwise fractious (Norfolk,[69] Isle of Man,[70] South Uist in the Outer Hebrides[71]), either by macerating the petals in the milk for the baby's bottle or dipping the rubber teat in the seeds. This was doubtless a once widespread practice in rural areas which enjoyed a recrudescence, or maybe independent development, in the cities when opium took over there from gin, its notorious predecessor in that function.

Cornfield poppies have served as a soporific in the Isle of Man[72] and the Scottish Lowlands.[73] However, they feature in the folk records much more often in their painkilling role. In Britain this has included treatment of toothache in Sussex,[74] earache in Somerset[75] and neuralgia in Montgomeryshire.[76] In Norfolk[77] wild poppies (*Papaver rhoeas* Linnaeus) have been known as 'headache flowers', the seeds being chewed there as a hangover cure. Poppies have been widely believed in Britain to be a *cause* of headaches as well. In Essex[78] fomentations have been applied to swollen glands and other inflammations, while in Dorset[79] the plants have been the source of an eye lotion.

Ireland's array of these subsidiary uses has been strikingly similar: toothache in Cavan,[80] Westmeath[81] and Co. Dublin,[82] earache in Tipperary,[83] neuralgia in Wicklow,[84] an ingredient in a mixture specifically for mumps in Tipperary[85] and a role as an eye lotion in 'Ulster'.[86] Only in the records for Wicklow have applications additional to those been uncovered: a cure for warts[87] and a syrup for coughs.[88]

Glaucium flavum Crantz
yellow horned-poppy
western and southern Europe, south-western Asia, North Africa;
    introduced into North America, Australasia

All parts of *Glaucium flavum*, like *Chelidonium majus*, exude a corrosive latex, which has predictably attracted some folk usage. Despite its wide distribution on coastal shingle, however, all but one of the records are from south-western England. The exception is Cumbria,[89] where the leaves were made into a poultice for bruises. In Dorset and Hampshire,[90] however, it was the root that was used for that purpose, whence its local names, probably Anglo-Saxon in origin, 'squat' (a bruise in West Country dialect) or 'squatmore'.[91] In the Isles of Scilly, however, the root had quite a different reputation: for the removal of pains in the breast, stomach and intestines as well as for disorders of the lungs. It was used to that end either as an emetic, in which case the root was scraped or sliced upwards, or as a purge, in which case the slicing had to be downwards.[92]

Chelidonium majus Linnaeus
greater celandine
Europe, north Asia; introduced into North America, New Zealand

Chelidonium majus has no claim to native status in the British Isles and is in fact normally found lingering in hedges in the vicinity of houses, so only marginally even ranks as a member of the wild flora; but it has been in Britain certainly since Roman times (as attested by finds in excavations in Dorset and Monmouthshire) and become so widely incorporated into folk use that it would be invidious to exclude it from mention.

Like other herbs with a highly corrosive latex, this plant has traditionally been used for warts above all (as recommended in several herbals and as reflected in various vernacular names) and very widely for corns, as in Som-

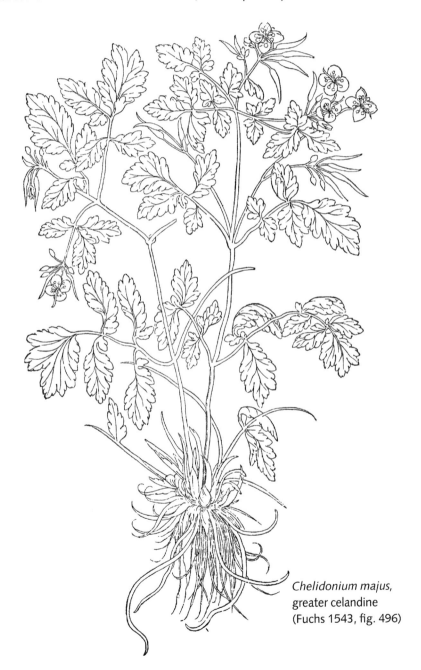

Chelidonium majus,
greater celandine
(Fuchs 1543, fig. 496)

erset[93] and Gloucestershire.[94] As an astringent it has found favour for removing wrinkles (East Riding of Yorkshire[95]) and suntan and freckles (unlocalised).[96] More drastic has been its role as an acrid spring purgative and kidney stimulant in the Isle of Man[97] and for treating cancer of the liver in Suffolk[98]—it was formerly much used for cancer in Russia. In Classical medicine, however, the main use of the latex seems to have been as an eye ointment, in deference to a myth that female swallows restored the sight of their young with it (whence the subsidiary name 'swallow-wort'). In unskilled hands that must always have been most dangerous, yet records from areas as widely separate as Sutherland,[99] Norfolk[100] and especially Devon[101] and Cornwall[102] (whence 'kenning herb' there) point to a once-frequent adherence to that belief; in Glamorgan, indeed, it has even been used for removing a cataract (one Welsh name of the plant is *llym llygaid*, 'sharp eyes').[103] William Withering noted that, when diluted with milk, the juice does indeed consume the white opaque spots on the eye familiarly known as kennings and opined, 'there is no doubt but a medicine of such activity will one day be converted to more important purposes.'[104]

The combination of yellow flowers and yellow juice has predictably brought greater celandine some currency as a jaundice cure as well. Though less popular than barberry (*Berberis vulgaris*), it has seemingly had quite a following for that even so, with records from the Isle of Wight,[105] Norfolk[106] and Berwickshire[107] as far as Britain is concerned.

Ireland can match that last use with records from Cavan,[108] Westmeath[109] and Cork.[110] In Westmeath it has additionally been used for eczema,[111] but otherwise applications of the plant feature noticeably more scantily than in Britain, probably reflecting a much slighter presence historically in that other island.

FUMARIACEAE

Fumaria Linnaeus
fumitory
temperate Asia, North Africa, Macaronesia; introduced into North and South America, Australasia

Fumaria was an astringent mainly in use for cosmetic purposes. Made into an infusion and mixed with milk and/or water, it had a high reputation in certain English country areas,[112] including Wiltshire,[113] Norfolk[114] and Suffolk,[115] for clearing the complexion of blemishes and cleansing the skin. A quite different application comes from far-off Orkney, where the juice was given to children to rid them of intestinal worms.[116]

Ireland has had at least one different use for the plant, too: in Cavan it was burnt and the smoke inhaled as a cure for stomach trouble.[117] Both the scientific and vernacular names are derived from *fumus,* the Latin word for smoke, so that is presumably an ancient practice, possibly even well pre-Classical.

Notes

1. for instance, Cameron
2. McNeill
3. IFC S 636: 191
4. IFC S 524: 11
5. Beith
6. IFC S 483: 329, 369
7. McNeill
8. for references, see under
   Potamogeton
9. Maloney
10. Withering 1787–92, 321
11. Sargent
12. IFC S 710: 49
13. IFC S 250: 35
14. Parkinson, 216
15. *Wiltshire Family History Society Journal,* 46 (1992), 6
16. Pratt 1857, 33
17. Henderson & Dickson, 45
18. Wood-Martin, 200
19. Gregory, 12
20. IFC S 968: 225; 959: 77; Logan, 51; Maloney
21. Friend 1883–4, ii, 368
22. Tongue
23. A. Allen, 178
24. Vickery MSS
25. Carmichael, ii, 280
26. *PLNN,* no. 26 (1992), 118
27. Vickery 1995
28. Johnston 1853, 27
29. Carmichael, ii, 280
30. Polwhele 1816, ii, 607; Davey, 10, 23
31. Bardswell
32. IFC S 672: 260
33. IFC S 589: 15, 62
34. IFC S 484: 41–2
35. Farrelly MS
36. Logan, 12
37. Ó hEithir
38. Barbour
39. IFC S 60: 302
40. Vickery MSS
41. IFC S 903: 448
42. Kermode MS
43. Pennant 1776, ii, 43
44. Johnston 1853, 28 footnote
45. Martin, 225
46. McNeill
47. Macpherson MS
48. Vickery MSS
49. Beith
50. McNeill
51. CECTL MSS
52. Freethy, 80
53. Pratt 1850–7
54. Hatfield, 43
55. Parkinson, 501
56. Hart 1898
57. IFC S 1075: 139
58. Henslow
59. MacFarlane
60. Beith
61. Henderson & Dickson, 80, 93
62. McNeill
63. Davey, 17
64. Lafont, 6, 70
65. Woodruffe-Peacock

66. Beith
67. Porter 1974, 52
68. Newman 1945
69. Hatfield, 40, 55, appendix
70. Fargher
71. Beith
72. Morrison
73. Simpson, 159
74. A. Allen, 43
75. Tongue
76. Evans 1940
77. Hatfield, 40, 61
78. Macpherson MS
79. Dacombe
80. Maloney
81. IFC S 736: 22, 24
82. IFC S 788: 145
83. IFC S 571: 208
84. McClafferty
85. IFC S 571: 208
86. St Clair, 79
87. IFC S 571: 208
88. IFC S 512: 523
89. Freethy, 45
90. John Aubrey, in litt. to John Ray, 5 Aug. 1691 (Lankester, 238)
91. Grigson
92. Borlase 1756; *Notes and Queries,* 10 (1854), 181
93. Tongue
94. Palmer 1994, 122
95. Vickery MSS
96. Tynan & Maitland
97. Quayle, 69
98. Taylor 1929, 118
99. Henderson & Dickson, 37
100. Haggard
101. Briggs 1872, 1880; Lafont
102. Davey, 23
103. Williams MS
104. Withering 1878–92, 316
105. Broomfield, 26
106. Taylor 1929, 119
107. Johnston 1853, 31
108. Maloney
109. IFC S 736: 136
110. IFC S 385: 55
111. IFC S 736: 136
112. Black, 230; Quelch, 89
113. Dartnell & Goddard, 55
114. de Castre
115. Withering 1787–92, 752
116. Spence
117. Maloney

CHAPTER 6

Elms to Docks

Dicotyledonous flowering plants in the orders (and families) Urticales (Ulmaceae, elms; Cannabaceae, hemp and hop; Urticaceae, nettles), Myricales (Myricaceae, bog-myrtles), Fagales (Fagaceae, beeches and oaks; Betulaceae, birches), Caryophyllales (Aizoaceae, dew-plants; Chenopodiaceae, goosefoots; Portulacaceae, blinks; Caryophyllaceae, pinks), Polygonales (Polygonaceae, knotweeds) and Plumbaginales (Plumbaginaceae, thrifts) are included in this chapter.

ULMACEAE

Ulmus glabra Hudson
wych elm
Europe, northern and western Asia; introduced into North
America
As the records for 'elm' remedies are almost exclusively Irish, it is probably safe to assume that it is to *Ulmus glabra* that they mainly and perhaps even wholly relate. For this is the only species accepted as indigenous in Ireland, where pollen evidence suggests that it was extremely widespread at earlier periods.

The commonest use appears to have been for scalds and burns. Caleb Threlkeld in 1726 identified the 'common elm' as the source of a slimy decoction of the inner bark which he found country people in the north of Ireland applying as a salve.[1] It was still in currency for that purpose, or remembered as such, in the 1930s in a band of counties stretching from Leitrim to Wexford. The mucilage has also been valued since Classical times for skin troubles in general; this, too, was a use formerly widespread in rural Ireland[2] which survived till more recently at least in Tipperary.[3] Like that of comfrey (*Symphytum officinale*) and royal fern (*Osmunda regalis*), the mucilage was also found effective for easing swellings and so had a reputation for curing sprains in Offaly[4] and Co. Dublin[5] as well as across the sea in Galloway.[6] The leaves were sometimes employed instead of the bark for swellings and inflammation.[7] Other, unrelated uses recorded have been to staunch bleeding in Cavan,[8] to cure jaundice in Kilkenny[9] and to counteract 'evils' (ulcers, cancer and the like) in Limerick.[10]

By contrast, the tree seems to have hardly featured at all in English folk medicine. Apart from an elm wood tea drunk for eczema in Hampshire,[11] the sole record traced is from the valley of the Upper Thames in Wiltshire, where for a cold or sore throat villagers stripped off the inner bark from young wands and either chewed that raw or boiled it down into a jelly eaten cold.[12]

CANNABACEAE

Humulus lupulus Linnaeus
hop
Europe, western Asia; introduced into North America,
    New Zealand

Opinions differ on whether *Humulus lupulus* is anywhere indigenous in the British Isles, but its pollen has been reported from deposits of prehistoric date, and though readily running into wild habitats from cultivation, it may be a genuine relic in fenny areas. Even so it must be considered doubtful whether any of the recorded folk uses of the plant antedate its cultivation as a crop.

Almost all those records are Irish. Apparently, Ireland alone has appreciated the alleged sedative effect of one or more of the plant's constituents. It has been used in Co. Dublin[13] and Clare[14] for calming the nerves and in Limerick as an antidote to insomnia.[15]

More intriguing is a practice reported from an unidentified part of England (the New Forest?): cleansing and curing ulcers and obstinate sores by means of a bread poultice on to which hops have been thickly sprinkled.[16]

URTICACEAE

Urtica dioica Linnaeus
common nettle
temperate regions worldwide

Urtica urens Linnaeus
small nettle
Eurasia, North Africa; introduced into other temperate
regions

With the possible exception of dandelions, elder and docks, no plants
have featured so extensively in folk
medicine in the British Isles as nettles.
Although there are one or two records
for the more vicious small nettle,
Urtica urens, almost always it
and *U. dioica* have not been dis-
criminated and they are accordingly treated here together.

Of a total of 311 localised records,
almost two-thirds (194) are accounted for
by use as a spring tonic to cleanse the blood
of impurities (and thus of boils, pimples,
sores of various kinds and clouded eyes).
'Three nettles in May keeps all diseases
away', at least for the rest of the year, was
once a widely quoted rhyme, firmly
believed in. Some of the 76 records for
rashes perhaps really belong in that category, too, but no fewer than 60 of these are represented by the practice of drinking nettle tea
to help clear measles rash, which is apparently
peculiar to Ireland and there largely restricted to
the border counties and the north-western
quadrant.

The two other major uses are as a counter-
irritant for rheumatic complaints (48 records),
which dates back at least to Roman times, and
for colds, coughs and lung trouble (29
records, 9 of them for consumption specifically). These exhibit no marked geographical patterns in their occurrence.

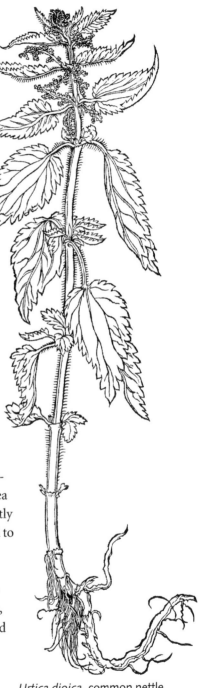

Urtica dioica, common nettle
(Brunfels 1530, p. 151)

Of the numerous ailments which crop up in the records much less commonly, two clearly owe their presence to the plant's astringent effect: bleeding, especially from the nose, and stomach upsets and diarrhoea (7 and 4 records, respectively). Three records of use as a skin-cleansing cosmetic belong here, too. Conviction that the plants are rich in iron have led to their being eaten for anaemia (5 records), while valuing of them for reducing swellings (7 records) has produced a particular targeting of mumps. Their claimed sedative property has also called forth a use for insomnia and 'nerves' (4 records), while by contrast the undoubted stimulus to the circulation imparted by the stings has encouraged their application to paralysed limbs and for heart trouble. Other uses for which, like these last, no more than three or four records at most have come to light include for jaundice, headaches, insect stings, dandruff, swollen glands (especially goitre), dropsy, ringworm, indigestion, ear infections, high blood pressure, shingles, piles, worms, epilepsy, cramp and corns. There is also a solitary record of the use of nettles to keep away flies.

Parietaria judaica Linnaeus
   P. diffusa Mertens & Koch
   pellitory-of-the-wall
   western and southern Europe, North Africa; introduced into North
      America, Australasia

(Folk credentials questionable) Though frequent in the British Isles and accepted as indigenous on cliffs, rocks and steep hedgebanks, *Parietaria judaica* also occurs widely in places associated with human activity. Both it and the related *P. officinalis* Linnaeus were once much valued for their diuretic action and consequently applied to dropsy and gravel complaints, but it is suspicious that the few records of folk use are virtually all, Irish[17] as well as English,[18] of use in the relatively sophisticated form of inclusion in 'cocktails' with various other standard diuretic herbs. That it is really a relic of the learned tradition in its entirety seems likeliest on the evidence.

MYRICACEAE

Myrica gale Linnaeus
   bog-myrtle, sweet gale, bog sally, black sallow, *roid, roideog, reileòg*
   Eurasia, North America

Like bogbean (*Menyanthes trifoliata*), essentially a plant of the peaty areas of the west, *Myrica gale* has enjoyed semi-sacred status in Irish lore and might have been expected to have occupied an equally central place medicinally, for lack of phytochemical efficacy does not seem to have been a barrier to the use of other herbal species lucky enough to have acquired a magico-religious halo. However, its role has been mainly the humdrum one of an insecticide: either to repel fleas and other insects, especially by being put in beds and linen (Caernarvonshire,[19] Isle of Man,[20] Galloway,[21] Islay and Jura[22]) or to destroy internal worms (most of the foregoing with the addition of the Highlands[23] and Western Isles[24] more generally). Despite the lengthy history of use for these purposes, the more recent, short-lived exploitation of the plant commercially as a midge repellent, under the fitting brand name Myrica, only came about through someone's chancing to notice in Scotland that midges avoid areas where this plant is plentiful.[25]

Two additional uses have been recorded in Britain: as an emetic in Caernarvonshire[26] and, combined with other herbs, as an inhalant to clear a blocked nose or sinuses in Cumbria.[27]

Ireland can add to those uses kidney trouble in Donegal,[28] measles in Sligo[29] and sore throats in Kildare.[30]

FAGACEAE

Fagus sylvatica Linnaeus
beech
Europe

Despite the prevalence of *Fagus sylvatica* in southern England, only one undoubted record of the use of this tree has been met with in the British folk literature: an infusion of the buds taken for boils or piles in Gloucestershire.[31] An Irish record from Meath[32] was probably a mishearing of birch, known to have been used there for the ailment in question.

Quercus petraea (Mattuschka) Lieblein
sessile oak
Europe

Quercus robur Linnaeus
pedunculate oak
Europe, Caucasus; introduced into Canada, New Zealand

The bark, leaves and acorns of both the native oaks, *Quercus petraea* and *Q. robur*, are rich in tannin and have therefore come into use for their astringent property. Despite the presence of both throughout the British Isles, records of the trees' use in folk medicine are predominantly Irish. These have all involved exploitation of the bark. Collected in spring from branches four to five years old, dried, chopped up and then boiled, this has been valued as a gargle for sore throats in Sligo[33] and Tipperary,[34] to counter diarrhoea in Meath[35] and for adding to a hot bath for sore or excessively perspiring feet (Donegal,[36] Meath,[37] Kilkenny[38]) or a sprained ankle (Offaly[39]). Because of its drying and constricting effect, the same decoction has found use for ulcers in Meath[40] and Sligo,[41] and for toothache and neuralgia in Wicklow.[42] It has also been deployed against pin-worms in Meath.[43] But for ringworm a decoction of six of the leaves has been the preferred treatment in Offaly.[44]

In Britain the properties of oaks have been valued noticeably more sparsely and for fewer though broadly similar ailments: for rheumatism in Essex,[45] diarrhoea in Suffolk[46] and sore throats in the Highlands.[47] That Suffolk use, though, has been unusual in involving a powder made from the acorns.

BETULACEAE

Betula pendula Roth
silver birch
Europe, western Asia, Morocco; introduced into North America,
  New Zealand

Betula pubescens Ehrhart
downy birch
Eurasia, Greenland; introduced into the rest of North America

Birch trees (*Betula pendula* and *B. pubescens*) have had two quite distinct roles in non-veterinary folk medicine, depending on whether the sap or the bark was utilised. The former has traditionally been prized over much of Europe for a tonic wine made from it, a tradition reflected in records in Britain from Lincolnshire[48] and the Highlands.[49] At least some of these British users have rated the wine highly as a treatment for rheumatism.[50] The method used to extract the liquid was to make an incision three to four inches wide in the trunk and funnel the resulting ooze through a hollowed-out piece of elder or a straw into a collecting container, limiting the procedure to just a day or two at most in order not to tap the tree to the point of exhaustion.

Use of the bark, on the other hand, appears to have been exclusive to Ireland, where it was considered effective for eczema; there are records of this from Meath,[51] Cork[52] and Kerry.[53]

Alnus glutinosa (Linnaeus) Gaertner   PLATE 3
  alder
  Europe, western Asia, North Africa; introduced into eastern
    North America
Because of the similarity in their names, elder (*Sambucus* spp.) is apparently
sometimes misrecorded as alder (*Alnus glutinosa*) by folklore collectors. To
judge from the ailments mentioned in such cases, two of the only four records
have resulted from confusions on this score. No such ambiguity, however, is
attached to one for the Somerset-Dorset border,[54] for in that case it was
explicitly a decoction of the ripe cones that was drunk daily as a cure for gout.
And in a Norfolk instance, too, the informant was quite definite that it was the
leaves of this tree, not that of elder, which were lightly crushed and laid on
burns; the locality in question is in any case one in which alders are plentiful.[55]

Corylus avellana Linnaeus
  hazel
  Europe, Asia Minor; introduced into North America
A tree so widespread and once even much commoner (to judge from the profusion of its pollen in subfossil peats), and with a semi-sacred status besides,
might have been expected to have given rise to a wide range of medicinal
uses. Only three folk records have been encountered for *Corylus avellana*,
however, and those all Irish: the ash from a burnt hazel stick was put on burns
in Monaghan,[56] the bark was applied to boils and cuts in Kerry[57] and in that
county also some unspecified part of the tree has formed a treatment for
varicose veins.[58]

AIZOACEAE

Carpobrotus edulis (Linnaeus) N. E. Brown

Carpobrotus acinaciformis (Linnaeus) L. Bolus
  Hottentot-fig
  South Africa; introduced into warmer temperate regions
Introduced into gardens from South Africa, species of the genus *Carpobrotus*
have escaped and become naturalised so plentifully in the far south-west of
Britain that in that relatively brief period they have acquired not only a new
vernacular name locally ('Sally-me-handsome', a corruption of *Mesembry-
anthemum*, the generic name formerly in use) but also earned the right to be
included in this account of the utilising of the wild flora for medicinal pur-

poses, contemporary though that utilising is, for in the Isles of Scilly the juice of the fleshy leaves is rubbed on to sunburn.[59]

CHENOPODIACEAE

Chenopodium album Linnaeus
fat-hen
temperate regions worldwide

Assuming *Chenopodium album* was the plant known there as 'lambs' quarters'—one of the alternative vernacular names of this species—a decoction of its stems was till relatively recently drunk in Co. Dublin for rheumatism.[60] Though now treated as a weed and generally disregarded, it was formerly valued as a nutritious food along with nettles and dandelions. It was, for example, added to soup in spring in Ayrshire,[61] perhaps semi-medicinally. Undoubtedly present in the British Isles in prehistoric times, that it was ever a native is open to question, however.

Salicornia europaea Linnaeus, in the broad sense
glasswort, marsh samphire
western Europe, North Africa, North America

Better known, like *Chenopodium album,* as a source of food, the gathering of *Salicornia europaea* from the saltmarshes of Norfolk has extended to its use there as an ointment for cracked hands and skin troubles more generally.[62] It has also been consumed in that county as a spring tonic.[63]

PORTULACACEAE

Montia fontana Linnaeus
blinks
temperate regions worldwide

A plant known in the Highlands as *fliodh Moire,* identified as 'marsh chickweed' and described as growing in pools and puddles,[64] was presumably *Montia fontana.* Its applications—heated and then placed on a festering hand or foot, and as a treatment for rheumatism—are ones for which common chickweed (*Stellaria media*) has been valued pre-eminently. In the Badenoch district of Inverness-shire[65] a distinction was carefully made between the chickweed of gardens and a kind growing on the moors, the latter regarded as superior. Only blinks, appears to fit this combination of features: it could be mistaken for chickweed, and, unlike that, is characteristic of moorland seepages.

CARYOPHYLLACEAE

Honckenya peploides (Linnaeus) Ehrhart
sea sandwort
Arctic and northern temperate zone
According to one of John Aubrey's correspondents in 1695, *Honckenya peploides* was one of several antiscorbutic herbs gathered in the northern parts of Orkney.[66]

Stellaria media (Linnaeus) Villars
common chickweed, *fliodh*
cosmopolitan weed
Perhaps because of their very commonness as weeds and therefore ready availability, *Stellaria media* and groundsel (*Senecio vulgaris*) are alike in having been employed for an impressive diversity of ailments, many of them the same ones. Chickweed, though, is remarkable for the very limited number of *ways* in which it has been applied. By far the commonest of those is in the form of a mat, as a hot and relaxing poultice. The reason why that so predominates is that it has been used on a quite disproportionately extensive scale for just one particular purpose: to reduce swellings, including those of sprains and mumps, and other forms of inflammation. The heavy concentration on that class of ailments, moreover, has been almost peculiar to Ireland, thus distorting matters even further. Out of sixty-eight records of use for that purpose in the British Isles as a whole, the only ones that are other than Irish are from Gloucestershire,[67] Berwickshire[68] and Orkney.[69]

In Britain, and England in particular, it is boils, abscesses and ulcers, rather, to which chickweed has been applied as a poultice: in Dorset,[70] Somerset,[71] Gloucestershire,[72] Norfolk[73] and the Highlands.[74] In Suffolk[75] 'sore legs' (leg ulcers?) have been similarly treated, and in the Isle of Man,[76] bruises. But whereas in Sussex[77] poulticing has been employed for rheumatism, in Inverness-shire[78] that and stiff joints, as also chilblains and rashes, have received the plant's benefits in the form of an ointment, while for sore eyes in Devon[79] and Somerset,[80] and eczema in Yorkshire,[81] that has been replaced in turn by a lotion. In Skye,[82] to procure sleep after a fever, the feet and knees were bathed with a chickweed wash preparatory to a warm poultice being placed on the neck and between the shoulders. A tea, though, has been found a sufficient remedy for insomnia in the Highlands,[83] and a rheumatism cure in Essex[84] has taken that form, too, while for 'water problems' in Durham[85] and for slimming in the Highlands[86] a variation on that has been to drink a decoction of the plant. A yet further approach is to eat the boiled leaves: to cleanse the system and improve the complexion in Northumberland[87] and, mixed with those of comfrey (*Symphytum officinale*), as a tonic and a treatment for diabetes in Liverpool.[88]

Though Ireland stands so sharply apart from Britain in that comparatively enormous use, especially in the border counties, of chickweed poultices for treating swellings and inflammation, a wide variety of subsidiary applications has occurred in both countries, some of them the same ones and employed to a similar extent. Seemingly special to Ireland, though, has been the treating of six afflictions not found mentioned in the records from Britain: sores (Louth,[89] Kildare,[90] Galway,[91] Kilkenny[92]), coughs and sore throats (Mayo,[93] the Aran Islands[94] and, mixed with elecampane, Limerick[95]), cuts (Offaly,[96] Tipperary[97]), jaundice (Galway[98]), burns (Donegal[99]) and colic (Cork[100]).

Stellaria holostea Linnaeus
greater stitchwort
Europe, south-western Asia, North Africa; introduced into North
  America, New Zealand

Stellaria holostea has traditionally had the reputation of relieving stitches and other muscular pains, whence the vernacular name. As recently as the 1930s, children in Somerset chewed the flowers for that purpose.[101] Under a Welsh name translating as 'herb for shingles' it is still in use in Caernarvonshire for that in a mixture with wood sage and navelwort.[102] But whether *tùrsairean*, a herb valued in the Highlands for a swollen breast, has correctly been identified as 'stitchwort'[103] must be considered doubtful, as that is an ailment for which chickweed (*S. media*) has pre-eminently been used.

In Ireland the same chewing of the flowers for stitches has been noted, and in the south of that country it has also been boiled down with sugar candy as a remedy for whooping cough under a name recorded as *thang-a-naun*.[104]

Spergula arvensis Linnaeus
corn spurrey
almost cosmopolitan weed

The only certain record of *Spergula arvensis* in folk medicine is John Parkinson's generalised 1640 statement: 'the country people in divers places say that they have had good experience' of speedily healing a cut by bruising the plant and then laying it on.[105] It is odd that there have been no later reports by folklorists of this use. One of the plant's vernacular names in Ulster is *grangore* or *glengore,* which, being Scots for syphilis, may imply a one-time venereal reputation.[106]

Lychnis flos-cuculi Linnaeus
ragged-robin
Europe, western Asia; introduced into North America, New Zealand
(Error suspected) As ragged-robin is also one of the vernacular names of red campion (*Silene dioica*), which is associated with snakes in western Wales folk beliefs to the extent that it bears a name, *blodwyn neidr,* 'snake flower' in Welsh,[107] the solitary record of *Lychnis flos-cuculi* in the folk medicine literature, an ointment made from it used for snakebites in Cardiganshire,[108] may probably safely be presumed to belong to that.

Agrostemma githago Linnaeus
corncockle
most temperate regions worldwide
(Error suspected) Two Wicklow records[109] of *Agrostemma githago* are surely misattributions of 'cockle', a common alternative name of burdock (*Arctium*). The species does not appear to have had a place in folk medicine in the British Isles.

Silene otites (Linnaeus) Wibel
Spanish catchfly
southern and central Europe, western Asia
(Error involved) John Ray, in his *Historia Plantarum* in 1695 (i, 1895), was misled (through being sent a specimen of the wrong plant) into identifying as *Silene otites* a herb known on Newmarket Heath in Suffolk as 'star of the earth' and renowned there at that period for curing the bites of mad dogs, as reported to him by Hans Sloane in 1687.[110] It was later shown conclusively that the plant with this reputation was in fact buck's-horn plantain (*Plantago coronopus*).[111]

Silene dioica (Linnaeus) Clairville
Lychnis dioica Linnaeus
red campion
Europe, western Asia, North Africa; introduced into North
      America, Australasia
Despite its general distribution throughout much of the British Isles, the only certain records traced of *Silene dioica* in folk medicine are exclusively southern English: the corrosive juice has been used for warts in Sussex,[112] for corns in Gloucestershire[113] and for both of those purposes in Somerset.[114] An oint-

ment made for snakebites used in Cardiganshire, however, was probably made from this and not ragged-robin (*Lychnis flos-cuculi*).

POLYGONACEAE

Persicaria bistorta (Linnaeus) Sampaio
bistort
northern and central Europe, mountains of southern Europe,
   south-western and central Asia

With a root rich in tannin and a powerful astringent, *Persicaria bistorta* might have been expected to feature in folk medicine at least as widely as its popularity for soup and spring puddings, though the latter also had a reputation for purifying the blood.[115] In Cumbria a tea made from it has been recorded as a headache cure[116] and it has also been used there as a vermicide.[117] In the Highlands it was valued for urinary complaints[118] and there is an unlocalised record ('in country places') of its use for toothache.[119] That is all. But what is the explanation of its subsequent discovery in cemeteries in both urban and rural areas in various parts of England and Scotland? Was it introduced into these to ensure a supply for the puddings connected with Easter, or because of some obscure medicinal belief, such as the one recorded in some of the sixteenth-century herbals, that it could aid conception?

Persicaria maculosa Gray
Polygonum persicaria Linnaeus
redshank
northern temperate zone; introduced into Australasia

Persicaria lapathifolia (Linnaeus) Gray
pale persicaria
northern temperate zone, Australia; introduced into North America

Oddly, the records for the folk use of the common weeds *Persicaria maculosa* and *P. lapathifolia* are exclusively Irish. A plant which from the verbal description is clearly one or the other has been used in Limerick to stop bleeding—on the strength of a belief that the blotch on the leaves is a drop of Christ's blood.[120] The name bloodweed has been recorded in Donegal as borne by a plant identified botanically as *P. lapathifolia*,[121] which suggests the same usage there as well; but whether this was also the 'bloodweed' similarly used in Tipperary[122] is uncertain, as that name has been given to a range of herbs allegedly with styptic properties. The joints of one or the other have also been recorded from an unspecific part of Ireland as eaten for a malady known as *brios bronn,*[123] perhaps the same as the *briose brún,* a name for a lameness in cattle apparently resulting from phosphorus deficiency.

Persicaria hydropiper (Linnaeus) Spach
water pepper
northern temperate zone, Australia; introduced into New Zealand
(Folk credentials questionable) The claim of *Persicaria hydropiper* to a place in the folk medicine repertory rests almost entirely on the assertion of just one author[124] whose data are unlocalised but appear to be based on first-hand information. According to this source, 'country people' (in Kent?) used the leaves for toothache; a stimulant plaster made from it also substituted for mustard poultices, while yet another practice was to lay the leaves on the skin to remove the blackness of bruises. It is possible, though, that most if not all these were derived from the learned tradition, in which the equating of this species with the *hudropeperi* of Dioscorides led to its being prescribed for a wide variety of ailments. The same could be said of Borlase's remark in his *Natural History of Cornwall* that 'arsesmart' (a widely used name for this plant in south-western England), when distilled 'has been found better for gravelly complaints than a great variety of drugs taken ... to little purpose.'[125]

Polygonum aviculare Linnaeus, in the broad sense
knotgrass
Eurasia, North Africa, North America; introduced into South
    America, Australasia
There is just one folk record of the use of the common plant *Polygonum aviculare:* in Somerset to staunch a nosebleed by rubbing it into the nostrils.[126] Its astringency gave it a reputation among the ancient writers as a styptic, but the equal availability for such purposes of the more readily obtained and more easily recognised yarrow (*Achillea millefolium*) doubtless caused the latter to be the normal stand-by.

Rumex acetosa Linnaeus
common sorrel, cuckoo sorrel, sour-dock, cow sorrel, red sorrel
Europe, temperate Asia, North America; introduced into New Zealand
There is considerable confusion between *Rumex acetosa* and wood-sorrel (*Oxalis acetosella*) in the folk records, especially in Ireland; but in at least one instance[127] the two are carefully distinguished by separate names and it would seem that 'cuckoo sorrel' normally denotes *R. acetosa* (which of the two is the much more often seen bearing so-called 'cuckoo spit', the excretion of Hemiptera insect species).

As with nettles (*Urtica*) and burdock (*Arctium*), one of the functions of sorrel has been to cleanse the blood of impurities and thereby clear up spots. To that end the juice has been drunk in the Isle of Man[128] and Berwickshire.[129] Rather similarly, the leaves have been eaten as a cure for scurvy in the Isle of Man,[130] Orkney[131] and Shetland[132]—and the Faeroe Islands,[133] too, a distribution thus seemingly Viking in origin. As a cooling herb the plant served in the Highlands as a digestive[134] and an appetiser[135]; its leaves were eaten by consumptives and infusions drunk by the fevered[136]; it has also enjoyed a reputation there for curing minor wounds and bruises.[137] A more esoteric reason for eating the leaves in Cumbria has been the belief that this relieved epilepsy.[138] The Isle of Man seems to have been alone in making use of the roots, to stimulate the kidneys.[139]

Ireland has shared most of these applications. It has been drunk to cleanse the system in Wicklow[140] and Carlow,[141] to help the kidneys and cool fevers in Clare[142] and, mixed with thistle tops and plantain heads, to cure consumption in Kildare[143]; similarly, the leaves have healed sores and bruises in Sligo[144] and Limerick[145] and staunched bleeding in Wicklow[146] and Cavan.[147] Other uses, though, emerge only from the Irish records. The leaves, in some cases crumbled and boiled first, have served in six of the south-eastern counties to poultice boils, septic sores and the pustules of chickenpox. Much more locally, the plant has been employed for jaundice and sore throat in Cavan,[148] cancer in 'Ulster',[149] burns in Meath,[150] warts in Waterford,[151] heart trouble in Tipperary (mixed with dandelions, *Taraxacum*)[152] and anaemia in some part of the country unidentified.[153]

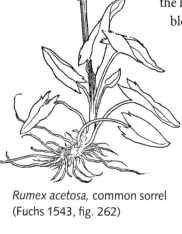

Rumex acetosa, common sorrel (Fuchs 1543, fig. 262)

Rumex hydrolapathum Hudson
water dock
western and southern Europe

With its very astringent roots, *Rumex hydrolapathum* formerly had a reputation as a cure for scurvy, especially when the gums had become spongy and black. In one district in Londonderry, where it grew in quantity, country doctors would come to gather it.[154] On the river Erne in adjoining Donegal, on the other hand, it was rated 'a grand blood purifier, as good as bogbean and burdock'.[155]

Those two Irish records stand on the authority of able botanists in each case, but elsewhere there may have been confusion with butterbur (*Petasites hybridus*), which is similarly valued for its roots and has been known as 'water docken' in Cumberland.[156] Perhaps it was that, and not *Rumex hydrolapathum*, whose root juice was drunk for colds and asthma in Cavan[157] (a known use of butterbur) or employed for cleaning the teeth in the Highlands, where *R. hydrolapathum* is very rare?[158] On the other hand, perhaps *R. hydrolapathum* was the 'bloodwort', a name borne by the plant in Cheshire,[159] whose roots were boiled in Wicklow and the liquid rubbed on parts pained by rheumatism and on mouth ulcers?[160]

Rumex crispus Linnaeus
curled dock
Europe, Africa; introduced into other continents

In Ireland, as 'yellow dock', one of its commoner alternative names, *Rumex crispus* is on record in folk use from Sligo,[161] Cavan[162] and Wexford.[163] In the last of these, the juice was squeezed out of the leaves and put on to a cloth which was then tied round a stone-bruise. In Cavan a decoction of the roots (which have been proved to have purgative properties) was drunk for constipation and liver trouble, and in Sligo for liver trouble, skin diseases and rheumatism.

Rumex conglomeratus Murray
clustered dock
Europe, Asia Minor, North Africa; introduced into North America

A decoction of a plant distinguished as 'narrow-leaved dock', presumably either *Rumex conglomeratus* or *R. crispus,* is on record from one village in Norfolk as a claimed cancer cure. The growth was steeped in the liquid and then poulticed.[164]

Rumex obtusifolius Linnaeus
broad-leaved dock
western and central Europe; introduced into North America,
Australasia

Probably the most general practice in all of folk medicine, occurring throughout the British Isles, is rubbing a dock leaf on to the skin to ease a sting. For
such a purpose, the wide leaves of *Rumex obtusifolius* most obviously suggest themselves, though they may be merely a quick and easy stand-in for the
more onerous but more certainly efficient practice of poulticing the sting
with the pulped root, sometimes every few hours, as in the Badenoch district of Inverness-shire.[165] In the case of most other uses, however, there has
probably been no consistent distinction drawn between it and the no less
common and generally distributed *R. crispus;* 'dock' or (less often) 'common
dock' may refer to either or both.

'Dock' in this more general sense has been used for all the ailments
appearing in records of a particular species, but predictably to a greater
extent. The complaints to emerge from the records with the next highest incidence after stings are burns and scalds, though only if the British Isles are
taken as a whole—the records traced from Britain alone are restricted just to
Cornwall,[166] Pembrokeshire[167] and South Uist in the Outer Hebrides[168] (in
other words the westernmost fringe). Third in popularity in Britain is applying a leaf to staunch bleeding from a cut, as a second-best to one from a plantain, near-universally favoured for that. That has been recorded from Essex,[169]
some part of Wales,[170] the Isle of Man[171] and Shetland.[172] That use in Essex
has involved soaking the leaf in brandy first, seemingly for lack of the petals
of Madonna lilies (*Lilium candidum* Linnaeus) which have been so widely
used, mixed with brandy, for the same purpose in many parts of the Eastern
Counties (or with whisky in Scotland or wine in the Mediterranean).

The leaves, roots and even seeds of docks have had many other applications besides just those. Most simply, the leaves have been used to absorb
moisture, as that of perspiring feet in the South Riding of Yorkshire,[173] or
when heated to alleviate headaches in Norfolk[174] or the pain of rheumatism
on the Dorset-Somerset border.[175] Slightly more advanced has been the use
of either the leaves or the roots as dressings for sores of a variety of kinds,
ranging from stone-bruises on the arms of Oxfordshire quarrymen[176] to
chapped thighs in Norfolk[177] and galled feet in Herefordshire[178] and Suffolk.[179] In Essex, one step further, the seeds have been boiled for drawing the
pus from a wound or a boil.[180] Docks have also been popular for rashes, but

whereas in Somerset[181] it has been deemed sufficient just to rub a leaf on one, elsewhere drinking an infusion made from the roots has been the preferred cure for those. In Merseyside,[182] for example, erysipelas has been treated with this infusion, and in Cornwall[183] it has been mixed with bramble juice and, with a suitable incantation, poured on the part of the body afflicted with shingles. Similarly, whereas in Hampshire[184] it has been the leaves that, mixed with lard, have produced an ointment for piles, elsewhere drinking a liquid processed from the roots has been regarded as a curative tonic: for cleansing the blood in Essex,[185] Oxfordshire[186] and Ayrshire[187] and for keeping scurvy away in the Highlands.[188] Still further uses of the plants have been for warts in Norfolk[189] and for obesity as well as anaemia in the Isle of Man.[190]

Ireland has not lagged behind in appreciating this range of virtues. Apparently peculiar to it has been the drinking of a decoction of the seeds for coughs of all kinds, colds and bronchitis. Records of this are virtually confined to the border counties (if veterinary uses for those purposes are added in, seven of them are represented in all). Similarly not met with in the records for Britain is the drinking of a decoction of the roots for liver trouble (Cavan,[191] Meath[192]) and jaundice (Monaghan,[193] Limerick[194]), and, in Wexford,[195] bathing cancerous sores in that liquid. Further ailments for which docks seem to have been employed in Ireland alone are heart trouble in Cavan[196] and corns in Limerick.[197] On the other hand, staunching bleeding with a leaf, though recorded from five widely separated counties (in one of them in combination with the dung of asses[198]) appears scarcely more widespread than the even more scattered records suggest that it has been in Britain. The two countries are also alike in the small use made of the leaves for alleviating rheumatism (Louth,[199] Westmeath[200]) or headaches (Kildare[201]).

In some places, particular potency has been ascribed to the whitish, slimy sheath at the base of an unfurling leaf. In Donegal[202] this was selected for poulticing ringworm, in Longford[203] for rubbing on a sting and elsewhere in Ireland[204] has constituted a remedy for 'a sore mouth' (chapped lips?). A marginal echo of the belief in Britain was the binding of the sheath over wounds in Shetland.[205]

Rumex palustris Smith
marsh dock
Europe, temperate Asia

There is a record from the marshland area of Norfolk of the use of the roots of a type of dock expressly named 'marsh dock', i.e. *Rumex palustris* (and 'with their feet in the water') as recently as the 1940s for bathing rashes, sunburn and the like.[206]

PLUMBAGINACEAE

Armeria maritima (Miller) Willdenow
thrift, sea pink
northern hemisphere; introduced into New Zealand

Though *Armeria maritima* is a common plant round most of the coasts of the British Isles, the only records of its use in folk medicine seem to be confined to the Orkney Islands and to South Uist in the Outer Hebrides. In the former, the thick, tuberous roots were sliced and boiled in sweet milk to produce a drink known as 'Arby', highly prized up to c. 1700 as a remedy for tuberculosis.[207] John Aubrey was also told by a medical correspondent that a cure for the ague in Orkney included drinking an infusion in which this plant was one of several herbal ingredients.[208] In South Uist, a sailor's remedy for a hangover was to boil a bunch of these plants complete with their roots and drink the liquid slowly when cooled.[209] The roots at least evidently contain a compound which induces heavy sweating.

Notes

1. Threlkeld
2. Purdon
3. IFC S 530: 51, 121
4. IFC S 811: 64
5. IFC S 787: 368
6. Mactaggart, 18
7. Ó Súilleabháin, 312
8. Maloney
9. IFC S 850: 56
10. IFC S 512: 445
11. Beddington & Christy, 212
12. Williams 1922, 275
13. IFC S 787: 37
14. IFC S 617: 333
15. IFC S 484: 41–2
16. Quelch, 99
17. Moore MS; Logan, 38
18. Vickery MSS (Co. Durham)
19. Pennant 1784, ii, 155
20. Paton, 46
21. Mactaggart, 217
22. Lightfoot, ii, 614; Vickery 1995
23. Johnson 1862
24. Goodrich-Freer, 206; Shaw, 50; Henderson & Dickson, 80; McNeill
25. *Independent*, 5 Aug. 1994
26. Pennant 1784, ii, 155
27. Freethy, 125
28. McGlinchey, 84
29. IFC S 171: 46
30. IFC S 771: 151
31. Palmer 1994, 122
32. IFC S 689: 103
33. IFC S 157: 314
34. IFC S 571: 239
35. IFC S 710: 48
36. McGlinchey, 84
37. Farrelly MS
38. IFC S 850: 166
39. IFC S 811: 65

40. Farrelly MS

41. IFC S 157: 314

42. McClafferty

43. Farrelly MS

44. IFC S 800: 219

45. Hatfield, 46

46. Emerson, 91; Taylor MS (Hatfield, 36); Jobson 1959, 144

47. Beith

48. Woodruffe-Peacock

49. Beith; A. Allen

50. *PLNN*, no. 37 (1994), 177

51. IFC S 710: 47

52. IFC S 385: 55

53. IFC S 475: 207

54. *PLNN*, no. 14 (1990), 63

55. Hatfield, 23

56. IFC S 932: 242

57. IFC S 475: 207

58. IFC S 476: 91

59. Vickery 1995

60. IFC S 787: 52

61. Hatfield MS

62. Hatfield, 48

63. Hatfield, appendix

64. Carmichael, vi, 75, 102

65. McCutcheon

66. Buchanan-Brown, 472

67. Palmer 1994, 122

68. Johnston 1853

69. Spence; Leask, 78

70. Dacombe

71. Tongue

72. Palmer 1994, 122

73. Hatfield, 33

74. Beith

75. Jobson 1959, 144

76. Fargher

77. Arthur, 45

78. Vickery 1995

79. Wright, 243

80. Tongue

81. *PlantLife* (Autumn 1997), 21

82. Martin, 223

83. Beith

84. Newman & Wilson

85. Vickery MSS

86. Beith

87. Hutchinson

88. Hatfield MS

89. IFC S 657: 217

90. IFC S 771: 170

91. IFC S 22: 402

92. IFC S 850: 78

93. IFC S 138: 465

94. Ó hEithir

95. IFC S 521: 150

96. IFC S 812: 440

97. IFC S 550: 278

98. IFC S 60: 302

99. IFC S 1090: 283

100. IFC S 287: 180

101. *PLNN*, no. 9 (1989), 39

102. Williams MS

103. Carmichael, vi, 143

104. Sargent

105. Parkinson, 562

106. *PLNN*, no. 23 (1992), 108

107. Vickery 1995

108. Jones 1930, 144

109. McClafferty

110. Lankester, 194

111. Steward 1739; Britten 1881a, 255

112. A. Allen

113. Palmer 1994, 122

114. Tongue

115. Vickery 1995

116. Newman & Wilson

117. Short 1746, 124

118. Beith

119. Pratt 1850–7

120. IFC S 498: 313

121. Hart 1898

122. IFC S 572: 92

123. Ó Súilleabháin, 310

124. Pratt 1850–7

125. Borlase 1758, 229

126. Tongue

127. IFC S 519: 115
128. Quayle, 69
129. Vickery MSS
130. Fargher
131. Buchanan-Brown, 472
132. Monteith, 77
133. Jóhansen
134. Carmichael, 123
135. Beith
136. Beith
137. Beith
138. Newman & Wilson
139. Fargher
140. Ó Cléirigh
141. IFC S 904: 474
142. IFC S 617: 335
143. IFC S 780: 243
144. IFC S 157: 174
145. IFC S 489: 169
146. IFC S 920: 74
147. Maloney
148. Maloney
149. Egan
150. IFC S 710: 42
151. IFC S 655: 266
152. IFC S 550: 280
153. Ó Súilleabháin, 309
154. Moore MS
155. Hart 1898, 388
156. Britten & Holland
157. Maloney
158. Beith
159. Britten & Holland
160. McClafferty
161. IFC S 157: 314
162. Maloney
163. IFC S 897: 81
164. Taylor 1929, 118
165. McCutcheon
166. Hunt, 413
167. Vickery MSS
168. Shaw, 48

169. Hatfield, 32
170. Hatfield MS
171. Vickery 1995
172. Jamieson
173. CECTL MSS
174. Hatfield, 39
175. Vickery MSS
176. 'E.C.'
177. Hatfield, 48
178. Jones-Baker, 101
179. Jobson 1959, 144
180. Hatfield, 32
181. Tongue
182. *PLNN*, no. 56 (1998), 269
183. Courtney, 154
184. Mabey, 111
185. Hatfield, 32
186. 'E.C.'
187. Hatfield MS
188. Beith
189. *PLNN*, no. 49 (1997), 239
190. Quayle, 68
191. Maloney
192. IFC S 710: 49
193. IFC S 932: 239, 312
194. IFC S 482: 344
195. IFC S 897: 236
196. Maloney
197. IFC S 488: 286
198. IFC S 269: 105
199. IFC S 657: 217
200. IFC S 736: 137
201. IFC S 780: 129
202. IFC S 1043: 266
203. *PLNN*, no. 22 (1991), 101
204. Ó Súilleabháin, 314
205. Jamieson
206. Hatfield, 50
207. Wallace; Neill, 59 footnote
208. Buchanan-Brown, 472
209. Shaw, 50

CHAPTER 7

St John's-worts to Primulas

Dicotyledonous flowering plants in the orders (and families) Theales (Clusiaceae, St John's-worts), Malvales (Tiliaceae, lime trees; Malvaceae, mallows), Nepenthales (Droseraceae, sundews), Violales (Cistaceae, rock-roses; Violaceae, violets; Cucurbitaceae, squashes), Salicales (Salicaceae, willows and poplars), Capparales (Brassicaceae, cresses), Ericales (Empetraceae, crowberries; Ericaceae, heaths) and Primulales (Primulaceae, primroses) are included in this chapter.

CLUSIACEAE

Hypericum androsaemum Linnaeus
tutsan
western and southern Europe, south-western Asia, North Africa;
   introduced into New Zealand

Medieval herbalists identified *Hypericum androsaemum* with the *agnus castus* of Pliny and it acquired its French-derived vernacular name tutsan (*toutsaine,* 'all-heal') in tribute to its supposed medicinal virtues. It is therefore hard to be sure whether its few appearances in the folk repertory are altogether innocent of that reputation in learned physic. In Buckinghamshire the pounded leaves were mixed with lard to produce an ointment for dressing cuts and wounds,[1] but in northern Wales, in both Merionethshire and Denbighshire, the plant's name in Welsh betrays that it was once a remedy for carbuncles.[2]

The lard ointment also features in the Irish records, from parts of Ulster[3] (including Londonderry[4]) and from Leitrim.[5] In the latter the plant went under the name 'touch-and-heal' and was employed 'to prevent a mark' more especially.

Hypericum perforatum Linnaeus; and other species: *H. tetrapterum* Fries, *H. humifusum* Linnaeus, *H. pulchrum* Linnaeus, *H. elodes* Linnaeus

St John's-wort

Europe, western Asia, North Africa, Macaronesia; introduced into Australasia, North America

In contrast to tutsan (*Hypericum androsaemum*), which is sufficiently differ-ent in appearance to have probably always enjoyed a place of its own in folk medicine, the five other species of the genus *Hypericum* that have been iden-tified botanically as in use in Britain or Ireland are on record for such broadly similar purposes as to suggest that no distinction has been made between them. They are therefore treated here as if they constituted a single entity. It is nevertheless worth noting that whereas 'St John's-wort' over much of low-land England is *H. perforatum,* in the regions to the north and west that name is borne largely or wholly by its more slender relation, *H. pulchrum.* The magico-religious status accorded to the latter has been in no way inferior and may in those regions antedate the arrival of Christianity which was respon-sible for the association of these plants with St John.[6] Though the range of ailments for which *H. pulchrum* is on record as having been used is consid-erably smaller, that may merely reflect the much greater exposure *H. perfora-tum* has had over the centuries to the learned tradition.

The principal cluster of applications that St John's wort—in the collective sense—has had as a folk herb has arisen from its astringency and its resulting power to staunch bleeding from scratches and more serious wounds. *Hyperi-cum perforatum* has been employed for these purposes in Somerset[7] and Kent,[8] and *H. pulchrum* in the Isle of Man[9] and the Highlands (in Glen Roy under a Gaelic name translating as bloodwort).[10] In the Isle of Man, *H. pulchrum* has also shared with *H. humifusum* a role in curing stomach upsets, the name *lusni-chiolg,* 'intestine herb', having been applied to both alike.[11] An infusion of 'St John's-wort' (species unstated) has also served as an old rustic remedy, in an unidentified part of England, for enuresis in children or the aged.[12]

Curiously, the property of St John's-wort which has lately won it much publicity, its mild antidepressant action, features very little in the folk records of the British Isles—seemingly only in the Isle of Man, where *Hypericum pul-chrum* has been widely in use for low spirits, nervousness[13] and as a general tonic,[14] and in the Highlands, where the herb was allegedly used by St

Columba, applied as a pad under the armpit or in the groin, to restore the sanity of a young shepherd after long hours alone on the hillsides. This legend gave rise to the Gaelic name translating as 'St Columba's oxterful'.[15] The plants' value for this purpose was trumpeted in the herbals—John Gerard recommended them for melancholia—and, despite the major place they have occupied in Germany allegedly as a folk cure, it may be that this particular use is wholly a legacy of the learned tradition and not truly a folk one at all.

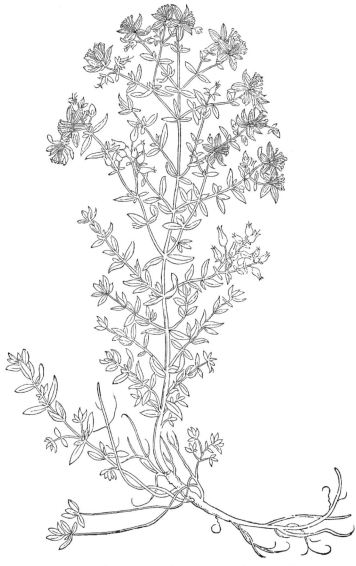

Hypericum perforatum, St John's-wort (Fuchs 1543, fig. 476)

Considering how generally disseminated an antidepressant could be expected to have been had this property been appreciated, that the rarity of that use in the British Isles records is real seems to be borne out by the considerable range of still further purposes for which St John's-wort has been employed. The most salient of those is for healing fractures and sprains—in the manner of comfrey (*Symphytum officinale*) and royal fern (*Osmunda regalis*); *Hypericum perforatum* has been used for those in Somerset,[16] *H. pulchrum* in the Highlands[17] and, mixed with goldenrod and heath speedwell, on Skye.[18] When cut and bruised, a resin-like substance can be extracted and has been applied as a protective coating to various afflictions as well: to burns in Somerset,[19] to bed sores in Norfolk[20] and the Westmoreland Pennines.[21] Probably related is its use for warts (Norfolk,[22] Wiltshire[23]). More surprising is the plants' serving as an infusion for coughs or catarrh in Somerset[24] and Fife,[25] and even more, in the first of those counties to make hair grow.[26]

In Ireland the main emphasis seems again to have been on the astringency. In 1697 John Ray was informed by a medical correspondent in Tipperary that under the Gaelic name *birin yarragh*, 'dysentery herb', a plant the latter was able to identify as *Hypericum elodes* was employed by the native Irish as a cure for diarrhoea. The correspondent had experimented with it himself, boiling it in milk, and claimed to have found it a highly effective astringent for fluxes in general.[27] *Hypericum elodes*, specifically, has also been recorded in use for diarrhoea in cows in Donegal,[28] so it may well be that it has a stronger potency in that direction than its British and Irish relatives. On the other hand, the member of the genus employed to staunch bleeding from wounds in Londonderry was identified by a botanist as another wet-ground species, *H. tetrapterum*.[29] Two further, but vague, Irish records of uses of St John's-wort in the collective sense have been to cure 'gravel' in 'Ulster'[30] and jaundice in some part of the country left unspecified.[31]

TILIACEAE

Tilia cordata Miller
Europe, western Asia; introduced into North America

Tilia ×europaea Linnaeus
lime
horticultural
An infusion of lime-tree flowers has been drunk for insomnia in Somerset[32] and for a headache in Norfolk.[33] Presumably the two native species, *Tilia cor-*

data and *T. platyphyllos* Scopoli, have been too scarce in recent centuries to have been drawn on for this purpose, and the hybrids between them, *T. ×europaea*, so generally planted, have necessarily stood in.

MALVACEAE

Malva sylvestris Linnaeus
mallow, hock
Europe, North Africa; introduced into North America, Australasia

Lavatera arborea Linnaeus
tree-mallow
southern and south-western Europe, North Africa; introduced into
    North America, Australasia

Althaea officinalis Linnaeus   PLATE 4
marsh-mallow
central and southern Europe, western Asia, North
    Africa; introduced into North America

Malva sylvestris, Lavatera arborea and *Althaea officinalis* are all mucilaginous in different degrees and have been utilised since ancient times more or less interchangeably, depending on which of them happened to grow most conveniently to hand. The common mallow, *M. sylvestris,* much the most generally distributed, is widely mis-called 'marsh-mallow', a name which properly belongs to *A. officinalis,* a relatively scarce plant of saltmarshes (though formerly much grown in cottage gardens). Tree-mallow, *L. arborea,* is similarly a coastal species but also very restricted in its range. These two last would doubtless have been preferred to *M. sylvestris* on account of their greater robustness and thicker leaves but over much of the British Isles would not have been available and

Malva sylvestris,
mallow (Green 1902, fig. 112)

M. sylvestris would have had to be accepted as an inferior substitute. Suggestively, in the Isle of Man, where tree-mallow occurs locally in quantity, the common mallow bore a name in Manx showing that it was regarded as merely a small version of that.

Whether *Malva sylvestris* itself was available prehistorically, however, is a matter of doubt, for everywhere in the British Isles it seems a follower of humans and seldom if ever occurs in the kinds of habitat which might give it a claim to be considered indigenous. Possibly some at least of its presence is the result of its introduction at different times expressly for medicinal purposes, for mallow held a prominent place in the learned tradition as well as in the folk one. In the Roman levels of a site excavated near Glasgow, about A.D. 150, pollen clusters of this species have been found unaccompanied by any of its seeds, suggesting that the flowers (and maybe other parts, which, unlike those, leave no remains) were utilised medicinally[34] in obedience to Pliny, who recommended a daily dose of the plant. Though mainly used for other purposes, at least in the folk medicine of the British Isles, there is a record from Norfolk of the fruits being chewed by children as a laxative,[35] while in three English counties (Wiltshire,[36] Hampshire,[37] Durham[38]) mallow has been in repute as a general cleansant of the system. Both of those uses may be dim echoes of Roman (or even pre-Roman) doctoring.

The Malvaceae have been prized in folk medicine for two applications far above all others, one of them general, the other more specific. Of 153 records logged in this study for the three species in question, these two uses account for 57 and 40, respectively. The general application was (and frequently still is) as a soothing poultice for sores, cuts, bruises, ulcers, boils, skin complaints and inflammation of any kind as well as to soften and disperse swellings. including those in mumps and swollen glands. In Radnorshire[39] a 'marsh-mallow' poultice has been held to be a certain cure for a limb that has become infected, while in Lincolnshire[40] *Malva sylvestris* has been found so helpful in cases of blood-poisoning that it has been planted in gardens as a stand-by. Usually the leaves, but sometimes the roots or even the flowers, were pounded and mixed with lard or goose grease to produce an ointment known in some areas as 'marsh-mallow salve'. Intriguingly, species of the family native to Africa are extensively used for this same purpose in tribal medicine there—like the ability of plantain (*Plantago*) leaves to staunch bleeding, this is evidently another group of plants valued for a particular healing property in widely separated parts of the world, perhaps as a result of quite independent discoveries. In the British Isles, mallow poultices feature in the folk records from most parts of Britain and Ireland with the conspicuous exception of the Scottish Highlands and most of Wales—from which all the species have probably been absent historically.

To a striking extent the main uses to which mallows have been put and the relative frequencies of those uses parallel those recorded for comfrey (*Symphytum officinale*). This strongly suggests that the two have served as alternatives, the mallows standing in for comfrey in areas where that much less generally distributed plant is rare or absent. Not only have both been valued for treating swellings (pre-eminently for sprains in the case of comfrey), but they have both been widely used as well, if to nothing like the same extent, for two other purposes. The more important of these, accounting for the 40 mallow records, is as a demulcent for coughs, colds, sore throats, asthma and chest troubles—chewed or sucked or infused and either drunk or gargled in the case of mallows. The other is for easing rheumatism, stiff joints or backache, though that category of complaints might equally well be subsumed within the main one of poulticed inflammation.

Other ailments against which mallows have been deployed in Britain include sore or strained eyes (Cornwall,[41] Somerset,[42] Gloucestershire[43]), varicose veins (those second two counties again), toothache and teething (Devon,[44] Caernarvonshire[45]), kidney and urinary troubles (Devon,[46] Lincolnshire,[47] Yorkshire[48]), dysentery (Devon,[49] Isle of Man[50]), corns (Norfolk[51]), gripes in children (unlocalised[52]) and gonorrhoea (Devon[53]).

Ireland departs from the general patterns in one very major respect. The practice of bathing a sprain or, much more rarely, a fracture with the liquid produced from boiling the leaves or roots receives at least seven times as many mentions in the records from there as in those from Britain, accounting for not far short of a third of all the records from the British Isles for the uses of poultices for swellings. Inexplicably, that application of mallows to sprains is strongly concentrated in Leinster, which is one part of Ireland in which these plants might have been expected to have been supplanted by comfrey for that purpose had the latter been a comparatively late introduction by settlers from England. That matters are not that simple is further shown by the use in Louth of a poultice of *both* (as if to be on the safe side) and by the fact that in the records for the western county of Limerick[54] mallow has been found mentioned only once but comfrey no fewer then twelve times. The impression that *Malva sylvestris,* rather, could have been the latecomer and not comfrey, as one might at first suppose, is supported further by the comparative paucity of Irish records for most of the rarer purposes for which mallows have been reported in use in Britain. Of these, only urinary complaints have been found recorded as a use from as many counties (Londonderry,[55] Cavan,[56] Westmeath[57]) as in Britain. Otherwise the Irish records have yielded only warts (Waterford[58]) and the cleansing of the system (Kerry[59]).

Malva moschata Linnaeus
musk-mallow

Europe, North Africa; introduced into North America, New Zealand (Name ambiguity suspected) A statement by David Moore, in his report on the botany of Londonderry,[60] that *Malva moschata* was generally mistaken there for the 'true marsh mallow' appears to have been a slip for *M. sylvestris.* The ailments to which he says it was applied are ones recorded from other Irish counties for the latter.

DROSERACEAE

Drosera Linnaeus
sundew

northern temperate zone

'Our Englishmen nowadays set very much by it, and holde that it is good for consumptions and swouning, and faintness of the harte, but I have no sure experience of this, nether have I red of anye olde writer what vertues it hath, wherefore I dare promise nothing if it.' So wrote William Turner in the sixteenth century in his *Herball*, without, unfortunately, leaving it quite clear that the uses he mentions were folk ones (as he seems to imply by saying he had encountered them in no written work). If indeed they were, though, they would appear to have disappeared without trace, for the only English use found recorded in recent times for *Drosera* has been for warts, in the North Riding of Yorkshire.[61] The juice is so acrid that just a droplet or two will burn off one of those, according to William Withering,[62] writing perhaps from first-hand experience. Presumably it was because of this acridity that sundew was valued in the Highlands for ridding the hair of lice.[63]

In Ireland, on the other hand, the plants have enjoyed a reputation in places if not for consumption at least for whooping cough and asthma. For the former, the leaves were boiled in milk (sometimes that of asses, for preference[64]), and that was given to the children to swallow, a procedure followed also when sundew served there, too, as a jaundice remedy—only in that case the drinking had to continue for ten days or more.[65] For asthma the leaves were chopped up finely and the juice squeezed out and bottled, a few drops being drunk when needed.[66] These last two are recorded from the area just south-west of the border, whereas it has been down south in Limerick[67] that the plants, known there as the 'Blessed Virgin's chalice', have had one at least of their local clusters of popularity as a treatment for whooping cough.

CISTACEAE

Helianthemum nummularium (Linnaeus) Miller

H. chamaecistus Miller

rock-rose

Europe, south-western Asia

(Name ambiguity) 'Rock Rose' features in a list of supposedly wild plants utilised for folk medicine in Limerick.[68] All the species of the family Cistaceae, however, are very rare in Ireland and unknown in that particular county. Unless one of the garden species was being alluded to, presumably some member of the genus *Rosa* was known by that name.

VIOLACEAE

Viola odorata Linnaeus   PLATE 5

sweet violet

Europe, south-western Asia, North Africa, Macaronesia; introduced
into North America, Australasia

Though at least some of the species in the same section of the genus *Viola* are known to share the same properties, 'violet' has probably done duty in folk medicine for all of them indiscriminately—when it has not been intended for butterwort (*Pinguicula vulgaris*), which was often known, confusingly, as 'bog violet'. Sweet violet, *V. odorata*, seems to have been the one normally singled out, if only because it was conveniently at hand in cottage gardens, cultivated for its scent—and once introduced, very difficult to eliminate.

The well-attested power of that scent to induce faintness or giddiness in people with a particular constitutional susceptibility to it, or when made into 'violet balls' to revive them, has probably been well known since very early times: the use of a decoction of the plant or a compress of it to ease a headache certainly goes back at least to the Dark Ages in the learned tradition and may be even older in the folk one, if the fact that its use is on record from the Highlands[69] is indicative of ancient survival. Against that, though, is the suspicious lack of any evidence of this elsewhere in Britain other than some part of the south-western Midlands, where dried flowers have been made into a pudding and eaten to cure 'giddyness of the head'.[70] The flowers, indeed, feature in the folk medicine records only exceptionally, the sole other instance traced being an Isle of Man one.[71] There they have been made into a soothing syrup, which is also sedative and mildly laxative.

The most widespread folk application of violets has been for cancerous tumours, either on their own or in combination with other herbs, either externally or internally, either by crushing the fresh leaves and laying them on as a poultice or eating them or drinking an infusion. That this is recorded predominantly from southern England (Somerset,[72] Dorset,[73] Kent,[74] Gloucestershire,[75] Oxfordshire,[76] Norfolk[77]) and otherwise in Britain only from Wales (unlocalised[78]) could be indicative of a borrowing from the learned tradition; on the other hand, that distribution does coincide suggestively with the part of Britain in which sweet violet is most plentiful as a presumed native, which could equally be evidence of a usage that is autochthonous. In two of these same counties (Oxfordshire,[79] Norfolk[80]) a poultice of the leaves has also been valued for treating an ulcer. The plants' astringency has led to their being applied to skin problems and as a beauty lotion in the Highlands[81] and presumably explains their use on stings, as a counter-irritant, in Dorset.[82]

Records from Ireland are markedly more restricted. The use for tumours is known there also (Westmeath,[83] Tipperary[84]); otherwise a poultice of the leaves for boils in Meath[85] and a decoction of them for 'a pain in the head' in Limerick[86] are the sole remedies that have been noted.

The one folk record that could credibly refer to the common dog-violet, *Viola riviniana* Reichenbach, rather than to the sweet violet, is the one brought back by Martin Martin from his visit to Skye in 1695: boiled in whey, it made a 'refreshing drink for such as are ill of fevers' under the name *dail-chuach*.[87]

Viola tricolor Linnaeus
wild pansy, heart's-ease
Europe, parts of Asia; introduced into North America, North Africa,
    New Zealand

(Name ambiguity suspected) The name heart's-ease was generally applied in Ireland to self-heal (*Prunella vulgaris*)[88] and all records almost certainly apply to that. A claim in Limerick[89] that 'wild pansies' produced a salve used for cuts and deeper wounds, an application otherwise unrecorded in folk medicine for any *Viola* species, probably arose from confusion with self-heal, too: that is a purpose for which that herb was particularly widely used.

CUCURBITACEAE

Bryonia dioica Jacquin

Bryonia cretica subsp. *dioica* (Jacquin) Tutin

white bryony

central and southern Europe, western Asia, North Africa;
introduced into North America, New Zealand

Because of its thick root, which grows deep in the ground, *Bryonia dioica* was popularly identified with mandrake (*Mandragora* spp.) by country folk, a

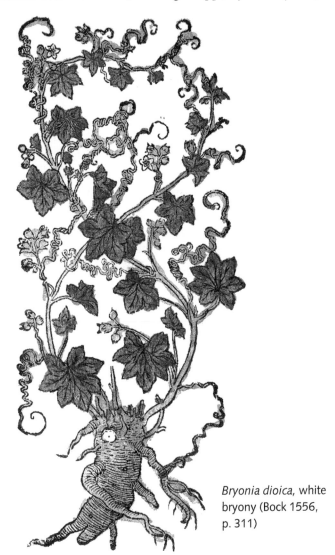

Bryonia dioica, white bryony (Bock 1556, p. 311)

belief which must by definition have come from learned medicine. The name still lingers on—or modified to 'English mandrake' by those wise to the confusion. A variant of the belief, surviving in the Fens of East Anglia[90] if not elsewhere, was that mandrake occurred in two forms, one of which was this species and the other the vaguely similar black bryony (*Tamus communis*). This notion came from the early herbals, whose authors took these species to be respectively the *ampelos leuke* and *ampelos agria* described by Dioscorides. As in similar cases in folk taxonomy where species were paired—one was assumed to be the expression of the male principle in nature, the other of the female one—mandrake had the reputation, preserved in the Forest of Dean in Gloucestershire,[91] of being a powerful aphrodisiac and a procurer of fertility. This found reflection medically in the restriction of the 'male' kind to the ailments of women and mares and of the 'female' one to those of men and stallions.[92] As the embodiment of the female principle, white bryony exerted the greater power, an assumption given added credence by the greater violence of its action (for which reason its use was reserved on the whole for animals). Its acrid juice is so strongly purgative and blistering that it can cause gastritis, and as few as a dozen of the berries may lead to death. As far as human beings were concerned, it was a herb to be used only with extreme caution: Dorset folk were therefore daring in taking it as a substitute for castor oil.[93] Indeed, the only other record of its application to a human ailment seems to be an unlocalised one for gout, reported by John Aubrey to John Ray in 1691: supposedly, an old woman had cured that after many years by employing the leaf of 'wild vine' (botanically identified as *B. dioica*).[94] People in Norfolk were surely sensible to close with the plant's powers no further than carrying a piece of the root in their pocket as an antidote to rheumatism.[95]

SALICACEAE

Populus alba Linnaeus
  white poplar
  eastern Europe, western Asia, North Africa; introduced into other
    temperate regions
(Folk credentials questionable) Although at least some of the poplars, including the native aspen (*Populus tremula* Linnaeus), resemble willows in having salicin in their bark, *P. alba* is the only member of the genus, an introduced species, for which records have been found in the folk medicine literature of the British Isles. They relate to north-eastern Somerset, where an infusion of the bark was held to be good for fevers and for relieving night sweats and

indigestion.[96] This can only have been a comparatively late use and may well have come from the written tradition.

Salix Linnaeus
willow, sallow, sallies
almost worldwide except Australasia and East Indies

Salix repens Linnaeus
Europe, western and central Asia

Because of a common failure by druggists no less than folklore collectors to distinguish between the species—let alone the hybrids—in the admittedly taxonomically difficult genus *Salix*, it is necessary for the most part to discuss these plants here only in a collective sense. Most if not all the taxa found wild in the British Isles, however, are probably similar phytochemically, with bark rich in tannin as well as in the all-important compound salicin.

The story is often repeated of the accidental discovery c. 1757 by a parson in the north of Oxfordshire, the Rev. Edward Stone, of the powerfully astringent property of the bark of white willow (*Salix alba* Linnaeus), which, he found, made it highly effective against 'agues' (including malaria) and other fevers.[97] Stone has consequently received the credit, and rightly, for first alerting the medical profession to this property and for thus starting science on the road which eventually led to the isolation of salicin and its clinical application, most notably in the form of aspirin, in the nineteenth century. However, those who relate the story are at fault in not pointing out to their readers that Stone had been plentifully anticipated in folk medicine in parts of the world as far apart as Burma (Myanmar), Africa and North America as well as Europe at least as early as biblical times. Before learned medicine adopted its disdainful attitude to folk tradition, knowledge of the effectiveness of willow 'juice' in allaying fevers was leaking up from that basic substratum into the late medieval literature and the syncretistic repertory of the physicians of Myddvai in south-western Wales.

The apparently age-old practice in folk medicine of drinking the bitter infusion known as willow-bark tea as a means of relieving fever, surviving into relatively recent years in Sussex[98] and the Fens of East Anglia,[99] has been attributed to a naive theory that because these trees grow in damp places they must be good for ailments caused by damp conditions. That explanation, however, must surely be fanciful in view of the large number of other plants characteristic of damp habitats which might equally well have been chosen for the purposes in question. There may be significance in the fact that the only records for drinking that infusion are from the south-eastern quarter of England—more widespread, alternative ways of ingesting the plant, at any rate for other afflictions for which aspirin would now be customary, are chewing the bark or a twig or sucking the leaves, for rheumatism in Surrey[100] and Herefordshire,[101] for arthritis in Norfolk[102] and for a headache or hangover in Norfolk[103] and Lincolnshire.[104]

Willows have also attracted a variety of applications in Britain arising from their astringency: staunching bleeding as well as reducing dandruff in Cumbria[105] and, combined with a soaking in vinegar, removing warts in Wiltshire[106] and corns in Norfolk.[107]

Ireland can boast at least one record of an aspirin-like use: the leaves of what a botanist found to be creeping willow (*Salix repens*) have been much prized for 'pains in the head' in one glen in Donegal.[108] Ireland has also known one use as an 'astringent': for diarrhoea in Leitrim[109] and Cork.[110] But mixing the ashes with some fatty substance to produce an ointment has enabled the virtues of 'sallies' to be extended to further and different kinds of conditions in that country: to ringworm in Westmeath,[111] erysipelas in Laois[112] and baldness in Galway[113]; it was doubtless the way in which the blossom of 'weeping willow' (strictly speaking the planted species *S. babylonica* Linnaeus, but usually hybrids of that) was used on burns in Tipperary, too.[114]

BRASSICACEAE

Sisymbrium officinale (Linnaeus) Scopoli
hedge mustard
Europe, south-western Asia, North Africa; introduced into North
and South America, South Africa, Australasia

(Folk credentials lacking) An ancient remedy for coughs, chest complaints and particularly hoarseness, *Sisymbrium officinale* appears to be unrecorded in any unambiguously folk context. Essentially a weed of waste places, the species is very doubtfully native in the British Isles and may indeed be only a relatively recent incomer. 'Blue eye', recorded as a jaundice remedy in Wicklow,[115] has been ascribed to it but must surely belong there to germander speedwell (*Veronica chamaedrys*).

Descurainia sophia (Linnaeus) Webb ex Prantl
Sisymbrium sophia Linnaeus
flixweed
Eurasia, North Africa; introduced into North and South America,
New Zealand

(Folk credentials lacking) The remains of the once popular medicinal herb *Descurainia sophia* have been detected in a Romano-British deposit,[116] but in the absence of any records for it in the folk literature, that occurrence seems safely attributable to an alien import by Roman settlers or Roman commerce.

Alliaria petiolata (M. Bieberstein) Cavara & Grande
garlic mustard, hedge garlic, Jack-by-the-hedge, sauce alone
Europe, south-western Asia, North Africa; introduced into North
America, New Zealand

As its vernacular names indicate, *Alliaria petiolata* functioned as an alternative to garlic. Though that was chiefly in cooking, its leaves also substituted for garlic's medicinally by being applied externally to sore throats in Kent (?)[117] and chewed for sore gums and mouth ulcers in Norfolk.[118] Rubbing the leaves on the feet was a cure for cramp in Somerset.[119] More surprising, though, has been its use for wounds (again in Kent?).[120]

The prevalence of ramsons, otherwise wild garlic (*Allium ursinum*), in the west of the British Isles, would explain the restriction of these records to the south-eastern quarter of England, to which this hedge plant may formerly have been mainly restricted. There has been a find of it in a Romano-British deposit.[121]

Erysimum cheiranthoides Linnaeus
treacle mustard
Europe, north Asia, North Africa; introduced into North America,
New Zealand

Under the name 'English wormseed' in the seventeenth century, *Erysimum cheiranthoides* was still 'much used by the country people where it groweth to kill the wormes in children, the seede being a little bruised and given in drinke or any other way.'[122] Rather over a century later, William Withering made an assertion to the same effect, though possibly just repeating the statement of that predecessor.[123] Curiously, though, no more recent records of this plant's use in folk medicine have been discovered.

Barbarea vulgaris R. Brown; and perhaps also *B. intermedia* Boreau
(western and south-western Europe; introduced into Australasia)
winter-cress
Eurasia, North Africa; introduced into North America, Australasia

(Folk credentials questionable) 'I had it shown to me as a secret cure of a sore leg, and nourished in the garden as a rare plant after it had done the feat.'

Thus Threlkeld wrote in 1726 of his experience in and around Dublin. The species involved could have been either the native *Barbarea vulgaris* or the introduced *B. intermedia* (which appears to have been a widespread cottage garden herb in the west of the British Isles). That no record of any more certainly folk use of this common herb has been found suggests that Threlkeld's informant took the idea from some learned source.

Rorippa nasturtium-aquaticum (Linnaeus) Hayek, in the broad sense
Nasturtium officinale R. Brown
water-cress; *biolar*
western and central Europe, western Asia, North Africa; introduced
into North America, Australasia, etc.

Although *Rorippa nasturtium-aquaticum* is so familiar a plant and so widely common, it appears to have been curiously little-used in Britain, and especially England, as a folk remedy, to judge from the paucity of records: as a tonic and general cleanser of the system in Norfolk[124] and the Highlands,[125] to allay fevers by cooling the blood in the Isle of Man[126] and (once extensively) the Highlands,[127] to act as an antiscorbutic (it is less bitter than scurvy-grass, *Cochlearia* spp.) in Mull and in the Inner Hebrides[128] and to correct barrenness among Highland women.[129] There is also an unlocalised record of its use as a wart cure.[130]

In Ireland, by contrast, this has occupied a central place in the folk repertory, and in two main ways, both on record from a goodly scattering of at least nine counties: as a purifying tonic and as a remedy for colds, coughs and chest complaints. Other, much more minor applications, all apparently unrecorded from Britain, have been to stomach trouble (Cavan,[131] Kildare,[132] Tipperary[133]), kidney ailments (Cavan,[134] Limerick,[135] Wicklow[136]) heart trouble (Donegal,[137] Sligo,[138] Longford,[139] Westmeath[140]), rashes (Mayo,[141] Galway,[142] Clare[143]), rheumatism (Cavan,[144] Roscommon[145]), cuts (Monaghan[146]), scrofula ('Ulster'[147]), swellings (Roscommon[148]) and sore eyes (Louth[149]). Though most frequently eaten raw, the plant has frequently been boiled instead, even though that allegedly weakens its efficacy.

Cardamine pratensis Linnaeus
cuckooflower, lady's-smock
Europe, north Asia, North America; introduced into New Zealand

Cardamine pratensis shared with mistletoe (*Viscum album*) a reputation for nervous afflictions, though by comparison with mistletoe apparently only a minor one. Claims by physicians that the flowering tops have powerful antispasmodic properties which are helpful in cases of hysteria, epilepsy and St Vitus' dance appear in the learned medical literature from the time of John Ray onwards, but evidence that this was also (and maybe originally) a folk remedy seems to be limited to the Highlands[150] and to one nineteenth-century author's sweeping assertion that 'the belief in their good effect in such cases is certainly very widely spread among the peasantry'[151] (of Great Britain, by implication). Had that been true, more records would surely have been picked up by folk collectors? As it is, the only other ones traced have been for other purposes: in the Highlands[152] to allay fevers and in Gloucestershire[153] to ease persistent headaches.

Erophila verna (Linnaeus) de Candolle, in the broad sense
  Draba verna Linnaeus
  whitlowgrass
(Folk credentials questionable) The use of *Erophila verna* as a cure for whitlows in Essex[154] in the 1920s may well have been inspired by a reading of the herbals. The lack of other and earlier records looks suspicious.

Cochlearia officinalis Linnaeus
  north-western and central Europe; introduced into North America

Cochlearia anglica Linnaeus
  scurvy-grass
  north-western Europe
As the vernacular name scurvy-grass advertises, *Cochlearia* was valued, in both folk and learned medicine, as an antiscorbutic *par excellence*, being particularly rich, as we now know, in vitamin C. John Parkinson in his 1640 herbal said the kind he knew as 'Dutch Scurvey-grass', i.e. *C. anglica*, was the more effective and the more frequently used for this purpose than the saltier 'English Scurvy-grass', i.e. *C. officinalis*.[155] That was a distinction probably too subtle, however, to have arisen within the folk tradition; such folk records as have been found of the use of these plants for scurvy all come in any case from the far north and west of the British Isles, where *C. officinalis* predominates. That the herb was also once valued for this purpose in the Faeroe Islands[156] suggests that its popularity in their neighbour, the Shetlands,[157] as a cure for skin complaints was an extension of use for scorbutic sores more specifically. The custom in Kent[158] of taking a daily draught of the drink in spring, as a means of cleansing the system, was clearly part of the same family of uses.

  When Martin Martin visited Skye in 1695, however, he noted this herb in favour only for colic, constipation and stitches; scurvy finds no mention.[159] Almost a century later, John Lightfoot in his turn was able to report it as esteemed in the Highlands only as a stomachic.[160] Other Highland records have been similarly unconnected with scurvy: as a poultice for cramps and boils[161] and for taking away water from the eyes.[162]

In Ireland, unlike Britain, scurvy-grass has also been found effective for cuts. On one of the islets off the coast of Donegal an ointment was made from it for that purpose.[163]

Capsella bursa-pastoris (Linnaeus) Medikus
shepherd's-purse
cosmopolitan weed

The astringency possessed by the very common weed *Capsella bursa-pastoris* (probably a native of Asia) has led it to be valued for stopping bleeding and for excessive menstrual discharge, uses which feature in the folk records from the Highlands[164, 165] and Essex,[166] respectively. A related function in the Isle of Man is as a cure for diarrhoea.[167]

For Ireland, however, as so often, applications seem to have been quite different: in Limerick it has been drunk as a tea or chewed for kidney trouble,[168] and there is a record of its use for rickets that has yet to be pinpointed geographically.[169]

Lepidium latifolium Linnaeus
dittander
Europe, south-western Asia, North Africa; introduced into
    North America

'The women of Bury [St Edmunds] in Suffolk doe usually give the juice thereof in ale to drinke to women with child to procure them a speedy delivery in travail'. This seventeenth-century report[170] by John Parkinson is the only known claim *Lepidium latifolium* has to be considered a possible folk herb. His contemporary, John Ray, despite his East Anglian background, could do no more than repeat the report without comment.[171]

Sinapis arvensis Linnaeus
charlock
Europe, western Asia, North Africa; introduced into other continents

Sinapis arvensis and its fellow weed of cultivated ground, wild radish (*Raphanus raphanistrum*), were drawn on in the Shetlands to keep scurvy at bay.[172]

In Ireland, if it is rightly identified as the 'corn kale' (which might equally be wild turnip, *Brassica rapa* Linnaeus), its juice was drunk in Limerick as a spring tonic to keep the system free of diseases for the rest of the year.[173] In the area just south-west of the border a preparation of the flowers was the usual cure for jaundice.[174]

Raphanus raphanistrum Linnaeus
wild radish
Europe, North Africa, Japan; introduced into North and South
    America, Australasia
See under charlock, *Sinapis arvensis*, preceding.

EMPETRACEAE

Empetrum nigrum Linnaeus
crowberry
Eurasia, North America
A locally abundant plant of moors, at one time regarded as a berry-bearing form of heather ('*Erica baccifera*'), *Empetrum nigrum* was found in use in the Inner Hebrides by Martin Martin in 1695 as a cure for insomnia, a little of it boiled in water and applied to the crown and temples.[175] It was presumably the 'kind of heath' claimed by a later author to be in use for the same purpose in 'the Highlands',[176] but the description of its application is so similar that the record may be an unacknowledged repeat of Martin's. Another record from the Inner Hebrides, from Colonsay, credits its juice with the power to heal sores that are festering.[177]

ERICACEAE

Daboecia cantabrica (Hudson) K. Koch
St Dabeoc's heath
south-western Europe; introduced into New Zealand
On his visit to the west of Ireland in 1700, when he added *Daboecia cantabrica* to the list of the wild plants of the British Isles, Edward Llwyd learned that on the moors of Mayo and Galway the women sometimes carried a sprig of it on them as a preservative against some mishap which, as ill luck would have it, is written only partly legibly in the letter in question.[178] Of possible alternative readings, 'incontinence' seems most likely, for other kinds of heath are on record as in folk use for similar-sounding trouble.

Arctostaphylos uva-ursi (Linnaeus) Sprengel   PLATE 6
bearberry
northern Eurasia and North America, and mountains to their south
(Folk credentials questionable) Featured in the older herbals, *Arctostaphylos uva-ursi* enjoyed a revival in eighteenth-century official medicine on being found effective against urinary problems (the result of containing arbutin, it has turned out). In the Highlands,[179] where it is specially frequent, the berries are credibly stated to have been 'used medicinally' but it is unclear whether this antedated the demand for the herb by physicians and apothecaries.

Calluna vulgaris (Linnaeus) Hull   PLATE 7
heather, ling
Europe, Morocco, Azores; possibly native to eastern North America;
  introduced into New Zealand

Erica tetralix Linnaeus   PLATE 8
cross-leaved heath
northern and western Europe; introduced into eastern North America

Erica cinerea Linnaeus
bell heather
western Europe, Madeira; introduced into eastern North America,
  New Zealand

The three common heath species in the British Isles (*Calluna vulgaris, Erica tetralix* and *E. cinerea*), let alone the rarer ones, are rarely if ever distinguished in the folk records. As the three are readily told apart at a glance, this has probably been due less to taxonomic myopia than because they were assumed to share the same medicinal virtues.

Considered a panacea in the Shetlands in the early eighteenth century,[180] 'heather' does indeed seem to have had a rather wide range of applications. Several of these, though, may have had a common derivation: faith in a relaxing or mildly soporific effect. In the Highlands,[181] for example, it has been valued for countering insomnia and soothing 'nerves' but also as a treatment for consumption. On the other hand, its employment for rheumatism (recorded in Britain from Cumbria[182]) is allegedly because of a muscle-toning property, while its astringency has clearly prompted its use for stomach upsets and diarrhoea (Cumbria,[183] too). A reputation as a diuretic has also made it a remedy in Dorset for ailments of a urological nature.[184]

In Ireland, the recorded uses of 'heather' are much the same: for a weak heart in Clare[185]; coughs in Wicklow[186] and asthma in Tipperary[187]; rheumatism in Cavan[188] and 'a bad stomach' in Limerick.[189] Employment for heartburn in Cavan[190] seems to be the only one not known from Britain.

For most purposes a tea was brewed from the young 'tops' or the flowers, but for heartburn the 'tops' were chewed and the juice swallowed, while in Limerick it was the seeds that were boiled, and in the Highlands a mat of the plant with which the temples were poulticed for insomnia.

Vaccinium oxycoccos Linnaeus
cranberry
northern Eurasia, northern half of North America

Once a common plant in the Fens of East Anglia before they were so largely drained, *Vaccinium oxycoccos* has been credibly suggested[191] as the identity of the 'fen-berries' or 'marsh whortles' said by Thomas Moffet in the seventeenth century to be in use in the Isle of Ely as an 'astringent'.[192]

Vaccinium vitis-idaea Linnaeus
cowberry
arctic and northern Eurasia, mountains of southern Europe, North
    America

In Cumbria[193] the leaves of *Vaccinium vitis-idaea* were one of the ingredients in a concoction that produced an inhalant for a blocked nose or sinuses. It is unexpected that this often abundant moorland species seems to be otherwise absent from the folk medicine records.

Vaccinium myrtillus Linnaeus
bilberry, blaeberry, *fraughan*
northern Eurasia, mountains of southern Europe; introduced into
    North America

The uses of the popular food-for-free *Vaccinium myrtillus* bear some similarity to those of 'heather', especially on account of its shared astringency. 'Blaeberry tea' has been widely valued in north-western Scotland for dissolving kidney stones and countering other ailments of the urinary tract.[194] There, too, but perhaps at one time much more widely still, in both the Highlands[195] and the Western Isles from Arran[196] at least north to Skye,[197] its berries seem to have rivalled tormentil (*Potentilla erecta*) as a treatment for diarrhoea. A further reputation enjoyed in the Highlands[198] was for its power to soothe pain, recalling the application of 'heather' to rheumatism. Yet again like 'heather' it has been found useful against symptoms accompanying colds:

in Wales[199] for poulticing a sore throat and in Cumbria[200] as an ingredient in an infusion helping to produce an inhalant.

In Ireland the focus has mainly been on the plant's ability as a diuretic to deal with kidney trouble (Wicklow,[201] Kilkenny[202]) and gravel stones (county unspecified[203]). It has also been employed there against jaundice in Cavan,[204] asthma in Carlow[205] (together with broom), measles in Monaghan[206] (together with nettles) and as an antidote to pain in Wexford.[207]

PRIMULACEAE

Primula vulgaris Hudson   PLATE 9
primrose
western and southern Europe, Asia Minor, North Africa; introduced
into North America, New Zealand

Perhaps because it is the commoner of the two and much the more generally distributed throughout the British Isles, the primrose, *Primula vulgaris,* has had three uses which particularly stand out in the folk records, whereas the cowslip (*P. veris*) has had only one. One of those three uses is predominantly English: made into an ointment to heal cuts, bruises, chapped hands or chilblains (Devon,[208] Dorset,[209] Hampshire,[210] Cumbria,[211] the Highlands[212]) or, combined with bramble tops, to clear up spots and sores on the face (Dorset[213]). That sounds like the ointment smeared on ringworm in Suffolk,[214] while a record from the Outer Hebridean island of Bernera of an application of the leaves to cure persistent boils on the legs[215] perhaps belongs in this category, too. Another group of uses, less prominent and more scattered, presumably comes from the plant's reputation as a relaxant. In Devon, drinking the juice has been the way to restore your voice should you lose it, and eating the raw leaves a remedy for arthritis.[216] In Suffolk a primrose snuff has been taken for migraine[217] (and in Cardiganshire, too, if a use with the leaves of betony recorded in an old household recipe book[218] was really a folk one). Doubtless for this reason, too, drinking the juice has been reckoned in Wales a sound treatment for madness[219] and a decoction of the leaves believed by many to help a failing memory.[220]

Except for records from Suffolk[221] and the Highlands[222] a primrose salve for burns appears to be exclusively Irish, while Ireland is evidently also alone in having valued the plant for jaundice. These are the other two main uses of the plant overall and the records for both are, curiously, all from that country's central belt. In Ireland, as a remedy for burns, the plant is combined with other herbs rather more often than it is employed on its own. In further sharp contrast to Britain, the only Irish record picked up of an application to cuts is one from Laois—and that merely as one of three ingredients, along with elder bark and ivy juice[223]; however, the root, chopped up and fried with lard, has served as a skin ointment in Westmeath[224] and the leaves have had a place in a poultice for erysipelas in Donegal.[225] More equally shared with Britain has been appreciation of the plant's relaxing property: toothache has been eased in Co. Dublin by rubbing with a leaf for about two minutes[226] and the juice drunk in Carlow to counter a pain in the stomach,[227] while in Cork a tea of both cowslips and primroses has doubtless been a doubly sure remedy for insomnia.[228]

Primula veris Linnaeus
cowslip
Europe, temperate Asia; introduced into North America

The role of *Primula veris* seems to have been mostly as a second-best: used for much the same ailments as the primrose (*P. vulgaris*), it is on record from some areas where the other is apparently not, despite the primrose being much the more generally distributed and in most regions much the more plentiful. A particularly striking anomaly is that the records for cowslip as a jaundice remedy are all English (Dorset,[229] Norfolk[230]) whereas the more numerous ones for that in the case of the primrose are all Irish. In that instance it seems the primrose has been second-best, the Irish forced to have recourse to that because of the great scarcity of the cowslip in large parts of that country (though widespread on the limy soils of its midlands).

Special to the cowslip, at least in Britain, has been its role as a folk cosmetic (the leaves and stalk avoided because those can seriously irritate certain skins). The plant is said to have enjoyed a great vogue in that capacity in the Highlands up to the eighteenth century,[231] and there are records also from Devon,[232] Wiltshire[233] and (perhaps) Kent.[234] Special to the cowslip, too, is its use for coughs in Norfolk[235] and to banish 'decline' (presumably tuberculosis) in South Wales, in parts of which there was once a well-known rhyme to that effect.[236] Otherwise the cowslip's recorded repertory echoes that of the primrose: insomnia in Devon[237] and Derbyshire,[238] wounds in Dorset,[239] backache in Wiltshire[240] and to 'strengthen the senses' in South Wales,[241] this last recalling the use of primrose in Lincolnshire to help a failing memory.

Ireland's chief distinction is the cowslip's wide popularity there for countering insomnia, with records from Cavan,[242] Co. Dublin,[243] Clare,[244] Limerick[245] and—combined with primroses, a unique use of those for this pur-pose—Cork.[246] With two exceptions the other uses traced for the plant in the records find no reflection in the British ones: to give goodness to the blood in Co. Dublin[247] and to cure dropsy in Limerick[248] and palsy in Lim-erick[249] and Wexford[250] (so popular for that in the last as to have locally acquired the name palsywort).

An ointment made in Wicklow[251] for wrinkles and spots, however, sounds too like the British cosmetic to be claimed as purely Irish, while if 'strengthen-ing the senses' embraced curing deafness, then that is the other exception. But whereas in South Wales the senses were strengthened simply by drinking cowslip tea or wine, the remedy for deafness recorded from several parts of Ireland was both different and elaborate. Best known from a classic description by Oscar Wilde's mother,[252] this required bruising the flowers, leaves and roots, pressing them in a cloth, adding honey to the liquid extracted and then putting a few drops of that into the nostrils as well as the ears while the patient lay prone. After a while the patient turned face upwards, bearing away 'whatever obstructives lay on the brain'. A later record of a deafness remedy from Mayo[253] repeats Lady Wilde's description so faithfully as to suggest a straight parroting of that, but another from Cork[254] is more convincingly independent.

Lysimachia nemorum Linnaeus
yellow pimpernel
western and central Europe, Caucasus

The flowers of *Lysimachia nemorum* have been boiled in Cavan as a cure for gallstones.[255] Otherwise the only record is from an untrustworthy source that, allegedly in Ireland somewhere, the plant has been used in conjunction with tormentil (*Potentilla erecta*) as a hypnotic for insomnia.[256] It may well be that it shares with cowslips (*Primula veris*) a soporific effect.

Lysimachia vulgaris Linnaeus
yellow loosestrife
temperate Eurasia; introduced into North America, Australasia

(Folk credentials questionable) A herb recommended by 'the Irish Aescu-lapius', the druid Diancecht (fl. 487 B.C.), for poulticing a sore throat has been identified, on unknown grounds, as 'yellow baywort',[257] a name which more probably belongs to *Lysimachia vulgaris* than any other. Though well enough distributed in both Britain and Ireland to be a likely plant to have had some place in folk medicine, it clearly cannot be admitted as a member on such evidence.

Anagallis arvensis Linnaeus
scarlet pimpernel
worldwide except tropics

Though a common weed over much of the British Isles and seemingly native in coastal habitats here and there (mostly in the far west), the records for *Anagallis arvensis* as a folk medicine are oddly restricted geographically, with a marked concentration in the south-west of Britain, albeit in use for a diversity of ailments there. This may well be a relic of the older cultural layer of that region associated with the speakers of the Cymric branch of Celtic. In Wales the plant allegedly had a magical aura, with a reputation for keeping away melancholy, to which end an infusion of it was once widely drunk.[258] Certainly 'pimpernel' features with impressive prominence in the recipes of the medieval physicians of Myddvai in Carmarthenshire, which may in this

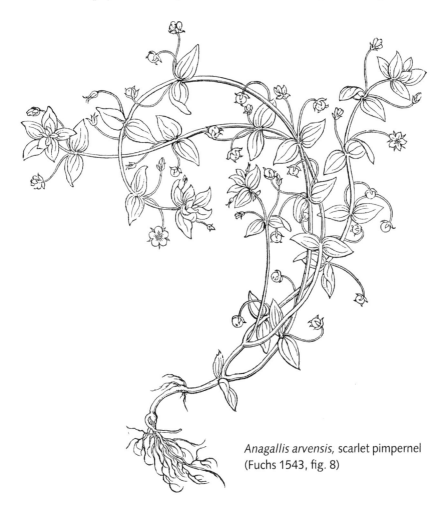

Anagallis arvensis, scarlet pimpernel
(Fuchs 1543, fig. 8)

case have been drawing on local folk usage (they recommended it for fevers, abdominal complaints, profuse menstruation and festering swellings); it is impossible to be sure, however, that it was this species they understood by this name. Indeed, paucity of the records for folk uses of *A. arvensis* and the absence of any focus in these on one ailment above all others hardly give the impression of a herb that was particularly highly valued. Two of the records are for an application for which numerous other species have been rated as effective and might equally well have served, namely the healing of warts (Somerset,[259] Sussex[260]). The plant is known to have a powerful diuretic property, and perhaps it was for that that an infusion of the plant was drunk as an 'alterative' (as determined by a medical practitioner) by cottagers in early nineteenth-century Devon.[261] Someone more recently found to be using this plant in Devon, however, was doing so to soothe stings and against sore eyes.[262] Possibly it came into its own more particularly as a counter-irritant, like nettles: in Glamorgan it was once a remedy for the bites of dogs and snakes, applied to the wound with a cloth.[263] In keeping with this general elusiveness, the one source which claims it as much prized in the Highlands fails to mention for what it was used there.[264]

Ireland has yielded very few records, by contrast. They add one further ailment for which this plant has been used: chronic or muscular rheumatism, in 'some places' in Ulster (?).[265] They also provide the sole certain evidence of advantage being taken of the diuretic property mentioned above, for in Sligo an infusion has been drunk for kidney trouble.[266]

Samolus valerandi Linnaeus
brookweed
cosmopolitan

Even had it not been a relatively uncommon species and mostly maritime, a combination of factors likely to have deterred herbal use, the extreme bitterness of *Samolus valerandi* would probably have repelled would-be exploiters, too. Not surprisingly, the sole folk use of it traced was as an external application, for eye troubles. The user in question, an Englishman living in Wales, knew the plant by the name kenningwort (from the ulcers popularly termed kennings) and had earned a reputation for achieving remarkable cures with it.[267] As 'kenning herb' was one of the names borne by greater celandine (*Chelidonium majus*) in Cornwall,[268] advertising that plant's similar function there, it would be tempting to postulate a misidentification did not the record stand on the authority of someone known to have been a competent field botanist. So sure indeed was the latter that it was this species being referred to (pointed out to him by a local farmer) that he was led to suggest that Linnaeus and others may have been right after all in supposing it to be the mysterious *samolus* mentioned by Pliny the Elder—despite the fact that it was specifically as a veterinary cure that that was described by the Roman author as much in use by the druids of Gaul.[269] While almost certainly unaware of the evidence supporting the claims of brookweed to herbal status, some later authors[270] have asserted that in some country parts of Britain this species is still considered a certain remedy for a particular disease of pigs (one of the two kinds of animals specified by Pliny). The source(s) of those assertions were, however, not disclosed, and even supposing they were correct, the probability is that brookweed was adopted as a cure for the disease in question merely because it was the plant bearing *Samolus* as part of its scientific name. It is too much to hope that the identity of the herb Pliny intended by that name will ever be established, and for the reasons rehearsed above unlikely that that was brookweed.

Notes

1. *Hardwicke's Science-gossip* (1866), 83
2. Williams MS
3. Purdon
4. Moore MS
5. IFC S 200: 75
6. Grigson; Vickery 1981
7. Tongue
8. Pratt 1850–7
9. Quayle, 69
10. Beith
11. Moore 1898; Paton MS
12. Quelch, 142
13. Moore 1898
14. Paton; Quayle, 69
15. Beith, 40
16. Tongue
17. Carmichael, iv, 208
18. Martin, 230
19. Tongue
20. Taylor MS
21. Duncan & Robson, 63
22. *PLNN*, no. 18 (1991), 84
23. Whitlock 1976, 164
24. Tongue
25. Simpkins, 133
26. Tongue
27. Lankester, 319
28. Hart 1898, 381
29. Moore MS
30. Egan
31. Sargent
32. Tongue
33. Hatfield, 39
34. Knights et al.; Dickson
35. Hatfield, 28
36. Wright, 239
37. Wright, 239
38. Vickery MSS
39. Howse, 206
40. Rudkin, 203
41. Vickery MSS
42. Tongue
43. Lafont
44. Lafont
45. *PLNN*, no. 43 (1996), 209
46. Collyns

47. Woodruffe-Peacock
48. Vickery MSS
49. Collyns
50. Quayle, 69
51. Hatfield MS
52. Quincy, 112
53. Collyns
54. IFC S 657: 160
55. Moore MS
56. Maloney
57. IFC S 747: 186, 187
58. IFC S 637: 142
59. IFC S 476: 91
60. Moore MS
61. Vickery MSS
62. Withering 1787–92, 191
63. Carmichael, vi, 77
64. Ó Súilleabháin, 315
65. Logan, 47
66. Logan, 26
67. IFC S 512: 115; 513: 558
68. IFC S 485: 191
69. Beith
70. Hughes, 95
71. Garrad 1985, 17
72. Tongue
73. Dacombe
74. Vickery 1995
75. Palmer 1994, 122
76. Hole
77. Hatfield, 26
78. Trevelyan
79. 'E.C.'; Hole
80. Hatfield MS
81. Beith
82. Dacombe
83. IFC S 747: 387
84. IFC S 560: 378
85. IFC S 710: 49
86. IFC S 500: 74
87. Martin, 223
88. Hart 1898, 377
89. IFC S 484: 41
90. Randell, 86
91. Palmer 1994, 122
92. Rudkin
93. Dacombe
94. Lankester, 238
95. Taylor 1929, 117
96. Tongue
97. Stone
98. A. Allen
99. Porter 1964, 9; 1974, 52
100. CECTL MSS
101. CECTL MSS
102. Hatfield, 46
103. Vickery MSS
104. Hatfield, 40
105. Freethy, 133
106. Whitlock 1976, 164
107. Wigby, 65; Hatfield 53
108. Hart 1898, 370
109. IFC S 226: 22
110. IFC S 385: 55
111. IFC S 736: 22, 24
112. Roe, 33
113. Logan, 116
114. IFC S 572: 71
115. McClafferty
116. Godwin
117. Pratt 1850–7
118. Hatfield, 52
119. Tongue
120. Pratt 1850–7
121. Godwin
122. Parkinson, 870
123. Withering 1787–92, 400
124. Hatfield MS
125. Beith
126. Fargher
127. MacFarlane
128. Vickery 1995
129. Carmichael, iv, 203
130. Dyer 1889, 295
131. Maloney
132. IFC S 777: 173
133. IFC S 571: 167
134. Maloney

135. IFC S 521: 149
136. IFC S 921: 90
137. McGlinchey, 86
138. IFC S 170: 203, 259
139. IFC S 770: 63
140. IFC S 736: 389
141. IFC S 93: 347
142. IFC S 59: 369
143. IFC S 616: 78
144. IFC S 975: 27
145. IFC S 251: 173
146. IFC S 960: 211
147. Egan
148. IFC S 268: 230
149. IFC S 658: 135
150. Beith
151. Johnson 1862
152. MacFarlane
153. Hopkins, 80
154. Hatfield, 35
155. Parkinson, 286
156. Jóhansen
157. Martin, 378; Hibbert, 541
158. Pratt 1850–7
159. Martin, 226, 229, 230
160. Lightfoot, 343
161. Beith
162. Carmichael, vi, 105
163. Sullivan & Stelfox
164. Beith
165. Polson
166. Hatfield, appendix
167. Vickery 1995, 352
168. IFC S 523: 268
169. Ó Súilleabháin, 313
170. Parkinson, 855
171. Ray 1690, 287
172. Tait
173. IFC S 504: 279
174. Logan, 46
175. Martin, 224
176. Polson, 34
177. McNeill
178. Campbell
179. Pratt 1850–7
180. Monteith, 25
181. Beith
182. Freethy, 124
183. Freethy, 124
184. Vickery MSS
185. IFC S 601: 183
186. IFC S 920: 69, 71, 72
187. IFC S 550: 288
188. Maloney
189. IFC S 480: 197
190. Maloney
191. IFC S 920: 69, 71, 72
192. Moffet
193. Freethy, 125
194. Beith; McNeill
195. Pennant 1776, ii, 42
196. Lightfoot, 201
197. Martin, 192
198. MacFarlane
199. Trevelyan
200. Freethy, 125
201. IFC S 914: 554, 555
202. IFC S 907: 212
203. Ó Súilleabháin, 312
204. Maloney
205. IFC S 838: 245
206. IFC S 932: 239
207. IFC S 897: 153
208. *Transactions of the Devonshire Association for the Advancement of Science, Literature, and Art*, 103 (1971), 269
209. Dacombe
210. Beddington & Christy, 212
211. Freethy, 87
212. Beith
213. Dacombe
214. Vickery 1995
215. Beith
216. Lafont, 69
217. Jobson 1967, 60
218. Jones 1996
219. Tynan & Maitland

220. *Notes and Queries,* ser. 8, 7 (1895), 86
221. Taylor 1929, 118
222. Beith
223. IFC S 826: 62
224. IFC S 746: 57, 64
225. McGlinchey, 83
226. IFC S 788: 92
227. IFC S 903: 625
228. IFC S 337: 77
229. Vickery 1995, 93
230. Taylor 1929, 119
231. MacFarlane
232. Lafont
233. Whitlock 1992, 106
234. Pratt 1850–7
235. Hatfield, 30
236. Trevelyan, 91
237. Lafont
238. Hatfield MS
239. Dacombe
240. Whitlock 1992, 106
241. Trevelyan, 97
242. Maloney
243. IFC S 794: 36
244. IFC S 617: 333
245. IFC S 510: 96
246. IFC S 337: 77
247. IFC S 794: 418
248. IFC S 498: 81, 313
249. IFC S 491: 40; 498: 127
250. IFC S 897: 217
251. McClafferty
252. Wilde, 42; Wood-Martin, 187
253. IFC S 138: 168
254. IFC S 287: 180
255. Maloney
256. Moloney
257. Maloney
258. Trevelyan, 97
259. Tongue
260. A. Allen, 178
261. Collyns
262. Vickery 1995
263. Trevelyan, 313
264. Carmichael, vi, 70
265. Purdon
266. IFC S 170: 258
267. Rootsey, 92
268. Davey, 23
269. Pliny, book 24, section 63
270. Pratt 1850–7; Johnson 1862

CHAPTER 8

Currants, Succulents and Roses

Dicotyledonous flowering plants in the order Rosales and families Grossu-lariaceae (currants), Crassulaceae (stonecrops), Saxifragaceae (saxifrages) and Rosaceae (roses) are included in this chapter.

GROSSULARIACEAE

Ribes rubrum Linnaeus
red currant
western Europe; introduced elsewhere

Ribes nigrum Linnaeus
black currant
northern Europe and Asia, and mountains to their south; introduced
elsewhere

Ireland has supplied the sole record of the herbal use expressly of 'wild cur-rant': in Cavan the leaf of that has been rubbed on parts affected by ringworm.[1] Whichever of the two species, *Ribes rubrum* or *R. nigrum* was meant—and it could have been either or both—'wild' must have meant merely bird-sown among native vegetation from some cultivated source. Chance, isolated bushes that spring up in this way have been traditionally regarded with a certain awe, as their origin seems mysterious, and that alone would be sufficient to account for a preference for wild-growing currants for medicinal purposes.

Though both black and red currants are very rarely found far from habi-tations in Ireland, that is less true of Britain. The much lengthier history of fruit-growing in the latter accounts for that in large part, but there is weighty botanical authority for the view that both species are also indigenous there in certain habitats, especially fens and wet woods. Even if that view is correct, however, the plants were probably always too scarce to have constituted a ready-enough source for medicine, a secondary use of them which would almost certainly have had to wait until they were grown for food.

While it is strictly speaking irrelevant to the theme of this book to cover folk medicine from plants in cultivation, there would seem to be a marginal case for making an exception in this instance. However, apart from a tea made from the dried leaves of either species used in East Anglia as a weaker alternative to the (more usual) one made from raspberry leaves for easing labour in childbirth,[2] it is black currant juice, from the fresh or jellied fruit, for coughs, colds and chest complaints that monopolises the folk records. That those records are from many parts of England but almost wholly from there is doubtless merely a reflection of the comparative incidence of fruit-growing— at any rate in the past.

CRASSULACEAE

Umbilicus rupestris (Salisbury) Dandy
Cotyledon umbilicus-veneris Linnaeus, in part
  navelwort, wall pennywort, pennyleaf
  southern and south-western Europe, North Africa, Macaronesia

Sempervivum tectorum Linnaeus
  house-leek, sengreen
  horticultural

It is convenient to consider *Umbilicus rupestris* and *Sempervivum tectorum* together, for the range of ailments to which their fleshy leaves have been applied is so broadly similar that they must surely have stood in for one another to no small extent. *Umbilicus* is rather tightly restricted to the west of the British Isles, where it is an abundant and unquestioned native. *Sempervivum*, on the other hand, is a sterile cultivar or hybrid of a mountain plant of central Europe, capable only of vegetative propagation and thus entirely dependent on deliberate introduction by humans; consequently, in the British Isles it is confined exclusively to the walls and especially roofs of old buildings, clinging on as a relic of long-forgotten introductions and for the most part sufficiently ignored and self-sustaining to be ranked as 'wild' by field botanists. A plant with strong magico-religious associations, allegedly sacred to the sky god and generally said to owe its presence to having been planted on roofs to protect houses from lightning bolts, *Sempervivum* may nevertheless have been treasured as much, if not more, for employment as a medicine. At what period or periods it was brought over from continental Europe can only be guessed at—as the common vernacular name for it, sengreen, is its Anglo-Saxon one (and the plant features in the *Lacnunga* as an ingredient in a cough medicine[2a]), the post-Roman invasions rather suggest themselves, but earlier and possibly even much earlier importations cannot be ruled out. Certainly it is no latecoming usurper of the place in folk medicine presumptively occupied previously by *Umbilicus,* for not only has its use in rural Wales and Ireland and even the Highlands been widespread and to all appearances deeply established, but it even bears names of its own in the Gaelic languages.

Because the folk uses recorded for *Umbilicus* are not found outside the western areas where that species abounds, those for *Sempervivum,* the range of which is not determined climatically, predictably far outnumber them; those for the latter are in fact twice as numerous, and perhaps partly thanks to its magical reputation they also extend to a greater diversity of ailments. The one outstanding difference between the two is the very much greater popularity of *Sempervivum* as a treatment for sore eyes. That constitutes indeed the single greatest use of the plant by a very wide margin, accounting for 41 of the 147 records traced. Most of those 41 are from a wide spread of Irish counties, but in proportion to their area Wales and south-westernmost England are also well represented. By contrast, *Umbilicus* has been recorded in use for the eyes solely from some unspecified part(s) of Wales[3] as far as Britain is concerned (but that use did not feature in a more recent field survey[4] of Welsh folk medicine in which this herb emerged prominently in connection with other ailments). *Sempervivum* also has a monopoly of the relatively few records of treating earache or deafness with drops of the juice and for the application of the leaves to staunch bleeding—both of which emerge as British rather than Irish practices, the former

Umbilicus rupestris, navelwort
(Green 1902, fig. 214)

very markedly so and particularly characteristic of southern Wales (Brecknockshire, Glamorgan and Carmarthenshire[5]) though reported also from Oxfordshire,[6] Norfolk[7] and the Highlands.[8] Peculiar to *Sempervivum* as well is its employment for cancerous growths, a use for which the only records traced are from two of the Eastern Counties, Essex[9] and Cambridgeshire.[10]

These exceptions apart, both plants have been valued in the main for soothing and healing soreness of the skin, whatever its cause, and as a treatment for various kinds of eruptions on it. The leaf might be applied as a poultice or reduced to a form in which it could be mixed with cream or fat and turned into an ointment. In both it has been corns, warts, burns and chilblains that have received this attention most frequently; but when the records for those uses are compared geographically, the surprising fact emerges that *Sempervivum* and *Umbilicus* are almost exactly mirror images of one another: the eleven counties in which *Umbilicus* has been employed for burns, for instance, are almost an entirely different set from the nine in which that use has been recorded for *Sempervivum*. While this lends support to the idea that the two functioned as stand-ins for one another, the pattern exhibited by that standing-in has evidently been extremely complex. In only two cases are the distributions neat and suggestive. The records of the use of *Umbilicus* for corns—the single commonest affliction for which that plant features (19 records out of 80)—are mostly from the northern half of Wales[11] and the rest from the southeastern corner of Ireland (Wicklow,[12] Wexford,[13] Carlow,[14] Cork[15]). And similarly, *Umbilicus* is on record for chilblains in four south-eastern Irish counties (Tipperary,[16] Carlow,[17] Wexford,[18] Wicklow[19]), the two Welsh counties (Pembrokeshire,[20] Cardiganshire[21]) facing the second two of those,

Sempervivum tectorum,
house-leek (Green 1902, fig. 218)

and more distantly, Devon.[22] Could these two distribution patterns be the legacy of population movement between Wales and Ireland?

Nowhere in the British Isles does there seem to have been such high regard for the virtues of *Umbilicus* as the Isle of Man—according to one source[23] it was esteemed throughout the island as late as 1860—but neither corns nor chilblains feature among the ailments for which is has been recorded there; instead, only bruises,[24] scalds,[25] felons[26] and erysipelas[27] find mention (though it may also have been the *lus-ny-imleig* valued for a womb ulcer[28]). Intriguingly, the inclusion of *Umbilicus* among the nine or ten ingredients in a special poultice for erysipelas[29] was shared by the island with Donegal.[30] In Skye,[31] where that plant was also valued for erysipelas, it was used in the belief that it drew out the 'fire' from the affliction.

As is usually the case with folk herbs enjoying a strong reputation for effectiveness for certain purposes, these two have also attracted to themselves a tail of miscellaneous other uses. *Sempervivum* is on record in Britain for insect and nettle stings in Kent[32] and Gloucestershire,[33] croup in Norfolk,[34] asthma in Lincolnshire[35] and fevers in the Highlands.[36] The only singleton for Britain produced by *Umbilicus*, on the other hand, is a record as a treatment for epilepsy in some unspecified part of the west of England[37]; though attributed to 'herb doctors', that record may have been derived from reports in the medical press a decade earlier by a general practitioner in Poole, Dorset, of a dramatic improvement in that affliction brought about by the juice of this plant.[38] Its use had been suggested to the general practitioner in question by someone who had read of this in a magazine article, which in turn presumably drew on a folk medicine source.

Surprisingly, the sole uses exclusive to Ireland in terms of the records traced are confined to that same miscellaneous tail. Surprisingly, too, though *Umbilicus* is by far the more plentiful of the two plants in that country, the Irish uses of that for which only single records have been turned up—for tuberculosis in Wicklow[39] and jaundice in Waterford[40]—are outnumbered by their *Sempervivum* equivalents: for headaches in Roscommon,[41] for worms as well as kidney trouble in Cavan[42] and as an abortifacient in Mayo.[43] Though *Sempervivum* has yielded the only Irish records of its employment for cuts (Cavan,[44] Carlow[45]), *Umbilicus* beats that with the only ones for its application to sore eyes (Leitrim,[46] Wicklow[47]) and as an earache cure (Mayo[48]). But as a treatment for lumps and swellings, *Sempervivum* not only has a monopoly of the records traced for Ireland but a widely scattered distribution in that role as well (Londonderry,[49] Leitrim,[50] Wicklow,[51] Carlow[52]).

Sedum telephium Linnaeus

Hylotelephium telephium (Linnaeus) Ohba
  orpine, live-long
  northern temperate zone

(Folk credentials questionable) Primarily a divinatory as a folk herb, *Sedum telephium* seems likely to have owed its medicinal uses in the British Isles entirely to the learned tradition of the books. Once widely grown in cottage gardens in England and southern Scotland as a wound plant (under the name 'orpies' or 'orpy-leaves'),[53] its recommendation to James Robertson in 1767 by a gardener in the remoteness of Sutherland as a remedy for the bite of a mad dog or an adder[54] is the closest to a hint of an alternative origin that has been discovered. In so far as the species can be considered a member of the native flora—and that only in Britain—it has probably always been too scarce to be drawn on in the wild for cures.

Sedum acre Linnaeus

  biting stonecrop, wall pepper
  Europe, north and western
    Asia, North Africa;
    introduced into North
    America, Australasia

The juice of *Sedum acre* has been more recently used in Norfolk to treat dermatitis[55] and has served in the past in Cardiganshire as an ointment for shingles.[56]

In Ireland a decoction of a plant known simply as stonecrop (a name which could apply to several species), said to grow on walls in one case and on thatched roofs in another, has been recorded from Cavan,[57] Leitrim[58] and Wex-

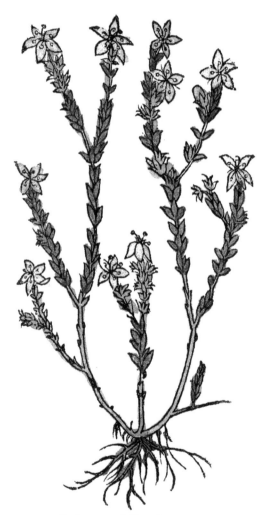

Sedum acre, biting stonecrop
(Bock 1556, p. 143)

ford[59] as a remedy for ridding the system of worms. It has also been valued in Westmeath for kidney trouble.[60]

Sedum anglicum Hudson
English stonecrop
Atlantic Europe, Morocco

A plant abounding in Colonsay, an island of the Inner Hebrides, and once there pounded with groundsel to produce a mixture to reduce swellings 'especially on horses' (but perhaps on people, too?) was botanically identified as *Sedum anglicum*.[61] It perhaps stood in for house-leek (*Sempervivum tectorum*) there.

SAXIFRAGACEAE

Saxifraga × urbium D. A. Webb
Londonpride
horticultural

In Carlow the often well-naturalised garden hybrid *Saxifraga × urbium* was a speciality cure of a local healer in 1928. Mixed with salt and rubbed on a rupture, it gradually reduced the swelling, it was claimed.[62]

Saxifraga granulata Linnaeus
meadow saxifrage
western and central Europe

(Folk credentials questionable) A plant bearing a Gaelic name identified in some dictionaries with *Saxifraga granulata* has been used as a decoction for kidney troubles in Westmeath.[63] The species was widely recommended in the learned tradition for treating gravel and stones (allegedly because of the resemblance of the root to those), but it is too great a rarity in Ireland, accepted as native only in the vicinity of Dublin, to make a very credible folk herb there. The record more probably relates to parsley-piert (*Aphanes arvensis*), a much more widespread Irish plant with a folk reputation for relieving similar ailments.

Chrysosplenium Linnaeus
golden-saxifrage
northern temperate zone

(Folk credentials questionable) According to an eighteenth-century physician in Nottinghamshire,[64] 'an ointment made from this [*Chrysosplenium* sp.] has been kept a secret among some glass-makers, who had experienced its virtues in curing burns by hot metal.' It is not clear whether this statement was referring to a local use or whether the information was second-hand, taken from some printed source, possibly even a German one (for the author was an immigrant from Germany).

ROSACEAE

Filipendula ulmaria (Linnaeus) Maximowicz
Spiraea filipendula Linnaeus, *F. hexapetala* Gilibert
meadowsweet
arctic and temperate Europe, temperate Asia; introduced into
eastern North America

Like willows, *Filipendula ulmaria* contains salicylate (it is the one from which salicylic acid was first made in 1835). It has been widely employed for the same range of complaints for which today we would use aspirin, and many claim it is free from aspirin's side effects. Back in 1691, John Aubrey wrote to John Ray about a woman in Bedfordshire who was achieving 'great cures' with the plant for agues and fevers, with the addition of some green wheat.[65] There are more recent records of its use for fevers, coughs, colds, sore throats or headaches in Devon,[66] Somerset,[67] the Highlands and/or Western Isles,[68] and South Uist in the Outer Hebrides.[69] But it has enjoyed a reputation for more then just those: for treating burning or itching eyes in Devon,[70] as a tonic in Devon also[71] (and in Nottinghamshire, too, to judge from the name 'Old Man's Pepper' recorded for it from there[72]), for curing diarrhoea, 'stomach cold' and pains in general in Somerset,[73] relieving sunburn or reducing freckles in Norfolk[74] and easing nervousness in the Isle of Man.[75]

In Ireland some of those uses are on record, too: for colds in Cavan,[76] for diarrhoea there[77] and in Cork,[78] as a seasonal tonic in Louth[79] and for nervousness in Westmeath.[80] But apparently peculiar to Ireland is a reputation for dropsy and kidney trouble in Cavan[81] and Sligo,[82] and for jaundice in children in Limerick.[83] In 'Ulster' alone a decoction of the plant seems to have been recorded as a drink for those with a tendency to scrofula.[84]

Rubus idaeus Linnaeus
raspberry
northern and central Eurasia, North America

An infusion of the leaves of *Rubus idaeus* drunk regularly during pregnancy to allay labour pain is recorded from many parts of England as well as from the Highlands.[85] Probably an age-old remedy, it has more recently received respect in official medicine and by the 1940s was in general use in one of the maternity hospitals in Worcestershire, preliminary tests having appeared to confirm the belief that the compound then called fragarine relaxes the womb muscles.[86] In the Highlands,[87] however, and more generally in folk medicine, the belief is that it strengthens them. Modern pharmacology, though, is indicating a story that, as so often with herbal remedies, is turning out to be much more complicated than at first supposed. Among raspberry's active constituents are a smooth muscle relaxant as well as at least two smooth muscle stimulants.[88] To further complicate the picture, it seems that the Worcestershire hospital studies may even have used the wrong plant, strawberry, in their study (hence the name fragarine, from *Fragaria,* the botanical name for strawberry).[89] This is one of many instances highlighting the need for co-operation between historians of folklore, pharmacognocists and medical practitioners.

Other traditional uses for raspberry include its use both for procuring abortion in Cambridgeshire during early pregnancy[90] and, in the Sheffield area of Yorkshire, preventing miscarriages, increasing the flow of maternal milk and, unsurprisingly, helping painful menstruation.[91] In the Black Country of Staffordshire[92] on the other hand, it is for preventing morning sickness that it has acquired a reputation. That is more likely to have come from the astringent properties that raspberry leaves share with those of blackberries and strawberries, which has made them an alternative remedy for diarrhoea in Suffolk,[93] southern Yorkshire[94] and Westmoreland.[95] Paradoxically, though, it is for curing constipation that they have been prized in Dorset.[96]

Raspberry leaf tea has also enjoyed a strong following in some areas for alleviating fevers, coughs, colds and sore throats (Wiltshire,[97] Norfolk,[98] South Riding of Yorkshire[99]); that aspirin-like usage presumably also accounts for its presence in a Yorkshire remedy for arthritis[100] and in a Devon one for consumption.[101] Another group of ailments for which raspberry has been valued in Devon is kidney stones and gravel, but for that it was a daily dose of the jam dissolved in a glass of gin and water that was rated effective.[102] Yorkshire's particularly wide range of uses has even included as a wash for sore eyes.[103]

Irish records, however, are strikingly scarce by comparison. Only a single one has been traced of the use of the plant in childbirth, and that a relatively recent one from Antrim,[104] but reticence on the part of adults about such matters could well explain their apparently total absence in that connection even from the very extensive Schools Survey of 1937–8. But even raspberry leaf tea has been little-known there, if the solitary record for that from Limerick[105] (for easing sore throats) is anything to go by. Yet raspberries certainly grow wild in Ireland quite widely and are accepted as native in at least upland areas there.

Rubus fruticosus Linnaeus, in the aggregate sense   PLATE 10
blackberry, bramble; briar (in Ireland)
Europe, North Africa, Macaronesia, North America; introduced
into Australasia

The leaves (or roots) of *Rubus fruticosus* have enjoyed the same reputation as that of raspberry and black currant for an astringency that has made them valuable against diarrhoea (Devon,[106] Essex,[107] Fife[108]) and coughs, colds, sore throats or asthma (Devon,[109] Somerset,[110] Hertfordshire,[111] Lincolnshire,[112] southern Yorkshire,[113] the Highlands[114]). Also prominent, but apparently almost exclusive to the south-west of England, has been their application to skin disorders in the widest sense, from shingles (Cornwall,[115] Devon[116]) and boils (Cornwall[117]) to spots and sores on the face (Dorset[118]) and burns and scalds (Cornwall,[119] Wiltshire,[120] Colonsay in the Inner Hebrides[121]). In the Chiltern Hills[122] and East Anglia,[123] cancers have been treated with a black-berry poultice. In Sussex a thorn in the finger was drawn out by moistening a leaf and leaving it on as a plaster for an hour or two,[124] in Devon an infusion of the leaves is still in currency as a tonic,[125] in Dorset chewing the tip of a shoot has been reputed an excellent cure for heartburn,[126] while in the Isle of Man the boiled leaves have soothed sore eyes.[127]

In Ireland much the most widespread use of the blackberry has been for staunching diarrhoea (and for that in cattle, too). All the other applications feature in the records only marginally by comparison: for cuts in Offaly[128] and Louth,[129] as a tonic in Limerick[130] and Cork,[131] for ulcers in Limerick,[132] burns in Louth,[133] kidney trouble in Kerry,[134] swellings in Wicklow,[135] indigestion in Carlow[136] and sore, swollen or sweaty feet in Leitrim.[137]

Potentilla anserina Linnaeus
Argentina anserina (Linnaeus) Rydberg
silverweed, goosegrass, wild tansy
northern half of Eurasia, North and South America, Australia

Of the few recorded uses of the mild 'astringent', *Potentilla anserina,* two are of interest for their lengthy continuity. One was as a cosmetic by young women, to cleanse the skin of spots, pimples, freckles or suntan—observed in an unstated part of England (probably the Bristol area) by the foreign botanists Pierre Pena and Matthias de l'Obel in the sixteenth century[138] and still current around the start of the nineteenth century in the Highlands,[139] where it was steeped in buttermilk. In Leicestershire it was used specifically to remove the disfiguring marks left by smallpox.[140] The other, no less time-honoured practice has been to wear the leaves in shoes or other footwear to prevent over-sweating leading to soreness, hence the names 'traveller's joy' and 'chafe grass'. In addition to pilgrims,[141] carriers in eighteenth-century Nottinghamshire[142] and schoolboys in nineteenth-century southern York-

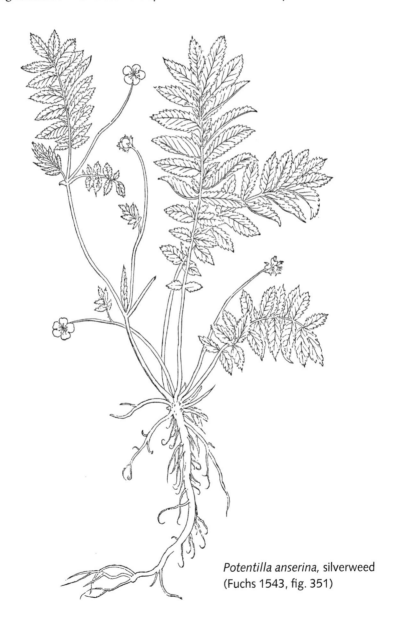

Potentilla anserina, silverweed
(Fuchs 1543, fig. 351)

shire[143] resorted to this, and it survived in rural parts of the Eastern Counties till the 1940s at least.[144] Similarly, the bruised leaves, mixed with salt and vinegar, were applied to the soles to allay the heat in fevers. Far away in Shetland, however, the plant has been found in use only for digestive complaints.[145]

In Ireland the plant has had very different applications: in Londonderry (as *mashcoms*) to staunch diarrhoea or bleeding piles,[146] on the Clare-Galway border for heart trouble[147] and in Co. Dublin 'for a man's health'—whatever that meant.[148]

Potentilla erecta (Linnaeus) Raeuschel
tormentil,[149] aert bark, tormenting root
Europe, western Asia, North Africa, Azores, Labrador

With the thickest roots, with a higher proportion of tannin in them, *Potentilla erecta* was the native species of the genus much the most widely employed as an 'astringent' (though because of its powerful effect it needed to be used with discretion). Pre-eminently a plant of acid, heathy ground, its records as a medicinal plant are correspondingly largely from the north and west of the British Isles, where it has served as the principal cure for diarrhoea above all, though also for cuts in Cumbria.[150] For its stimulating effect, on the other hand, it has been valued as a tonic in Norfolk[151] and Shetland,[152] for fevers in Devon[153] and as a gargle for enlarged tonsils and throat trouble in Norfolk.[154] In South Uist in the Outer Hebrides it was a multi-purpose herb, curing any suppurating sore, a corn or even indigestion.[155] In the Highlands it has been an antidote for worms,[156] in Perthshire a lotion for sunburn[157] and in Gloucestershire an alternative to silverweed (*P. anserina*) and blackberry (*Rubus fruticosus*) as a balm for the feet.[158]

In Ireland the lesser uses recorded are fewer but similar: for cuts in Cavan,[159] for obstructions or other trouble in the liver in 'Ulster'[160] and for burns and scalds in some unspecified county (or counties).[161]

Potentilla reptans Linnaeus
creeping cinquefoil
Europe, North Africa, western Asia; introduced into North and
    South America, Australasia

Potentilla reptans has owed its place in folk medicine to its being mistaken for the more potent tormentil (*P. erecta*)[162] or being used in its stead in regions with little or no acid ground suitable for that. In Gloucestershire it was one of three ingredients in a tea much drunk as a remedy for 'red rash' (erysipelas?),[163] while in Essex a tea made wholly from it has been esteemed as a digestive.[164]

In Ireland it has been recorded as much valued for 'ague' in Cavan.[165]

Fragaria vesca Linnaeus   PLATE 11
wild strawberry
Europe, western and central Asia, Macaronesia, eastern North
   America; introduced elsewhere
Another 'astringent', *Fragaria vesca* resembles silverweed (*Potentilla anserina*)
in having been valued as a cosmetic: in Cornwall girls rubbed their faces with

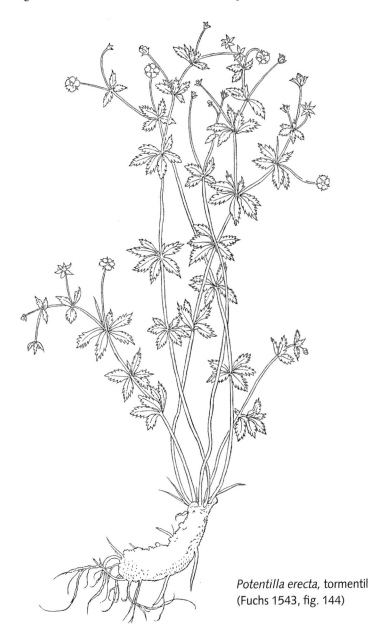

Potentilla erecta, tormentil
(Fuchs 1543, fig. 144)

its leaves to improve their complexions, a use reflected in a folk song fragment in Cornish collected in 1698.[166]

Ireland has produced the only other record of a non-veterinary use: from Antrim, of a belief that excessive ardour can be cooled with strawberry-leaf tea[167]; but the leaves for that may have come from a garden species and not this native one.

Geum urbanum Linnaeus   PLATE 12
herb-Bennet, wood avens
Europe, western Asia, North Africa, Australia; introduced into
   North America, New Zealand

Though long a prominent member of the learned repertory, the widespread, easily distinguished and readily accessible *Geum urbanum*, in places an inextinguishable garden weed, was almost completely neglected in British and Irish folk medicine, if the near-absence of records for it is a fair reflection of the reality. For Britain there is just an isolated record from Bedfordshire of the use of 'green benet', which has been identified as this species. The plant was stewed with vinegar and, when cold, used to soothe sore eyes.[168]

Assuming it is correctly identified as the 'evans' employed for kidney trouble in Cavan,[169] that is the only reliable record traced from Ireland, similarly. The species does receive mention in another Irish source, as in use for chills,[170] but in that case the record is neither localised nor unambiguously a folk one.

Agrimonia eupatoria Linnaeus
agrimony
Europe, south-western Asia, North Africa, Macaronesia; introduced
   into North America

Agrimonia procera Wallroth
fragrant agrimony
Europe

Though *Agrimonia eupatoria* is a common plant of the lowlands and its popularity as a medicine goes back at least to Galen and Pliny, it may resemble house-leek (*Sempervivum tectorum*) in having been taken over for herbal use in the British Isles from an intrusive tradition: its seeds have been detected in Norse levels at York and it also features in the Anglo-Saxon manuscripts. That the records of its folk use come preponderantly from areas in the west particularly associated with Norse settlement is therefore suspicious.

Principally taken in the form of a tea, as a mild tonic and stimulant, *Agri-*

monia eupatoria is one of several herbs to have gained a reputation as a general prophylactic and purifier of the system. As such it is on record as having been drunk, on its own or combined with other herbs, in many parts of England as well as south-eastern Scotland. It has also been valued more specifically as a treatment for sore throats and the heavier kinds of colds and

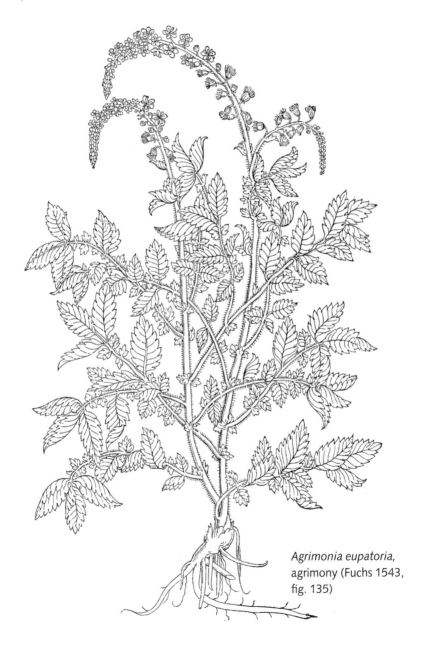

Agrimonia eupatoria,
agrimony (Fuchs 1543,
fig. 135)

coughs—in Devon,[171] Gloucestershire[172] and Suffolk[173]—as well as for various rheumatic complaints in three of the Eastern Counties,[174] the East Riding of Yorkshire,[175] Cumbria[176] and Montgomeryshire.[177] In the last of these, though, the 'backache' for which use of a poultice of the herb is recorded may have been a misnomer for kidney pain (as have proved to be the case in some other instances[178]): a weak infusion of the dried leaves has long had a place in folk medicine, too, for chronic disorders of the liver, kidneys and bladder. Employed (as recommended by Galen) for liver complaints in Norfolk[179] and the Highlands[180] and for jaundice in Norfolk[181] and the Isle of Man,[182] it has been applied to kidney trouble unambiguously in Pembrokeshire,[183] Worcestershire[184] and Caernarvonshire.[185] But despite John Quincy's assertion in 1718 that 'the country people use the herb bruis'd, or its juice, in contusions and fresh wounds',[186] that use has not been encountered among the localised folk records and may therefore have become rare or extinct. The same applies, at least in Britain, to a claim a century later that agrimony was a favourite application to ulcers 'in some rural districts'.[187]

Ireland has had echoes of those uses for colds and liver complaints (both in Clare[188]) and jaundice (in Londonderry[189]), while the plant's diuretic effect has led to its use to treat enuresis in children in Wicklow.[190] In Londonderry it was also much used at one time in cases of scurvy and sometimes for old ulcers, too.[191] Hard to understand, though, is a botanist's report that agrimony was popular in Donegal[192] for treating sore eyes, for eyebright (*Euphrasia officinalis*), so generally favoured for that elsewhere, can surely never have been scarce in that county?

There is evidence that the rarer species, the fragrant agrimony, *Agrimonia procera,* may often have been preferred. In the Isle of Man it is the only one occurring as an obvious relic of herbal use.[193]

Sanguisorba minor Scopoli
Poterium sanguisorba Linnaeus
salad burnet
central and southern Europe, Caucasus, North Africa; introduced
　　into North America, Australasia

(Folk credentials questionable) As the allusion to blood in the scientific name indicates, *Sanguisorba minor* had a place in the written tradition as a wound plant. That only a solitary record of an allegedly folk use for that purpose (in Sussex[194]) has been traced makes it look unlikely that this was a genuine member of that rival repertory.

Alchemilla vulgaris Linnaeus, in the broad sense
  lady's-mantle
  Europe, northern and western Asia, eastern North America,
    Australia; introduced into New Zealand
Like several other herbs, *Alchemilla vulgaris* is not a single entity but (in this case) a composite of a number of distinct microspecies which reproduce

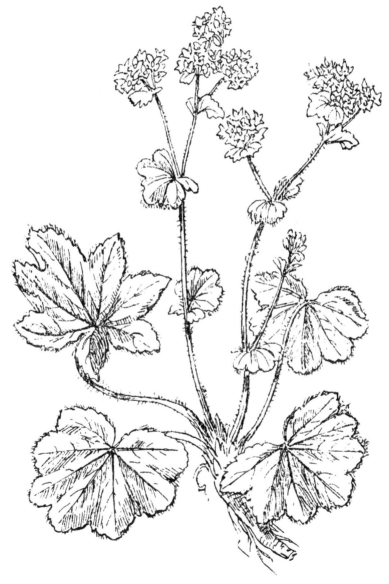

Alchemilla vulgaris, lady's-mantle (Green 1902, fig. 189)

asexually. Most of these are characteristic of upland hay-meadows, a habitat in which some are considerably plentiful. Upper Teesdale, in the Pennines, has more of the different kinds than anywhere else in the British Isles, three of which have distributions there so strongly associated with human activity as to suggest they were introduced at some period in the past, either intentionally for medicinal purposes or accidentally as weeds.[195] No English records of the use of lady's-mantle in folk medicine, however, have been traced: indeed the sole British ones are from the Highlands, where they were in use for sores and wounds.[196]

Rather, it is Ireland that seems to have made use of these herbs very largely. The mysterious, dew-like appearance of the expressed juice evidently gave them there a semi-magical reputation,[197] though they presumably possessed some demonstrable styptic action quite apart from that to have proved popular for cuts and nosebleeds in Londonderry[198] and, especially, Wicklow,[199] and perhaps a diuretic one, too, to have recommended themselves for kidney trouble in Cavan[200] and Kerry.[201] Other applications recorded are for burns and scalds in Cavan,[202] for 'incurable diseases' in Galway[203] and for sore heads (impetigo?) under the name 'thrush ointment' in Kildare.[204]

Aphanes arvensis Linnaeus, in the broad sense
parsley-piert
Europe, south-western Asia, North Africa, Macaronesia; introduced
into North America, Australasia

As its former name 'parsley breakstone' advertised, drinking a decoction of *Aphanes arvensis* was once much in favour for countering gravel in the kidneys or bladder—for example among the poor in Bristol, as noticed by two foreign botanists in 1571, who expressed surprise that the plant was nevertheless not well known to the herbalists.[205] Half a century later, Thomas Johnson found it being brought in from the countryside by herb women for sale under that name in London's Cheapside.[206] That a Herefordshire name for the plant at much the same period was 'colickwort'[207]—colic being a term used for the pain caused by a kidney stone—strengthens the impression that its use for that complaint was well established at the folk level, as does the further fact that a name in Irish, *minéan Merr* (for *Muire?*), has survived for it in that same connection in Westmeath.[208] The only other evidence of its persistence in folk use in Ireland into the nineteenth and twentieth centuries seems to be from Londonderry,[209] and in England records of a similar age, still as 'parsley breakstone', have been traced only from Suffolk[210] and Birmingham.[211] Cities feature too much in this account for there not to be some suspicion that that may nevertheless be a herbal use originally derived from the learned tradition. Against that is parsley-piert's *alter ego* as 'bowel-hive grass', a name equally indicative of the ailment at which it has been also targeted specifically: inflammation of the bowels or groin in children. A localised record of the plant in use for that is known from Berwickshire.[212]

Rosa Linnaeus
wild rose
northern temperate and subtropical zones; introduced into
   Australasia

It is hard to believe that treating colds and sore throats with rose-hip syrup[213] and cuts with the crushed leaves in Essex[214] can be the sole English records of the use of the common and familiar roses in folk medicine; nothing else, however, has been traced. A herbal mixture employed in the Highlands to poultice erysipelas has been recorded as including a decoction of the wood and leaves of roses,[215] but that may have arisen through common figwort's (*Scrophularia nodosa*) being so generally known in folk parlance as 'the rose', for, suspiciously, it is the latter that has been a remedy for erysipelas in Donegal.[216]

In Ireland, wild roses and brambles are too commonly called 'briars' interchangeably to allow any appearances of that word in the folk medicine records to be referred with confidence to either. In Donegal, however, the juice of a plant expressly named as *rós* has been a cough cure.[217]

Rosa rubiginosa Linnaeus
sweet-briar
Europe, western Asia; introduced into North America, Australasia

Readily told from other wild roses by its distinctive scent and widely grown in cottage gardens for that, *Rosa rubiginosa* has been recorded from Longford as taken as a decoction for jaundice.[218] It is possible that the bushes that served as that source were wild ones, but if so they would only have been derived from gardens in that particular county. The species is considered a possible native in some other parts of Ireland, however.

Prunus spinosa Linnaeus
blackthorn, sloe
Europe, south-western Asia; introduced into North America, Australia

A geographical curiosity thrown up by *Prunus spinosa* is the restriction of its widespread use for warts virtually to the southern half of England (Dorset,[219]

Herefordshire,[220] Buckinghamshire,[221] Essex,[222] Suffolk,[223] Norfolk,[224] Cambridgeshire[225]) despite the tree's general distribution through much of the British Isles. The sole non-English record for that ailment is from Denbighshire.[226]

The strong astringency of the berries and inner bark has also made the plant an alternative to tormentil (*Potentilla erecta*) or blackberry (*Rubus fru-*

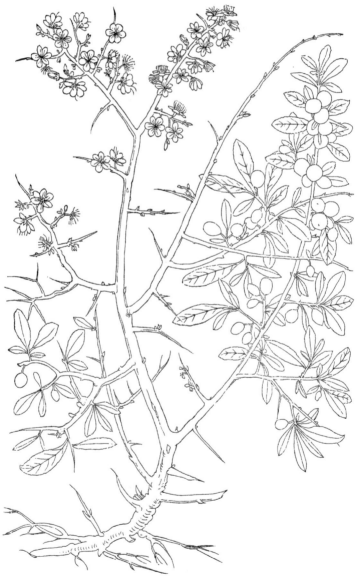

Prunus spinosa, blackthorn (Fuchs 1543, fig. 227)

ticosus) for countering diarrhoea, in Cornwall,[227] Dorset,[228] Hertfordshire,[229] Leicestershire[230] and if 'internal disorders' is a euphemism for that at least in part, in Sussex,[231] Northamptonshire[232] and Lancashire,[233] too. That same property could explain the making of a jelly from the berries for treating 'a relaxed throat' in the Isle of Man.[234] Paradoxically, though, the tree has also been credited with a relaxing effect: in Wiltshire an infusion of the inner bark has been drunk for piles,[235] and in the Highlands the flowers have provided a laxative.[236]

A third group of complaints for which blackthorn has been valued comprises coughs (Norfolk,[237] Denbighshire 'and elsewhere'[238]), sore throats (Norfolk[239]) and fevers (the Highlands[240]). In Suffolk, sloe wine has also been esteemed as a cure for colic,[241] and in Anglesey the berries and leaves have been chewed to lower blood pressure.[242]

Irish records are inexplicably scarce. The antidiarrhoea use widely recorded in England is known also from 'Ulster', but there as an infusion made from the thorns.[243] In Cavan, sloe gin has been reckoned good for the kidneys,[244] while in Tipperary a decoction of the bark has been given as a daily dose to children troubled with worms.[245]

Prunus avium (Linnaeus) Linnaeus
wild cherry, gean
Europe, western Asia, North Africa; introduced into North America,
    New Zealand

Though the naturalised morello cherry (*Prunus cerasus* Linnaeus) is nowadays as widespread as the native species and tends not to be distinguished from it by non-botanists, of the two, only *P. avium* would have been available in earlier times for use in folk medicine. As its scientific name implies, *P. avium* is also sometimes called 'bird cherry', a name which more properly belongs to another native species, the more northern *P. padus* Linnaeus. Though *P. padus* has been exploited for medicine in Fennoscandia, the sole folk remedy using it in the British Isles that has been traced is a veterinary one.

The only use of *Prunus avium* in folk medicine seems to have been for colds or coughs, for which records have been traced from three widely separated areas: Norfolk[246] and the Highlands[247] in Britain, and Mayo[248] in Ireland. The record from the Highlands, though, sounds suspiciously like a learned rather than a strictly folk use in that it involved dissolving the gum (as recommended by Dioscorides) in wine, which was hardly a liquid to be found in the average croft.

Malus sylvestris (Linnaeus) Miller
crab apple
north-western Europe

Only where a record specifically mentions crab apple (or 'crab') in the generic sense can it be taken to relate to apple trees of the kind most likely to be native to the British Isles and thus alone available before the sweet cultivated kinds were introduced (though that was well before Roman times, according to the latest authoritative opinion). Of such records there are only three, and two of them Irish: one a vague and unlocalised one of the use with buttermilk for a relaxed throat and hoarseness,[249] the other from Sligo of a treatment for internal cancer[250] (boiling the leaves and drinking the juice). The sole British record involved the juice, too: for bruises in Suffolk.[251]

More often, the kind of apple is not identified, leaving it to be assumed that any variety will serve (including those of the cultivated and introduced *Malus pumila* Miller). Not all apples with small, sour fruits are the true crab apple (*M. sylvestris*), and forms or derivatives of *M. pumila* may have sometimes stood in for that in folk usage. However, as it is the acid juice that is valued for some of the purposes featuring in folk medicine, a preference in these cases for kinds possessing that in the fullest and most powerful degree can be inferred. William Withering found what country people called 'verjuice' was used extensively on recent sprains[252] (but unfortunately failed to say in which part of England that was). In the East Riding of Yorkshire a piece of the fruit rubbed on a wart is reputed to turn it black and eventually cause it to drop off,[253] so strong is the astringency.

No less prized for their ability to soothe have been hot poultices of rotten apples. Applied to 'any sore places' in Norfolk,[254] these have been a treatment for earache in Wiltshire,[255] small boils in the East Riding of Yorkshire[256] and 'rheumatism in the eye' in some area(s) unspecified.[257] According to this last source, decoctions of the flowers or fruit were also once used by young women as an astringent cosmetic. The sole record that can be added to that list is an application in Antrim to chilblained toes.[258]

Sorbus aucuparia Linnaeus
rowan, mountain ash
Europe, south-western Asia, Morocco; introduced into North America, New Zealand

As a tree with much magico-religious lore attached to it in the Gaelic-speaking parts of the British Isles (in the uplands of which it is also commonest),

Sorbus aucuparia has predictably been deployed against a variety of ailments—though not nearly as widely as one might have expected. In seventeenth-century Wales the berries were eaten for scurvy,[259] in the eighteenth century a purge was derived from the bark in Moray[260] and in the nineteenth century some unstated part of the tree was valued in Aberdeenshire for toothache.[261] A gargle made from the boiled berries[262] is on record from the Highlands as well.

Ireland's greater tradition of utilising the bark of trees for medicinal purposes finds reflection in the boiling of that for a cough cure in Louth[263] and its inclusion in a herbal mixture taken for 'the evil' (i.e. scrofula) in Sligo.[264] In Cavan the leaves have served as a poultice for sore eyes, and the berries have been eaten raw as a cleansing tonic for the blood[265]; the berries, too, have been eaten in 'Ulster' to rid the body of worms.[266]

Crataegus monogyna Jacquin   PLATE 13
hawthorn, quick, mayflower, whitethorn
Europe, western Asia, North Africa; introduced into North America, Australasia

Crataegus laevigata (Poiret) de Candolle
C. oxycanthoides Thuillier
midland hawthorn
western and central Europe; introduced into North America
Like the rowan (*Sorbus aucuparia*) and elder (*Sambucus nigra*), fellow trees bearing sprays of white blossom, hawthorns have had strong magico-religious associations down the millennia, associations which have hung on in rural Ireland till relatively recent years. Today, by far the commoner of the two species native to the British Isles, *Crataegus monogyna* may formerly have been the rarer in southern England, for its degree of interfertility with the midland hawthorn, *C. laevigata,* is so great that it must once have been isolated from it ecologically in order to have survived as a separate species. Biometric studies have shown that present-day hawthorn populations consist of an admixture of the two to a much greater extent than previously suspected, the product not only of hybridisation in the wild but probably also of much planting in the past of nursery stock of hybrid origin. *Crataegus laevigata* is essentially a woodland plant of clay soils, while *C. monogyna* was probably originally confined to open scrub on limestone and chalk, and to fens. *Crataegus laevigata* seems the more likely to have attracted awe, for it is the only one reliably in flower on Old May Day in southern England and alleg-

edly the only one with blossoms emitting a powerful odour of rotting flesh.[267] Distinguishing between the species, however, has probably always been a feat confined to botanists—in folk culture all hawthorns were doubtless regarded as belonging to a single entity.

Compared with the tree's prominence in folk beliefs its role in folk medicine appears to have been but slight. Both the flowers and the berries have enjoyed a reputation as a heart tonic in Devon[268] and the Isle of Man,[269] while in the Highlands[270] hawthorn tea has been drunk as a 'balancer' for either high or low blood pressure. In the Isle of Man[271] and the Highlands,[272] too, the plant has provided a remedy for sore throats. In Derbyshire an infusion of the leaves served to extract thorns and splinters[273] and in East Anglia a decoction of them substituted for those of raspberries (*Rubus idaeus*) to ease labour in childbirth.[274]

The sole Irish records picked up are both from Leitrim: as a toothache cure[275] (involving steeping the bark in black tea and holding the liquid in the mouth for a few minutes) and as an ingredient in a remedy for burns.[276]

Notes

1. Maloney
2. Newman & Newman, 186
2a. Cockayne 1864–6; Grattan & Singer 1952
3. Johnson 1862
4. Williams MS
5. Williams MS
6. 'E.C.'
7. Hatfield MS
8. Beith
9. Hatfield MS
10. Porter 1974, 47
11. Williams MS
12. IFC S 925: 6
13. IFC S 897: 217
14. IFC S 903: 624
15. IFC S 338: 223
16. IFC S 572: 70
17. IFC S 903: 624
18. IFC S 898: 82, 85
19. IFC S 925: 6
20. Williams MS
21. Williams MS
22. Lafont, 66; *PLNN*, no. 61 (1999), 289
23. *Phytologist*, n.s. 4 (1860), 167
24. Fargher
25. Roeder
26. Roeder
27. Roeder
28. Moore 1898
29. Roeder
30. McGlinchey, 83
31. MacCulloch, 90
32. Pratt 1850–7
33. Vickery MSS
34. Taylor 1929, 119
35. Hatfield MS
36. Beith
37. Johnson 1862
38. Salter
39. McClafferty
40. IFC S 655: 265
41. IFC S 268: 118

42. Maloney
43. Vickery 1985
44. Maloney
45. IFC S 904: 256
46. IFC S 191: 88
47. IFC S 921: 69, 89
48. IFC S 138: 168
49. Moore MS
50. IFC S 190: 342
51. McClafferty
52. IFC S 903: 624
53. Johnston 1853
54. Henderson & Dickson, 94
55. Hatfield, 50
56. Williams MS
57. Maloney
58. IFC S 225: 360
59. IFC S 888: 294
60. IFC S 736: 190
61. McNeill
62. O'Toole
63. IFC S 736: 389
64. Deering, 199
65. Lankester, 238
66. Lafont
67. Tongue
68. Beith
69. Beith
70. Lafont
71. Lafont
72. Grigson
73. Palmer 1976, 113
74. Hatfield, 50
75. Fargher
76. Maloney
77. Maloney
78. IFC S 385: 55
79. IFC S 637: 216
80. IFC S 736: 137
81. Maloney
82. IFC S 157: 314
83. IFC S 504: 279, 376
84. Egan
85. Beith

86. Whitehouse
87. Beith
88. Newall, 226
89. Newman 1948
90. Hatfield MS
91. Vickery 1995
92. CECTL MSS
93. Chamberlain 1981, 214
94. Vickery 1995
95. Wright, 243
96. Dacombe
97. Whitlock 1976, 167
98. Hatfield MS
99. Vickery 1995
100. Vickery MSS
101. Lafont
102. Lafont
103. Vickery 1995
104. Vickery MSS
105. IFC S 524: 10
106. Lafont
107. Hatfield MS
108. Simpkins, 411
109. Lafont
110. Tongue
111. Ellis, 366
112. Gutch & Peacock
113. Vickery MSS
114. Beith
115. Courtney, 154
116. Lafont
117. Baker
118. Dacombe
119. Hunt, 413; Davey, 143; Hole, 65
120. Whitlock 1992, 105
121. McNeill
122. D. Hart-Davis, in litt. Feb. 2000
123. Taylor MS (Hatfield, 77)
124. Arthur, 45
125. Lafont
126. Dacombe
127. Fargher
128. Barbour
129. IFC S 672: 211

130. IFC S 522: 197
131. IFC S 385: 54
132. IFC S 505: 148
133. IFC S 672: 211
134. IFC S 476: 91
135. McClafferty
136. IFC S 907: 208
137. IFC S 190: 169, 171, 172
138. Pena & de l'Obel, 308
139. Pratt 1852, i, 32
140. Bethell; Friend 1883–4, ii, 371
141. *North Western Naturalist*, n.s. 2 (1954), 322
142. Deering, 162
143. *North Western Naturalist*, 14 (1939), 217
144. Newman 1945
145. Jamieson
146. Moore MS
147. Gregory
148. Colgan 1904, 301
149. strongly accented on the second syllable (*Scottish Naturalist*, 1 (1871), 54)
150. Freethy, 127
151. *Norfolk and Norwich Notes and Queries*, vol. 1 (answer to query 544)
152. Jamieson; Vickery 1995
153. Bray, i, 274
154. Pigott
155. Shaw, 47–8
156. Beith
157. Barrington, 103
158. Vickery MSS
159. Maloney
160. Egan
161. Ó Súilleabháin, 310
162. Moore MS
163. Britten & Holland, 559
164. Newman & Wilson
165. Maloney
166. Deane & Shaw
167. Vickery MSS
168. English Folklore Survey, 195
169. Maloney
170. Moloney
171. Collyns; Lafont, 6, 70
172. Vickery MSS
173. Jobson 1967, 57
174. Newman & Wilson; Parson MS; Harland, 82
175. Vickery MSS
176. Newman & Wilson
177. Evans 1940
178. Williams MS
179. Taylor MS (Hatfield, appendix)
180. Beith
181. Hatfield, 42
182. Fargher
183. Williams MS
184. Archer, xiii
185. Williams MS
186. Quincy, 121
187. Johnson 1862
188. IFC S 617: 334
189. Moore MS
190. McClafferty
191. Moore MS
192. Hart 1898, 365
193. Allen 1986, 117
194. A. Allen, 185
195. Bradshaw
196. Beith
197. Meehan, 207–8
198. Moore MS
199. IFC S 920: 69, 71, 76
200. Maloney
201. IFC S 413: 228
202. Maloney
203. IFC S 5: 163
204. IFC S 771: 171
205. Pena & de l'Obel, 324
206. Johnson 1633, preface
207. Merrett, 92
208. IFC S 736: 389
209. Moore MS
210. Jobson 1959, 144

211. Vickery MSS
212. Johnston 1853
213. Vickery MSS
214. Hatfield MS
215. Beith
216. McGlinchey, 83
217. IFC S 1043: 71
218. IFC S 752: 10
219. Udal 1922, 260
220. CECTL MSS
221. Vickery MSS
222. Newman & Wilson
223. Glyde, 175
224. Hatfield MS
225. Parson MS
226. *Hardwicke's Science-gossip* (1872), 282–3
227. Vickery MSS
228. Vickery MSS
229. Ellis, 359
230. Wright, 243
231. Friend 1883–4, ii, 372
232. Friend 1883–4, i, 185
233. *Hardwicke's Science-gossip* (1882), 164
234. Fargher
235. Macpherson MS
236. Beith
237. Hatfield, 30, 89
238. Friend 1883–4, ii, 372
239. Hatfield, 29
240. Beith
241. *Folk-lore,* 35 (1924), 356
242. Vickery MSS

243. Buckley
244. Maloney
245. IFC S 571: 8
246. Hatfield, 30, 89
247. Beith
248. IFC S 93: 528
249. Moloney
250. IFC S 171: 47
251. Emerson
252. Withering 1787–92, 296
253. Vickery MSS
254. Hatfield, 52
255. Macpherson MS
256. Gutch, 69
257. Hole, 18
258. Vickery MSS
259. Ray 1670, 290
260. Pennant 1771, 311
261. *Phytologist,* n.s. 2 (1858), 415
262. Beith
263. IFC S 672: 76
264. IFC S 171: 53
265. Maloney
266. Egan
267. Allen 1980
268. Lafont
269. Quayle, 70
270. Beith
271. Quayle, 70
272. Beith
273. Vickery MSS
274. Newman & Wilson
275. IFC S 191: 91
276. IFC S 225: 30

CHAPTER 9

Legumes, Spurges and Geraniums

Dicotyledonous flowering plants in the orders (and families) Fabales (Fabaceae, legumes), Myrtales (Lythraceae, loosestrifes; Thymelaeaceae, mezereons; Onagraceae, willowherbs), Santalales (Viscaceae, mistletoes), Celastrales (Celastraceae, spindles; Aquifoliaceae, hollies), Euphorbiales (Buxaceae, boxes; Euphorbiaceae, spurges), Rhamnales (Rhamnaceae, buckthorns), Linales (Linaceae, flaxes), Polygalales (Polygalaceae, milkworts) and Geraniales (Oxalidaceae, wood-sorrels; Geraniaceae, crane's-bills) are included in this chapter.

FABACEAE

Anthyllis vulneraria Linnaeus
kidney vetch
Europe, North Africa; introduced into North America, Australasia
(Folk credentials questionable) Despite a reputation throughout Europe as a vulnerary, the only allegedly folk use traced of *Anthyllis vulneraria* has been in the Highlands, where, under two alternative Gaelic names, it is said to have been used in the past for cuts and bruises.[1] Caleb Threlkeld observed it being sold in markets in eighteenth-century Ireland, under the name 'stench'.[2] This rarity of records for a species so widespread in the British Isles and locally quite plentiful makes it likely that it was a borrowing from herbals.

Lotus corniculatus Linnaeus
bird's-foot-trefoil
Europe, Asia, mountains of North and East Africa; introduced
    into North America, Australasia

Another ancient wound herb like *Anthyllis vulneraria, Lotus corniculatus* also features hardly at all in the folk records despite its prevalence as a plant of the British Isles. That the only record of use—as an eyewash—comes from South Uist in the Outer Hebrides,[3] however, makes it a more convincing candidate for genuine folk status.

Lathyrus linifolius (Reichard) Bässler

L. montanus Bernhardi

bitter-vetch

Europe

Under the name carmele, a contraction of the Gaelic *corra-meille* (and no connection with caramel), dried root tubers of *Lathyrus linifolius* have had an age-old reputation in the Highlands and Western Isles for their property of allaying the pangs of hunger on long journeys, if chewed at frequent intervals.[4] Martin Martin[5] and James Robertson[6] also found a deep-rooted belief in Skye and Mull, respectively, that if chewed before drinking strong liquor, they prevented intoxication. A cure for diseases of the breast and lungs[7] as well as for indigestion[8] was further credited to the tubers. They were found to keep for many years, and a supply was often laid in for future use.

In Ireland, interestingly, knowledge of the plant's value extended to Donegal, where in the mid-nineteenth century it had some renown as making 'an excellent stomach drink'.[9] A 'vetch' from which a decoction of the roots has been used as a rub for backache in Wicklow[10] is as likely to have been this plant, too, as any of the species of *Vicia*.

Trifolium dubium Sibthorp

lesser trefoil

Europe; introduced into North and Central America, Australasia

Trifolium repens Linnaeus

white clover

Europe, north and western Asia, North Africa; introduced into North and South America, eastern Asia, South Africa, Australasia

(Folk credentials questionable) Studies by botanists[11] have shown that the plant most often identified as the mythical *seamróg* is the lesser trefoil, *Trifolium dubium,* or, rather less often, white clover, *T. repens.* It may be that both these species are phytochemically inert. Nevertheless, one or the other is most likely to have been the 'shamrock' recorded in use in folk medicine for coughs in Kerry,[12] liver ailments in Cavan[13] and toothache (for which it was smoked in a pipe) in the Isle of Man.[14]

Trifolium pratense Linnaeus
red clover

Europe, western and central Asia, North Africa; introduced into
North and South America, South Africa, Australasia

As so frequently seems to be the case, the uses of *Trifolium pratense* attributed to 'country people' by one of the early writers do not find reflection in the more recent folk records. According to John Parkinson, 'in many places' at the time he wrote (1640) the juice was applied to adder bites and to clear the eyes of any film beginning to grow over them or to soothe them when hot and bloodshot.[15] He makes no mention of coughs and colds, for which the plant has since been used in mixtures with other herbs in Norfolk[16] and Cumbria.[17] In the latter it has also been applied to rashes, in the form of a lotion produced by infusing the flowers and leaves.[18] Further, if this is what has been recorded simply as 'clover', a tea made from it has been drunk in Caernarvonshire for the nerves[19] and the leaves chewed in the Isle of Man to relieve toothache.[20]

In Ireland the plant's role as a cough remedy is more widely recorded than in Britain—from Cavan,[21] Wicklow,[22] Clare[23] and Kerry[24]—but exclusive to that country is the application of the leaves to bee stings in Offaly[25] and the drinking of an infusion of the flowering tops for cancer in Wicklow[26] and for stomach cancer specifically in Meath.[27]

Cytisus scoparius (Linnaeus) Link
Sarothamnus scoparius (Linnaeus) Wimmer ex Koch
broom

western and central Europe, Macaronesia; introduced into North
America, Australasia

Cytisus scoparius is one of the few herbs employed in folk medicine with general and emphatic confidence for one particular property: containing sparteine, a very powerful diuretic which triples renal elimination, an infusion or decoction of the young green 'tops' has been recorded from most parts of the British Isles as in use for dropsy and kidney ailments of all kinds. In modern herbalism the plant is used to slow and regulate the heart rate, but no evidence of that has been found in the folk records, by contrast. Instead, the only other uses in folk medicine which emerge at all widely are for rheumatic complaints (Essex[28] and Cumbria,[29] though predominantly Irish) and as a purgative, for liver troubles (Herefordshire,[30] Isle of Man[31]), jaundice (Norfolk[32]) and piles (Devon[33]). The Isle of Man has seemingly been unique in employing the plant for swellings[34] and to procure an abortion[35] as an alternative to gin.

Ireland's employment of the 'tops' for rheumatic complaints is on record from Leitrim,[36] Westmeath,[37] Co. Dublin,[38] Wicklow[39] and Limerick,[40] while a use for neuralgia in Kilkenny[41] is clearly cognate. But though the plant has featured as a liver remedy only from unspecified part of Ulster,[42] the country has made up for that with a remarkable diversity of other minor applications apparently exclusive to itself: for coughs and colds in Mayo[43] and Roscommon[44] or, combined with bilberry tufts, for asthma in Carlow[45]; for abscesses in Cavan[46] and boils in Carlow[47]; for erysipelas in Wexford[48] and rashes in Tipperary[49]; and for sprains in Kildare,[50] heartburn in Wicklow[51] and toothache in Carlow again.[52] Broom tips also anciently took the place occupied by juniper in the Scottish Highlands, being burnt as a fumigant.[53] An intriguing sidelight is the belief, reported from Cornwall[54] and Donegal,[55] that broom was one of those plants with a 'he-kind' and a 'she-kind', each held to be more potent (as a diuretic) if taken by the opposite sex. In other cases, separate and even quite unrelated species have been the recipients of this taxonomic twinning, but information is lacking on whether the distinction was made between broom and some other plant (dyer's greenweed, *Genista tinctoria* Linnaeus, perhaps) or merely between different growth states of broom itself.

Ulex gallii Planchon
western gorse
south-western Atlantic Europe

Ulex europaeus Linnaeus
gorse, furze
Atlantic Europe; introduced widely elsewhere

The recorded uses of gorse in folk medicine all come from those parts of the west of the British Isles where *Ulex gallii* is the only one certainly native and where *U. europaeus*, the common one over much of England, bears a name in Gaelic or Welsh indicative of comparatively recent introduction, for hedging and forage.

Apart from a veterinary use in the Isle of Man, the records come from Ireland without exception. The principal application there has been for coughs, colds, sore throats and hoarseness (Down,[56] Londonderry,[57] Donegal,[58] Wicklow,[59] Waterford[60]), including consumption (Limerick[61]). In Londonderry,[62] Wicklow[63] and Kilkenny[64] it has also featured as a tonic, especially for cleansing or 'increasing' the blood, while in parts of Ulster[65] and in Wicklow[66] and Wexford[67] it has been favoured for heartburn or hiccups. In Cavan[68] and Limerick[69] decoctions of the flowers or 'tops' have been given for jaundice and in Cavan[70] for heart trouble, while in parts of Ulster[71] it has been applied to ringworm and dermatitis and in Meath (with daisy roots) for a whitlow[72] or a swelling.[73] Widely employed for ridding livestock of worms, that use has also been extended to children in Antrim[74] and Sligo.[75]

LYTHRACEAE

Lythrum salicaria Linnaeus
purple-loosestrife
Europe, temperate Asia, North Africa, Australia; introduced into
   North America

Lythrum salicaria is another plant for which the evidence as a folk remedy is wholly Irish. Though the Gaelic name in general use for it in the west and south-west of Ireland[76] translates as 'wound herb', the present study bears out the experience of Michael Moloney that that finds no reflection in the folk records of recent centuries. Other *Lythrum* species in other parts of the world are, however, known to be wound plants, so that purple-loosestrife once served that purpose is not unlikely. As an 'astringent', though, there are generalised statements in the literature that it was popular among the Irish peasantry for curing diarrhoea,[77] and Caleb Threlkeld in 1726 recorded that a preparation of it cured a patient of his of a seemingly fatal case of dysentery. That no mentions of this common and conspicuous plant were picked up in an extensive trawl of the Irish Schools Survey of 1937–8 is therefore very surprising. Could use of it really have died out in the course of the previous hundred years?

THYMELAEACEAE

Daphne mezereum Linnaeus
mezereon
Europe, temperate western Asia; introduced into North America
(Folk credentials questionable) The berries of a plant known as 'mazeerie' are recorded as eaten in Lincolnshire as a cure for piles,[78] but as those of *Daphne mezereum* are highly poisonous the record must surely belong to *D. laureola*. The true mezereon—a name of Arabic origin, probably current only in the written and learned tradition—has undoubtedly been grown in cottage gardens, but as a wild plant it has probably always been much too rare ever to have had a place in the unwritten tradition.

Daphne laureola Linnaeus
spurge-laurel, wood-laurel
western and southern Europe, Asia Minor, North Africa, Azores;
   introduced into North America, New Zealand
Described by William Withering as 'a brisk and rather severe purgative',[79]
Daphne laureola finds a mention in Chaucer as a cottage garden laxative and
what is probably a Lincolnshire use in that capacity is mentioned under *D.
mezereum,* preceding. In the West Riding of Yorkshire 'the poor people' in
the eighteenth century employed *D. laureola* as a vomit.[80] In Herefordshire,
on the other hand, it was mixed with mistletoe and given for epilepsy.[81] No
records have been found of any seemingly true folk uses, however, of the purposes for which the druggists are said to have most valued it, namely as a
horse medicine and as a cure for venereal disease and both benign and malignant cancers. The herb collectors, who often sold it as 'mezereon',[82] are
described as scouring woods in Berkshire[83] and Sussex[84] for its roots in the
first half of the nineteenth century and greatly reducing its large populations
there as a result. While that shows that it existed as a wild plant in England in
sufficient abundance locally to have constituted a potential member of the
unwritten herbal tradition (unlike *D. mezereum*), the available evidence
makes it look more likely that its use was wholly a product of the learned
works and their followers.

ONAGRACEAE

Epilobium Linnaeus
   willowherb
   temperate zones
(Name ambiguity suspected) The Rev. Hilderic Friend[85] records having heard
'the small *Epilobium*'—whatever species he understood by that—called 'eyebright' in Somerset. That could imply that it has substituted for *Euphrasia
officinalis* as an eyewash; alternatively, it may have been merely an erroneous
transfer of the vernacular name.

Circaea lutetiana Linnaeus
   enchanter's-nightshade
   Europe, western and central Asia, North Africa, North America
Though *Circaea lutetiana* features in the Anglo-Saxon herbals as a plant of
semi-magical potency, its sole use in British folk medicine appears to have
been in the Highlands (where it could have been *C. ×intermedia* Ehrhart, its

widespread hybrid with the rare *C. alpina* Linnaeus) as an aphrodisiac, given by girls to their lovers without their knowing. The plant was claimed, when placed in water, to make it bubble.[86]

VISCACEAE

Viscum album Linnaeus
mistletoe
Europe, central Asia, Japan, North Africa; introduced into
North America

Formerly in great repute, *Viscum album* 'is now very much disregarded; and indeed its sensible qualities promise but little. Some remains of Druidical

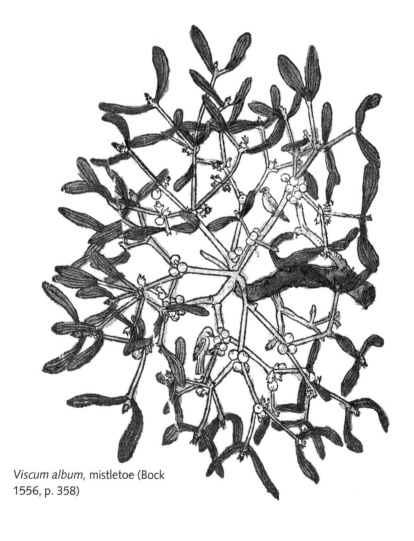

Viscum album, mistletoe (Bock
1556, p. 358)

superstition probably gave birth to its medical fame.'[87] So wrote the otherwise enlightened William Withering, dismissively. Attitudes now, however, are very different, and mistletoe is taken increasingly seriously by present-day medical science as an important source of therapeutic chemicals, both actual and potential. Even those Druidical superstitions hardly deserved Withering's contempt, for *Viscum* was one of three herbs mentioned by Pliny the Elder in his *Natural History* as held in high esteem by the contemporary Gauls—and, as it was a plant well known to the Romans, there can hardly be doubt about its identity. Pliny says the Druids believed it an antidote for all poisons and called it 'all heal', and that has survived as one of its vernacular names in both Wales and Scotland.

Since ancient times it has been known that the plant produces a substance which has a relaxing effect on the nervous system. That is the property that finds principal reflection in the folk records (naturally concentrated in the southern half of England, the only part of the British Isles in which mistletoe occurs in any quantity). Employment in that connection ranges from controlling the involuntary muscle contractions characteristic of chorea ('St Vitus' dance') in Wiltshire,[88] Hampshire,[89] Sussex,[90] Gloucestershire[91] and Lincolnshire[92] and those of epilepsy in Suffolk,[93] Herefordshire[94] and Lincolnshire,[95] to calming hysteria in Herefordshire[96] and heart palpitation in Inverness-shire.[97] Because of the control the plant is believed to exert over blood pressure as well, there is also a contemporary Essex record of eating a leaf daily to guard against a stroke.[98]

A secondary use of mistletoe in the more distant past has been for fevers, a practice surviving into the eighteenth century in Moray.[99] Relics of that presumably are its deployment against measles (to bring out the spots) in Somerset[100] and whooping cough in Norfolk.[101]

In Ireland the plant has enjoyed a reputation in Cavan[102] and Meath[103] for soothing the nerves in general, and in Limerick[104] and Cork[105] for palliating epilepsy and hysteria specifically.

CELASTRACEAE

Euonymus europaeus Linnaeus
spindle
Europe, western Asia; introduced into New Zealand
One of the vernacular names for *Euonymus europaeus*, 'louseberries', recorded from Gloucestershire, Warwickshire and Cumbria, is a relic of the once widespread decoction of the leaves or bark or powder employed against head lice

in children. Though mentioned by several other earlier writers, a record from Cumbria[106] is the only localised one that has been encountered in the folk literature.

A tea made from the bark has been a jaundice remedy in Essex,[107] but that sounds suspiciously like a carry-over from learned medicine, in which the plant has had a reputation for curing liver ailments.

AQUIFOLIACEAE

Ilex aquifolium Linnaeus   PLATE 14
  holly
  western and central Europe; introduced into North America,
    New Zealand

Though the tree *Ilex aquifolium* is common over much of the British Isles, its recorded use in folk medicine is very largely confined to central and southern England, and to one affliction mainly: chilblains. By beating those with a sprig of holly till they bled, it was believed that the circulation was improved (or, as an Oxfordshire theory had it, it let the chilled blood out).[108] For the same reason that was the way to relieve arthritis or rheumatism, people maintained in Somerset.[109] But if the rationale of applying a counter-irritant was considered to dictate too painful a procedure, chilblains could equally well be treated with an ointment made from mixing lard with the powdered berries (Wiltshire,[110] Essex[111]), or rheumatism relieved with an infusion of the leaves (in Devon).[112] A whooping-cough cure in Hampshire involved drinking new milk out of a cup made from the wood of the variegated variety of the tree.[113]

The Irish peasantry disregarded chilblains, it would seem. Instead, holly leaves were applied to burns in Meath,[114] and a stiff neck cured in Waterford[115] by beating it with a sprig from the tree.

BUXACEAE

Buxus sempervirens Linnaeus
  box
  southern Europe, North Africa; introduced into North America
    and elsewhere

(Folk credentials questionable) It has become accepted in more recent years that boxwoods on steep chalk or limestone slopes here and there in southern England today are native and not the product of ancient introduction, as formerly assumed. Potentially, therefore, they could have served as a source for medicinal use. *Buxus sempervirens* has been grown so widely as an ornamental, though, that the leaves in the case of the only folk records traced, for ridding the body of worms (human bodies in Suffolk,[116] horses' in Dorset[117]) are likely to have been taken from bushes ready to hand, for which reason this cannot be classed on present evidence as a wild herb.

EUPHORBIACEAE

Mercurialis perennis Linnaeus
dog's mercury
Europe, south-western Asia, Algeria

Records of *Mercurialis perennis* in the folk medicine literature must mainly belong to good-King-Henry (*Chenopodium bonus-henricus* Linnaeus), a formerly widely grown vegetable which was commonly known as 'mercury' at one time. Dog's mercury is highly acrid and for that reason unlikely to have been used for the healing purposes specified. If the botanist John Lightfoot was correctly informed, however, it *was* the species that the inhabitants of Skye took to induce salivation, under the name *lus-glen-Bracadale*.[118] Though very local on that island today, the ease and persistence with which the plant spreads tend to make for abundance wherever it occurs and it could thus have been present in sufficient quantity to be used herbally. Good-King-Henry, moreover, is not on record from Skye. It is nevertheless possible that dog's mercury was used there in all innocence in error for its harmless namesake.

Euphorbia helioscopia Linnaeus
sun spurge, wartweed
Europe, central Asia, North Africa; introduced into North America, Australasia

Euphorbia helioscopia, sun spurge (Fuchs 1543, fig. 465)

Euphorbia peplus Linnaeus
petty spurge, wartweed
Europe, north-western Asia, North Africa, Azores; introduced into
  North America, Australasia

Euphorbia hyberna Linnaeus
Irish spurge
south-western Europe

Euphorbia paralias Linnaeus
sea spurge
southern and Atlantic Europe, Siberia, North Africa; introduced into
  North America, Australia

Euphorbia lathyrus Linnaeus
caper spurge
southern and central Europe, Morocco, Azores (status doubtful);
  introduced into North America, Australasia

Euphorbia amygdaloides Linnaeus
wood spurge
central and southern Europe, Algeria; introduced into
  New Zealand

The corrosive milky juice of several of the species of the genus *Euphorbia* found in the British Isles is credited well-nigh universally with the ability to remove warts. Sun spurge (*E. helioscopia*) is the one most often cited in that connection, but petty spurge (*E. peplus*), the commoner as a garden weed, has probably often substituted for it. In southern and western Ireland, Irish spurge (*E. hyberna*) enjoyed a reputation as the most efficacious for the purpose,[119] in Scilly sea spurge (*E. paralias*) is known to have served instead,[120] while in north-eastern England[121] caper spurge (*E. lathyrus*) and in Limerick[122] some species surely misidentified as wood spurge (*E. amygdaloides*) have been yet further alternatives. In general, though, the species resorted to was probably immaterial; whichever happened to be handy was used. The one exception may have been *E. hyberna*, for a medical correspondent of John Ray's, writing from Tipperary in 1697, reported that the root of that was sometimes boiled in Ireland to produce a purge but was liable to give rise to severe convulsions followed by early death.[123] By the nineteenth century it seems to have become accepted that it was suitable for giving only to livestock for that purpose and its use for human beings was confined to practical joking: one man in Galway who was dosed with it 'ran up and down the street like a madman, and swelled so big that his friends had to bind him round with hay-ropes lest he shall burst.'[124]

Horseplay also found a use for *Euphorbia helioscopia* in the Isle of Man,[125] but in that case arising out of a different property of the juice: the ability to make the head of the penis swell. As an aid to sexual excitement this was sufficiently well known to have given rise to a name for the plant in Manx descriptive of the effect, and that 'Saturday-night-pepper' was one of the names borne by spurge in Wiltshire[126] suggests that it may have had this role in many other areas as well.

Like the Irish, the Manx also knew of the purgative power of spurges[127]; another of the plants' names in their language identified it as a herb for urinary purposes, too.[128] Contrariwise, in at least one part of Ireland *Euphorbia hyberna* has enjoyed a reputation as an infallible cure for diarrhoea.[129] In north-eastern Scotland *E. helioscopia* was employed against ringworm,[130] while in Lincolnshire[131] and (perhaps) Kent[132] the plant served to poultice adder bites and other venomous wounds. More unexpected is the infusion made from it in Northumberland and drunk twice daily to relieve the pain of rheumatism.[133]

RHAMNACEAE

Rhamnus cathartica Linnaeus
buckthorn
Europe, western Asia, north-western Africa; introduced into
North America

Though *Rhamnus cathartica* was once a standard purge for constipation, especially in children, even the supposedly mild dose of twenty berries acted so violently and produced such intensive griping pain that from the eighteenth century onwards, physicians advised against its use. Nevertheless, the berries were still collected in the Chilterns for druggists as late as the 1880s.[134] Though it was plentiful and accessible enough to have formed part of the folklore repertory, the virtual absence of records from the folk literature suggests that its use was either derived from learned medicine or abandoned so early that memory of it had become forgotten—at any rate as a human remedy: it is on record as one for cattle in Ireland.

Frangula alnus Miller
alder buckthorn
Europe, north Asia, north-western Africa; introduced into
North America
(Folk credentials questionable) According to John Gerard, 'divers countri-men' among his sixteenth-century contemporaries used an infusion of the inner bark of *Frangula alnus* as a purge and emetic.[135] But it is unclear whether by those words he meant the folk whom elsewhere he carefully dis-tinguishes as 'the country people', the followers of practices to which he tended to refer only rarely and then merely on account of their quaintness.

LINACEAE

Linum catharticum Linnaeus
fairy flax, purging flax
Europe, south-western Asia; introduced into North America
Evidence of *Linum catharticum*, a well-known purge and emetic, has been excavated from deposits in Britain as early as the Late Bronze Age, invariably from sites associated with cultivation. This may or may not indicate medici-nal use; there are, however, folk records from widely scattered and remote parts of the British Isles to suggest that its history as a purge goes back a very long way. In the Celtic-speaking regions it has also enjoyed a reputation as a cure for menstrual irregularities: in the Highlands, where it bore a name to that effect in Gaelic, this was apparently its principal use[136]; it is also indi-cated with greater or lesser explicitness from the Isle of Man[137] and Skye.[138] Its very power as a purge, evacuating 'viscid and watery humours from the most remote lodgments', was why it commended itself to 'the common peo-ple' for rheumatism as well, according to John Quincy, who nevertheless rated it 'only for very robust strong constitutions'.[139] There are more recent but, regrettably, unlocalised British records for its use for that purpose, too.[140]

Ireland supplies one further application: for urinary complaints in Cavan.[141]

Radiola linoides Roth
allseed
Europe, temperate Asia, Macaronesia, mountains of East Africa
(Name confusion suspected) A herb recorded in use in the Isle of Man for ruptures has been referred to *Radiola linoides*.[142] However, it is too rare on that island for the identification to be credible, and it is unlikely to have been cultivated.

POLYGALACEAE

Polygala vulgaris Linnaeus   PLATE 15
  common milkwort
  Europe, western Asia, North Africa; introduced into North America,
    Australasia

Polygala serpyllifolia Hose
  heath milkwort
  western and central Europe; introduced into North America,
    New Zealand
(Folk credentials questionable) Hopefully identified as the 'polygala' (much milk) of Classical authors, *Polygala serpyllifolia* and *P. vulgaris* were in consequence so particularly commended in the medieval herbals to nursing mothers for promoting the flow of milk after childbirth that their presence in the unwritten tradition seems doubtful at best. The near-absence of ostensibly folk records of that use is indeed suspicious, the sole one, from Norfolk,[143] being of a relatively recent date. Though it has been suggested that a herb used in the Isle of Man which bore a name translating as nipplewort[144] may have been *P. serpyllifolia* or *P. vulgaris* (both widespread there), that identification is by no means certain. It is true that species of *Polygala* have been known in the vernacular as 'milkwort' in the north of England and the Borders,[145] but that name could have been taken from the herbals; it is not necessarily evidence of a one-time widespread use for that same purpose quite independent of learned medicine. It is further suspicious that a herb valued for the ability of its 'milk' to cure warts, which must surely be spurge (*Euphorbia*), has also borne that name in parts of England, particularly the Eastern Counties.[146] It was doubtless spurge, too, that was the 'milkwort' recorded as used in some part(s) of Wales for slight bites by dogs, cats and 'venomous animals',[147] for that is one of the subsidiary applications featuring in the folk records for *E. helioscopia*.

OXALIDACEAE

Oxalis acetosella Linnaeus
  wood-sorrel
  Europe, northern and central Asia, allied species in North America
Because of its frequent confusion with 'cuckoo sorrel', which seems to have been normally *Rumex acetosa*, as well as its long-standing competition with *Trifolium* species for the honour of being the 'shamrock' of Irish legend, folk

records of *Oxalis acetosella* need to be sifted with more than ordinary care. Luckily, in some cases 'wood-sorrel' is named specifically, while in others that this species was doubtless the one intended can be deduced from the medicinal application mentioned. The possibility remains, however, that because of the similarity of their vernacular names, some transferring of applications between this and *R. acetosa* has taken place over the centuries in all innocence.

Even after excluding records likely to belong to other species, we are still left with a suspicious-looking pattern made up of applications recorded mostly from a single area only: to bruises just in Devon,[148] for instance. However, because the identity of the herbs recorded as employed in remedies in the island of Colonsay in the Inner Hebrides was checked by a botanist allegedly in all cases, it may be safe to accept that it was this plant that formed a main ingredient in plasters applied to scrofula there.[149] But though several authors have repeated the respective statements of the botanist John Lightfoot and his companion Thomas Pennant that a whey or tea of it was employed to allay the heat of fevers in Arran,[150] those two did not set eyes on the herb in question, which could therefore have been something else.

In Ireland 'wood-sorrel' explicitly has been recorded in use for diarrhoea in Mayo[151] and Wicklow,[152] as a blood tonic in Cavan,[153] as a heart tonic in Wicklow[154] and for countering palsy in Limerick.[155] Because clovers have been brought to bear on cancers in other parts of Ireland, it is probably also safe to assume that it *was* this plant, with its clover-like leaves, and not *Rumex acetosa* that was eaten for stomach cancer in some unstated part of 'Ulster'.[156]

GERANIACEAE

Geranium pratense Linnaeus
   meadow crane's-bill
   northern and central Eurasia; introduced into North America,
      New Zealand

(Folk credentials questionable) The astringency shared with other members of the genus by *Geranium pratense* brought great repute to a country herb doctor in early-Victorian Berwickshire for its effectiveness against diarrhoea, especially in teething children.[157] That this is the sole record traced of this widespread and conspicuous English plant makes it likely that it belongs to the learned tradition rather than to the oral folk one. Significantly, the species was strongly recommended as a vulnerary in the 1542 herbal of Leonhard Fuchs.

Geranium robertianum Linnaeus
  herb-Robert, (foetid) crane's-bill, bloodwort, red Roger;
   crobh dearg (Irish)
  Europe, southern temperate Asia, North Africa, Macaronesia;
   introduced into North and South America, New Zealand

Formerly known to every owner of cattle in Ireland as the standard remedy for red-water fever, a disease of farm animals especially prevalent in that country,

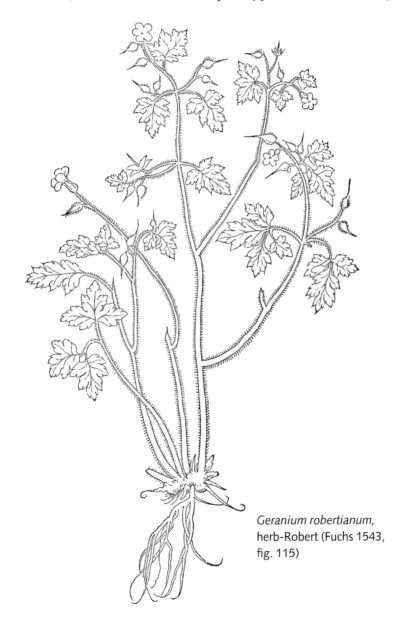

Geranium robertianum,
herb-Robert (Fuchs 1543,
fig. 115)

the consequent familiarity of *Geranium robertianum* gave it a particularly strong following there for human ailments as well. Foremost of those was kidney trouble, to judge from the number of records for that, which are Irish exclusively: from Cavan,[158] Meath,[159] the Aran Islands,[160] Limerick,[161] Carlow,[162] Kerry[163] and, if 'pain in the back', as so often, meant that, in Waterford,[164] too. Similarly an Irish monopoly, it appears, has been using the plant to ease sore throats and coughs of all kinds (Wicklow,[165] Carlow,[166] Limerick[167]). Almost as much of an Irish speciality, too, rather surprisingly given herb-Robert's recommendation as a vulnerary in the early herbals, has been the prizing of it for staunching bleeding; but in this case the restriction of records mainly to eastern coast counties (Down,[168] Cavan,[169] Meath,[170] Wicklow[171]) possibly hints at a tradition imported from Britain. Other, more localised applications in Ireland have been for rheumatic pains[172] and for a gripe in the stomach[173] in Tipperary, for gravel in Londonderry[174] and urinary retention in the Aran Islands,[175] and for gallstones[176] and diabetes[177] (the plant allegedly lowers the blood sugar level) in parts of the country left unspecified.

In sharp contrast, skin troubles, including skin cancer and especially erysipelas, appear to feature in the records only in Britain: in Devon,[178] 'South Wales',[179] Gloucestershire,[180] Yorkshire[181] and various parts of the Highlands.[182] In several of these areas that finds reflection in a vernacular name. Otherwise, Britain has no roles for this plant that appear to be at all widespread. This residue includes gout in Devon[183] and 'North Wales',[184] and stomach upsets in Devon[185] and the Isle of Man.[186] In this last, further uses have been for mouth sores and inflammation[187] and as a wash for the complexion.[188] The Highlands,[189] though, have produced the sole British counterpart of the widespread Irish reputation the plant has had for staunching bleeding. Finally, in one part of Gloucestershire a belief has been recorded that the two sides of the leaf have different therapeutic functions: one draws out the injurious matter, the other heals.[190]

Notes

1. MacFarlane
2. Threlkeld
3. Shaw, 49
4. Pennant 1774, 310; Grant
5. Martin, 226
6. Henderson & Dickson, 80
7. Lightfoot, 389; Pennant 1774, 310
8. Martin, 226
9. Hart 1898, 370
10. McClafferty
11. Colgan 1892; Nelson
12. IFC S 476: 91
13. Maloney
14. Moore 1898
15. Parkinson, 1112
16. Bardswell

17. Freethy, 112
18. Freethy, 112
19. Vickery MSS
20. Gill, 298
21. Maloney
22. McClafferty
23. IFC S 617: 333
24. IFC S 476: 91
25. IFC S 812: 441
26. McClafferty
27. IFC S 710: 49
28. Newman & Wilson
29. Newman & Wilson; Freethy, 123
30. Jones-Baker, 101
31. Moore 1898
32. *Folk-lore,* 36 (1925), 257
33. *Woodbine,* Autumn 1992
34. Moore 1898
35. Fargher
36. IFC S 191: 95
37. IFC S 737: 107
38. IFC S 787: 52
39. McClafferty
40. IFC S 483: 207; 512: 97
41. IFC S 907: 212
42. Egan
43. IFC S 137: 135
44. IFC S 269: 254
45. IFC S 903: 297
46. Maloney
47. IFC S 907: 299
48. IFC S 903: 298
49. IFC S 571: 7
50. IFC S 771: 241
51. McClafferty
52. IFC S 903: 297
53. Moloney
54. Davey, 111
55. McGlinchey, 83
56. St Clair
57. Lucas, 185
58. IFC S 1043: 71
59. McClafferty
60. Lucas, 185

61. IFC S 523: 272
62. Lucas, 185
63. IFC S 920: 74
64. IFC S 861: 212
65. St Clair
66. Lucas, 185; McClafferty
67. Lucas, 185
68. Maloney
69. IFC S 500: 76
70. Maloney
71. St Clair
72. IFC S 710: 43–4
73. Lucas, 185
74. Vickery 1995
75. Lucas, 185
76. Colgan 1911
77. Johnson 1862; Henslow
78. Rudkin
79. Withering 1787–92, 233
80. Anon. in Watson 1775, 737
81. Bull
82. Garner, 368
83. Lousley, 208
84. Bromfield
85. Friend 1883–4, ii, 363
86. Carmichael, vi, 102
87. Withering 1787–92, 609
88. Macpherson MS
89. Fernie, 320
90. Arthur, 45
91. Palmer 1994, 122
92. Gutch & Peacock, 120
93. Jobson 1959, 144
94. Bull, 335 footnote
95. Woodruffe-Peacock
96. Bull, 335 footnote
97. Beith
98. Hatfield, 91
99. Beith
100. *PLNN,* no. 24 (1992), 112
101. Haggard, 16
102. Maloney
103. IFC S 710: 48
104. IFC S 484: 43

105. IFC S 385: 55
106. Freethy, 100
107. Hatfield, 42
108. 'E.C.'
109. Tongue
110. Whitlock 1976, 167
111. Hatfield, 27
112. Lafont
113. *Notes and Queries,* ser. 1, 4 (1851), 227
114. IFC S 690: 39
115. IFC S 637: 21
116. Jobson 1959, 144
117. *PLNN,* no. 23 (1992), 103
118. Lightfoot, ii, 621
119. Sargent
120. *PLNN,* no. 27 (1992), 123
121. Vickery MSS
122. IFC S 498: 127
123. Lankester, 319
124. Hart 1873
125. *PLNN,* no. 6 (1989), 25
126. Dartnell & Goddard
127. Moore 1898
128. Kermode MS
129. Logan, 33
130. Gregor, 47
131. Britten & Holland, 274
132. Pratt 1850–7
133. Vickery MSS
134. Boulger
135. Gerard, 1287
136. Beith
137. Fargher
138. Henderson & Dickson, 93
139. Quincy, 175
140. Pratt 1850–7; Johnson 1862
141. Maloney
142. Henderson & Dickson, 93
143. Hatfield, 89
144. Moore 1898
145. Britten & Holland
146. Newman & Wilson; Taylor 1929; Parson MS
147. Trevelyan, 314
148. Lafont
149. McNeill
150. Lightfoot, 238; Pennant 1774, 175
151. Vickery MSS
152. IFC S 920: 75
153. Maloney
154. McClafferty
155. IFC S 524: 5
156. Egan
157. Johnston 1849
158. IFC S 975: 27
159. Farrelly MS
160. Ó hEithir
161. IFC S 482: 155
162. IFC S 907: 299
163. IFC S 412: 96
164. IFC S 655: 150, 267, 353, 355
165. McClafferty
166. IFC S 907: 268
167. IFC S 483: 21, 330, 369
168. Barbour
169. Maloney
170. IFC S 710: 49
171. IFC S 914: 549
172. IFC S 572: 89
173. IFC S 550: 279
174. Moore MS
175. Ó hEithir
176. Logan, 38
177. Moloney; Ó Súilleabháin, 311
178. Lafont
179. *Hardwicke's Science-gossip* (1869), 191
180. Britten & Holland
181. Britten & Holland
182. Gregor, 47; Polson, 32; MacFarlane; McCutcheon; Beith
183. Lafont
184. Pratt 1850–7
185. Lafont
186. Quayle, 69
187. Moore 1898
188. Paton
189. Cameron
190. Palmer 1994, 122

CHAPTER 10

Ivy and Umbellifers

Dicotyledonous flowering plants in the order Apiales and families Araliaceae (ivies) and Apiaceae (parsleys) are included in this chapter.

ARALIACEAE

Hedera helix Linnaeus
ivy

western and central Europe, south-western Asia; introduced into
North America, New Zealand

Few other herbs have been resorted to so generally—virtually throughout the British Isles—for one ailment in particular as *Hedera helix* has been for corns (or, much more rarely, bunions or verrucas). Usually the leaves were soaked in vinegar to soften them and then bound on as a poultice; less often, they were boiled and the resulting liquid rubbed in; more simply still, the leaves were worn inside a sock. Reputedly, the corn dropped off in a matter of days, without any pain.

The reputation for curing corns extended to warts (Essex,[1] Somerset[2]) and 'cold sores' or tetters (Berwickshire[3]), and from those it seems to have been a logical progression to skin disorders of a variety of kinds, of which British examples are rashes in Dorset[4] and ringworm in Berwickshire.[5] A special treatment in that connection has been the placing of a cap made from the leaves on the head of a child with eczema, apparently exclusive to parts of Scotland (Fife,[6] Colonsay[7] in the Inner Hebrides) and even more parts of Ireland. A remarkably similar distribution to that is shown by the records for treating burns and scalds with ointment made from the boiled leaves mixed with fat, but in this case the Scottish instances (Ayrshire,[8] the Highlands[9]) are joined by one from Devon.[10] Other uses which seem to have been predominantly Irish likewise crop up in the English records just here and there: the plant's reputed ability to staunch bleeding has led to its inclusion in an ointment for suppurating wounds in Herefordshire,[11] while as a treatment for inflammation it has found an outlet in Devon in the form of an infusion of the leaves and berries taken for mumps.[12] Irish faith in the berries as a cure for aches and pains is reflected by their being valued in Gloucestershire as very good for the nerves,[13] just as Ireland's valuing of the plant for coughs and colds is seemingly echoed in a belief in Shropshire that an infallible remedy for whooping cough is to drink from cups made from its wood.[14]

Ivy has either been more especially an Irish herb or its former uses have persisted there more obstinately than in Britain. No fewer than five of the plant's principal recorded uses—for corns, burns, eczema in children, inflammation and cuts—are known from many more counties in Ireland; moreover, except in the case of the last, the distribution of which seems to be confined to the country's central belt, the records are so widely spread as to suggest that they were more or less general in the not-too-distant past. In addition, ivy would seem to have been brought to bear on a considerably wider range of ailments than in Britain. Uniquely Irish, apparently, has been as a treatment for boils and abscesses: recorded from Cavan,[15] Longford,[16] Wicklow[17] and Limerick[18] as well as from Monaghan, where one side of a heated leaf was relied on to draw out the pus and the other to do the healing,[19] a procedure known from Donegal[20] and Leitrim[21] but applied there to extracting thorns from fingers. A boiled leaf also poulticed chilblains in Meath[22] and Wicklow,[23] bad sprains in Donegal[24] and warts in Laois.[25] In Waterford,[26] on the other hand, a leaf had its outer skin scraped off and applied to sore lips. So great was the plant's reputation for healing skin disorders that its use extended to ringworm in Leitrim,[27] measles in Tipperary[28] and skin cancer in the region east of Sligo.[29]

That the berries were eaten in Offaly and its neighbours[30] for aches and pains hints at an action akin to aspirin, which could account for the plant's popularity in Wicklow[31] and Kerry[32] for easing coughs and colds or, in another part of the country,[33] for clearing the chest in bronchitis. It could also account for the use of an extract of the leaves in Wexford[34] and Limerick[35] for back pain, though that could mean kidney trouble, for which the plant has also had its value in Roscommon[36] and for both that and jaundice in Cavan.[37]

In one application alone, and that a minor one, does Ireland seem to have been overtaken by Britain: the procuring of an infusion from the leaves as a lotion for sore eyes. Records of this have been traced only from Limerick,[38] but in Britain it is known from as far apart as Hampshire,[39] Suffolk[40] and Fife.[41]

Finally, there is a use of particular interest of which only a solitary record has come to light: a preparation of the leaves drunk as an abortifacient. This was a practice well known at one time to women in a village in (?) Wiltshire.[42]

APIACEAE

Hydrocotyle vulgaris Linnaeus
marsh pennywort
Europe, North Africa

(Identification uncertain) *Hydrocotyle vulgaris* seems the likeliest identity of the plant whose 'penny leaves that are got in the bog' were rated by two Limerick informants as excellent for dressing a burn.[43] Bog pondweed (*Potamogeton natans*), however, must also be considered a possibility.

Sanicula europaea Linnaeus FRONTISPIECE
sanicle
Europe, southern, central and eastern Asia, Africa

An ancient panacea, *Sanicula europaea* was praised so highly in the old herbals that its folk use cannot escape suspicion of being wholly derived from the written tradition. John Parkinson in his *Theatrum* of 1640 says the country folk applied an ointment made from it to their hands 'when they are chapt by the winde', but the uses recorded in the more recent folk literature mostly reflect the haemostatic property claimed for the plant. It seems to have enjoyed a particularly wide vogue in the Highlands[44] for healing infected wounds (as well as ulcers[45]), while the curing of haemorrhages and dysentery (as well as bruises and fractures) has been claimed for it in the Isle of Man.[46]

In Ireland, similarly, it has been valued for bleeding piles in parts of Londonderry.[47] In Donegal, however, the authority on that county's flora found it much prized as a treatment for consumption.[48]

Eryngium maritimum Linnaeus
sea-holly
coasts of temperate Europe; introduced into North America

The name eryngo, by which herbalists mainly understood *Eryngium campestre* Linnaeus, a species of mainland Europe very rare in Britain, was shared by the common *E. maritimum* of sandy shores, and at least some of the virtues claimed for the bitter root of the other were attributed to this one as well. The roots had to be dug from a depth of six feet or more, were then peeled, boiled and cut into slivers which were twisted like barley sugar and covered in a very strong syrup. The resulting 'eryngo-root', for which the town of Colchester enjoyed a particular reputation for centuries, was much prized for coughs and colds[49] as well as, in popular lore, as an aphrodisiac. Physicians thought highly of it as a tonic, too.

The plant was recorded by Roderic O'Flaherty as in use medicinally in 1684 in the remoteness of the Aran Islands, where it was still employed in the 1920s to rid children of worms and as a general prophylactic.[50] In the formerly hardly less remote Isle of Man, the root was also valued for its anti-irritant property,[51] and ear infections treated with juice squeezed from the leaves.[52] Yet the prominent place the species occupied in learned medicine together with the lack of records of putative folk use elsewhere in the British Isles make it more probable than not that even in those areas it owed its presence in the healing repertory to the written tradition originally.

Anthriscus sylvestris (Linnaeus) Hoffman
cow parsley
Europe, north Asia, North and East Africa; introduced into
 North America

Several wild species with umbels of white flowers and similarly finely cut leaves have traditionally been called 'parsley' in combination with one prefix or another (and shared other vernacular names as well, including 'keck', 'Queen Anne's lace' and even 'hemlock'). *Anthriscus sylvestris* is by far the commonest of them, at any rate in England—in the north and west of the British Isles it tends to be much scarcer—though its abundance may have come about only in recent centuries, as a consequence of the multiplication of roadside verges.

Whether or not records for 'wild parsley' or 'hedge parsley' belong to *Anthriscus sylvestris,* one or more herbs passing under those names have at any rate enjoyed a reputation in Gloucestershire (in the recipe book of a barely literate farmer[53]) and the Isle of Man[54] as a cure for kidney or bladder stones or gravel. As that was one of the virtues also credited to the parsley of gardens (*Petroselinum crispum* (Miller) Nyman ex A. W. Hill), however, the exploitation of the wild relative(s) may merely have been a carry-over from the cultivated species. More convincingly folk in origin was the use of a 'wild parsley' known as *tath lus* in the Outer Hebrides, where, especially in Eriskay, a preparation of that was once valued by women crofters as a sedative.[55] *Anthriscus sylvestris* is known to occur in those islands, though very sparsely.

In Ireland 'wild parsley' is similarly on record from Cavan[56] and Westmeath[57] as a remedy for kidney trouble. In the case of Westmeath, garden parsley has also served as a source of the preparation in question.

Scandix pecten-veneris Linnaeus
shepherd's-needle
central and southern Europe, western Asia; introduced into North
   and South America, North and South Africa, Australasia
A plant known as 'Adam's needle', one of the alternative names recorded for *Scandix pecten-veneris*, has been used in Tipperary for toothache.[58]

Myrrhis odorata (Linnaeus) Scopoli   PLATE 16
sweet cicely
upland Europe; introduced (?) into Chile
A contemporary use of *Myrrhis odorata* for coughs is known in Suffolk.[58a] There is one veterinary record, from Teesdale, also.

Smyrnium olusatrum Linnaeus
Alexanders
south-western and southern Europe, Canary Islands
Once widely eaten as a vegetable as an alternative to celery and common in many coastal areas, mainly in the west, *Smyrnium olusatrum* enjoyed a reputation, especially among seafarers, of 'clearing' the blood and preventing scurvy. Crews of ships used to put ashore in Anglesey specially in order to gather it.[59] On the Isle of Portland in Dorset it was known as 'helrut', credibly assumed to be a corruption of heal-root.[60] It was perhaps as a relic of its consumption for this general prophylactic purpose that the remains of the plant have turned up in a level of Roman age in South Wales.

Two more specific uses of it have been recorded, however. On one of the islands in the Outer Hebrides a broth made from lamb in which this and lovage had been boiled was reckoned to be good for consumptives.[61] And in the Isle of Man, where it was known as *lus-ny-ollee* and is still used by veterinary doctors there for animals with sore mouths,[62] it at one time came in handy as well when people had toothache.[63]

Conopodium majus (Gouan) Loret
pignut
south-western and Atlantic Europe

Well-known for its nut-like roots, *Conopodium majus* has been employed in the Isle of Man as a diuretic.[64]

In Ireland the plant has been valued in Donegal for cleansing the blood.[65] A tea substitute has been made from it in Fermanagh, but whether that was a medicinal use in unclear.[66]

Pimpinella saxifraga Linnaeus
burnet-saxifrage
Europe; introduced into North America

Although the acrid root of *Pimpinella saxifraga* once had the reputation, when chewed, of promoting the flow of saliva, causing it to be used for toothache and as a gargle, while its astringency made it popular for cleansing the skin of freckles, one assertion that these were long-established practices of 'country people'[67] (in England) is left no less ambiguous in other sources.[68] The only specific, allegedly folk record traced is from Aberdeenshire, where James Robertson in 1768 was told it was a cure for indigestion pains.[69] Most probably this was a legacy of learned medicine.

Sium latifolium Linnaeus
greater water-parsnip
temperate Europe

(Name confusion) 'Water parsnip' has been referred to *Sium latifolium* in one Irish list,[70] but clearly in error for hemlock water-dropwort (*Oenanthe crocata*), for which that has been in use as an alternative name.

Crithmum maritimum Linnaeus   PLATE 17
rock samphire
Atlantic and southern Europe, Black Sea, North Africa, Macaronesia

In Cornwall *Crithmum maritimum* was once 'thought to help digestion' when pickled.[71]

Oenanthe fistulosa Linnaeus
tubular water-dropwort
Europe, south-western Asia, north-western Africa

An infusion of the plant known to the informant as 'water fennel' has been recorded from Wicklow as a treatment for rheumatism.[72] That strictly speaking is the book name of the related species *Oenanthe fluviatilis* (Babington)

Coleman, which is, however, very rare in the county in question, where *O. fis-tulosa* on the other hand is locally common.

Oenanthe crocata Linnaeus
hemlock water-dropwort
south-western Europe, Morocco

There are numerous reports scattered throughout the medico-botanical literature of people mistaking the extremely poisonous *Oenanthe crocata* for wild celery or parsnips and dying within just an hour or two. In the west of the British Isles, where it is common, the local country people would normally have learned from childhood to leave it strictly alone; the fatalities have typically been of incomers unaware of the plant's identity and danger—for example, a group of French prisoners of war on parole in Pembrokeshire.[73] The poison resides in the dark, viscous resin and may act on the heart and nervous system simultaneously.

Unexpectedly, despite the seemingly total avoidance of deadly nightshade (*Atropa belladonna*), both *Oenanthe crocata* and the true hemlock (*Conium maculatum*) have been utilised in folk medicine, though presumably always with great caution and for external application only. Of the sole two records traced of the use of *O. crocata* outside Ireland, however, one dates from as far back as the early eighteenth century, when under the name 'five-fingered root' the plant is said to have been extensively employed for poulticing the severer kinds of 'felons'.[74] The other is from the Isle of Man, where it has been prized, apparently down to a more recent period, as a treatment for skin cancers.[75]

Oenanthe crocata, hemlock water-dropwort (Green 1902, fig. 266)

That Manx use has found fuller expression in Ireland, where only a plant of such virulence has apparently been rated an effective-enough weapon to deploy against tumours. As late as the 1840s it was still frequently used for those in Cork and other southern counties,[76] and if those were the 'external swellings' known under the name 'tahow', in Londonderry also.[77] The 'water parsnip' and 'water hemlock' reported more recently to have been applied in Ireland to scrofulous swellings in the neck[78] sound like this plant, too. It is probably also the 'water parsnip' that has been reckoned to cure boils in Cork.[79]

Foeniculum vulgare Miller
fennel
South Europe, North Africa; introduced into most temperate regions
(Folk credentials questionable) Well naturalised in parts of the British Isles, especially near coasts, *Foeniculum vulgare* may conceivably be native but is more probably wholly derived from cultivation. Only four records have been traced of its use in folk medicine, and that two of those also involve the cultivated sage strongly suggests that this has been a garden herb exclusively.

Silaum silaus (Linnaeus) Schinz & Thellung
pepper-saxifrage
northern and western Europe, western Siberia
'English saxifrage' (as he called it) 'our English women phisitians have in great use . . . against the stone', wrote John Gerard.[80] Half a century later, John Parkinson strengthened the claim of *Silaum silaus* as a folk herb by describing it as 'much used by country people' to help break and expel the stone, provoke urine and expel wind and colic as well as 'much given to sucking children for the frets, as women call it, which is winde in their bodies and stomackes.'[81] There are no localised records for it, however, nor any of more recent date in the folk literature. This rather suggests that herb women had taken it up from learned sources.

Meum athamanticum Jacquin
spignel, baldmoney
western and central Europe
Dubiously identified with a herb featured by Dioscorides, *Meum athamanticum* became familiar as 'meu' to apothecaries, among whom its aromatic and acrid roots had a reputation as a cure for flatulence. Latterly, the wild populations of the plant in the Pennines were raided, to the point of near-extinction, when snuff became fashionable and the roots were in demand for a scent for that.[82]

Hiding behind those herbalists' uses, however, may be some more purely folk ones. The curious alternative vernacular name which the species bears in Britain has been explained away as denoting that the plant was sacred to the god Balder, but in fact it appears to be a euphemism of the books for 'bawd-money', the version which seems to feature invariably in the folklore records. Could that be hinting at the use as an abortifacient for which 'Baudminnie' is said to have enjoyed a reputation in Galloway?[83] Disappointingly, other early Scottish records, from the Highlands[84] and Aberdeenshire,[85] respectively, are only of the chewing of the roots for flatulence; that the plant bore the name in the Highlands of 'micken',[86] however, may possibly be evidence that that use is an ancient one there, independent of the lore of the learned.

Conium maculatum Linnaeus   PLATE 18
hemlock
Europe, western and central Asia, North and East Africa, Canary
   Islands; introduced into North and South America, Australasia

Although most white umbelliferous plants are commonly miscalled 'hemlock' and in the south of Scotland that name has been applied especially to wild angelica (*Angelica sylvestris*) and hogweed (*Heracleum sphondylium*), the true plant is sufficiently distinctive by reason of its spotted stems to be readily recognisable by anyone interested in applying it medicinally. It seems safe to assume that specialists in herbal treatments, however unlettered, were normally sure of its identity, whatever the misnomers perpetrated by the uninformed. However, an extra layer of uncertainty is caused by the greater prevalence in the west of the British Isles of the even more poisonous *Oenanthe crocata*, which though quite different in appearance has 'hemlock' in its vernacular names and has had similar medical applications. The plant recorded under that name in the Aran Islands as used for poulticing what was either scrofula or abscesses has been referred to *Conium maculatum* without question,[87] yet botanists have noted that species there only once and the record is much more likely to belong to *O. crocata*, therefore.

The true hemlock is known as a macrofossil from Roman sites in Wales, and that fact taken together with its well-known use in Classical medicine and presence in the Anglo-Saxon herbals suggest that it has had many centuries to infiltrate any older, indigenous tradition of its use that may have existed here. Much of its distribution as a wild plant in the British Isles today may indeed be a legacy of its cultivation for medicinal purposes. The situation, though, has been complicated by the trumpeting of hemlock juice as a cure for cancer in the mid-eighteenth century by the much-respected Viennese physician Anton Storck, which despite much scepticism in higher medical circles in Britain following ambiguous reports of its efficacy (suspected by William Withering to have resulted at least in part from using the wrong plant[88]) led to some percolating of the remedy downwards. Though the orthodox treatment took the form of swallowing pills made from a decoction of the leaves, a blacksmith in Cornwall is on record as having believed he had cured himself of a cancer by drinking immense quantities just of the juice over a period of three years.[89] The normal practice in folk medicine, however, seems to have been the less daring one of poulticing external cancers with the leaves (as in Suffolk[90] and Angus[91]), which was merely a version of the hemlock poultice in widespread use for sores and swelling more generally (as in Cambridgeshire,[92] Berwickshire[93] and the Isle of Man[94]). In the Isle of Man[95] and the Highlands,[96] though, cases of a drastic and much more painful alternative are known that involved extracting a tumour by its roots by means of a plaster—provided that was done at an early stage. It was no doubt the plant's particular virulence that also caused it to be combined with pennyroyal (*Mentha pulegium*) and rue (the wholly cultivated *Ruta graveolens* Linnaeus) in a pill given at one time in the Cambridgeshire Fens for the purpose of inducing abortions.[97]

In Ireland, on the other hand, though hemlock poultices have been similarly in widespread use, especially in the north of the country,[98] for treating swellings and bad sores of all kinds, no records have been traced of their being applied to cancers. They have, however, been valued there additionally for rheumatism (Wicklow[99]), burns (Kilkenny,[100] Limerick[101]) and—unless 'hemlock' in this case refers to hogweed—wounds.[102] Quite unrelated to any of the foregoing, though, has been the reputation the plant has enjoyed in certain (unspecified) parts of Ireland as a means of curing giddiness.[103]

Apium graveolens Linnaeus
wild celery, smallage
central and southern Europe, southern Asia, North and South Africa,
    South America; introduced into other temperate regions

In Ireland the exceptional quantity in which the mainly scarce *Apium graveolens* of coastal marshes occurs in Co. Dublin has earned it a particularly wide and various use in that county as a medicine: above all for 'felons' and rashes,[104] but also for rheumatism,[105] boils[106] and for cleansing the blood of impurities.[107] It has also been favoured for rheumatism in Wicklow[108] next door. Similarly, its presence round the Shannon mouth has allowed it to be utilised in Limerick, too, for poulticing boils and abscesses.[109] Someone in Wicklow who valued it for kidney trouble,[110] though, may have learned of the diuretic property for which the related *A. nodiflorum* (Linnaeus) Lagasca (fool's water-cress, marshwort) has been exploited in Italy.

The only British records traced are from Devon, where a healer reputedly cured bad burns and infected breasts with a decoction of the plant applied as a plaster,[111] and from Essex, where a tea or decoction of the fruits or an infusion has been drunk for rheumatism.[112]

Petroselinum segetum (Linnaeus) Koch
corn parsley, honewort
western and southern Europe, Asia Minor, North Africa, Canary Islands
A maidservant observed c. 1620 by John Goodyer gathering *Petroselinum segetum* in a field in Hampshire told him she had learned during her upbringing in the Isle of Wight of its effectiveness in treating a chronic swelling on the cheek then known as a 'hone'. A handful of the pounded leaves was put in half a pint or more of beer, which was then strained and drunk for two weeks after fasting.[113] This is the only known record.

Ligusticum scoticum Linnaeus
lovage
northern Europe, eastern North America
A speciality of the Western Isles of Scotland, *sionnas* or *shunnis* in Gaelic, *Ligusticum scoticum* was once much valued there especially for diseases of cattle and sheep. Eaten raw first thing in the morning, it was also believed to preserve a person from infection for the rest of the day[114]; the root was reckoned good for flatulence[115] and the plant had a reputation (like celery) as an aphrodisiac.[116] On Lingay in the Outer Hebrides it was boiled with Alexanders (*Smyrnium olusatrum*) in a lamb broth and drunk 'against consumptions'.[117] In the Faeroe Islands it had a further use as a sedative,[118] but of that no Scottish record has been traced.

Angelica sylvestris Linnaeus
wild angelica
Europe, northern and south-western Asia; introduced into Canada
Less rich in active properties than garden angelica (*Angelica archangelica* Linnaeus), the common native counterpart, *A. sylvestris,* may have served as a poor man's stand-in for that. Considering how strongly garden angelica was recommended in the herbals and official medicine, however, folk records for

the wild plant are surprisingly few, yet surprisingly various: for lung and chest complaints in Londonderry,[119] for rheumatism[120] and corns[121] in Norfolk and as a spring tonic (under the name 'horse pepper') in Suffolk.[122] But was it really so neglected in the north and west or has its presence in the records from there lay hidden behind unidentified names?

Peucedanum ostruthium (Linnaeus) Koch
masterwort
central and southern Europe; introduced into temperate regions
(Folk credentials questionable) Though undoubtedly a relic of deliberate introduction (from southern Europe), *Peucedanum ostruthium* has been around so long—its seeds have been detected in a rath in an excavated ringfort in Antrim dated about A.D. 850–950—and under the name felon-grass it has achieved such a wide presence in hill farms, more especially in the Pennines, that it should not pass entirely without notice. Mainly a veterinary herb, its bitter acrid juice has been prized by country people in Kent (?) for toothache.[123] In the Isle of Man it shared with ribwort plantain (*Plantago lanceolata*) the name *slan lus*, 'healing plant'.[124]

Heracleum sphondylium Linnaeus
hogweed
Europe, western and northern Asia, north-western Africa; introduced
into North America, New Zealand
Though often called 'wild parsnip' (a name shared with elecampane, *Inula helenium*, and restricted by botanists to *Pastinaca sativa* Linnaeus) and, more vaguely, 'hemlock', *Heracleum sphondylium* can safely be accepted as correctly identified in the folk records by virtue of bearing a name special to itself both in Irish Gaelic and Manx. In the Isle of Man, where it is common (at any rate today), the seeds and roots have been boiled and the liquid drunk for jaundice and other liver troubles.[125] In Norfolk, on the other hand, hogweed juice has featured as a wart cure,[126] while in Mull, in the Inner Hebrides, James Robertson in 1768 found the tender shoots, stripped of their outer skin, enjoyed a reputation as a digestive.[127]

That this is the 'wild hemlock' whose pollen has been used in Essex[128] like puffball spores to staunch cuts slow to stop bleeding is seemingly confirmed by a record of that same use in Tipperary (under the plant's Gaelic name).[129] The only other Irish record traced, however, is a vague one from Westmeath: the drinking of a preparation of the plant for some unidentified sickness.[130]

Daucus carota Linnaeus
wild carrot
Eurasia, North Africa; introduced into most other temperate and
  many tropical regions

Contrary to what one might expect, the folk records on the whole carefully
distinguish wild *Daucus carota* from the cultivated plants in this particular
instance. This may be because the wild plant has been found to be the more
efficacious for some ailments at least. The majority of uses reported show
that it has been valued pre-eminently as a diuretic, for treating dropsy, gravel
or kidney complaints (Dorset,[131] Somerset,[132] Berwickshire[133]). As it was the
fruitlets that were usually employed to that end (though a decoction of its
rootstock was an alternative), that was presumably the unspecified function
they have performed 'medicinally' in the Isle of Man as well.[134] More localised
has been the making of a poultice from the mashed and boiled rootstocks
for applying to wounds and malignant, especially cancerous sores: in Britain
apparently confined to the Highlands,[135] where, mixed with oatmeal, it has
been a favourite remedy for 'lung disease', too.[136] In Dorset, on the other
hand, a traditional treatment for a burn has been to douche that in cold water
first to stop the pain and then apply scrapings from the rootstock to prevent
a blister forming and hasten the healing process.[137]

Irish records for the diuretic uses come from Co. Dublin,[138] Cork[139] and
Kerry,[140] while the carrot poultice just described has been applied to sores
and wounds in Antrim,[141] and in cases of earache in some part(s) of the
country left unspecified.[142]

Notes

1. Newman & Wilson
2. Tongue
3. Johnston 1853
4. Hole, 207
5. Johnston 1853
6. Simpkins, 411
7. McNeill
8. Hatfield MS
9. Lightfoot, 1094; Beith
10. Lafont
11. Vickery MSS
12. Lafont
13. Gibbs, 57
14. *Notes and Queries*, ser. 1, 7 (1853), 128
15. Maloney
16. IFC S 751: 118
17. McClafferty
18. IFC S 505: 148
19. IFC S 932: 239; 960: 211, 283
20. IFC S 1099: 224
21. IFC S 226: 484
22. IFC S 690: 41, 114
23. IFC S 920: 79

24. IFC S 1099: 224
25. IFC S 825: 72
26. IFC S 654: 244; 655: 268
27. IFC S 191: 90
28. IFC S 571: 357
29. Logan, 81
30. Barbour
31. IFC S 920: 70
32. IFC S 476: 460
33. Logan, 81
34. IFC S 898: 82
35. IFC S 510: 95
36. IFC S 250: 273
37. Maloney
38. IFC S 504: 18, 133
39. Beddington & Christy, 22
40. Jobson 1967, 59
41. Simpkins, 411
42. Humphries & Hopwood, 317
43. IFC S 483: 329, 369
44. Grant, 313; Beith
45. MacFarlane
46. Quayle, 70
47. Moore MS
48. Hart 1898, 387
49. *Essex Naturalist*, 1 (1887), 30–3
50. Ó Síocháin
51. Garrad 1985, 44
52. Fargher
53. Gloucestershire Record Office, MS P218.MI.1
54. Fargher
55. Goodrich-Freer, 206
56. Maloney
57. IFC S 747: 386
58. IFC S 530: 192
58a. *PLNN*, no. 77 (2003), 378
59. Quelch, 200
60. Barnes, 71
61. Martin, 145
62. Garrad 1985
63. Moore 1898
64. Fargher
65. IFC S 1098: 138

66. Glassie, 308
67. Pratt 1850–7
68. e.g. Withering 1787–92, 184
69. Henderson & Dickson, 155, 166
70. Moloney
71. Borlase 1758, 232
72. McClafferty
73. Watson 1746, 228
74. Watson 1746, 228
75. Fargher
76. Pickells
77. Moore MS
78. Moloney
79. IFC S 385: 80
80. Gerard, 890
81. Parkinson, 908
82. Edmondson
83. Mactaggart, 50
84. Lightfoot, 1095
85. Henderson & Dickson, 155, 166
86. Lightfoot, 1095
87. Ó hEithir; IFC S 1: 196
88. Withering 1787–92, 161–3
89. Polwhele 1816, 76
90. Taylor MS (Hatfield, 24)
91. Gardiner
92. Porter 1974, 43
93. Johnston 1853
94. Fargher
95. Gill, 188
96. Carmichael, ii, 257, 266; iv, 201
97. Porter 1969, 11
98. Moore MS; Hart, 378; Maloney; Foster 1951, 61; etc.
99. IFC S 920: 73
100. IFC S 849: 319
101. IFC S 484: 92
102. Ó Súilleabháin, 311
103. Barbour
104. IFC S 787: 53, 102, etc.
105. IFC S 787: 279
106. IFC S 787: 283, 364
107. IFC S 786: 204
108. McClafferty

109. IFC S 523: 130, 133, 166
110. McClafferty
111. Lafont, 83
112. Newman & Wilson
113. Johnson 1633, 1018; Gunther, 53
114. Dillenius, 114
115. Martin, 226; Lightfoot, 160
116. Beith
117. Martin, 145
118. Svabo
119. Moore MS
120. Hatfield, 46
121. Hatfield MS
122. Hatfield, 56
123. Pratt 1850–7
124. Kermode MS
125. Fargher
126. Taylor MS (Hatfield, 57)
127. Henderson & Dickson, 80
128. Hatfield MS
129. IFC S 550: 272
130. IFC S 746: 456
131. *Phytologist*, 3 (1848), 264
132. Falconer
133. Johnston 1853
134. Paton
135. Pennant 1776, ii, 42
136. Beith
137. Vickery 1995
138. IFC S 794: 36
139. IFC S 385: 55
140. IFC S 476: 91
141. Vickery MSS
142. Wilson

CHAPTER 11

Gentians and Nightshades

Dicotyledonous flowering plants in the orders (and families) Gentianales (Gentianaceae, gentians; Apocynaceae, periwinkles) and Solanales (Solanaceae, nightshades; Convolvulaceae, bindweeds; Cuscutaceae, dodders; Menyanthaceae, bogbeans) are included in this chapter.

GENTIANACEAE

Centaurium erythraea Rafn

C. umbellatum of authors, *C. minus* of authors

centaury

Europe, western Asia, North Africa, Azores; introduced into North
   America, Australasia

Less liable to upset the digestion than most vegetable bitters and so a preferable alternative to 'gentian' (under which name, or as 'red gentian', it has passed in some areas), *Centaurium erythraea* has been recorded very widely in the British Isles for use as a tonic. Like most tonics it has sometimes been prized for 'cleansing the blood' (hence the name bloodwort recorded for it in Shropshire[1]) or 'strengthening the nerves' (in the Isle of Scilly[2] and in South Uist in the Outer Hebrides[3]), while in the Highlands it has had the special role of promoting appetite in tubercular patients.[4]

   Centaury has also enjoyed some subsidiary popularity as an indigestion remedy (Yorkshire,[5] Lancashire,[6] Cumberland,[7] the Highlands[8]) and as a cure for biliousness (Isle of Man[9]). In Cardiganshire,[10] on the other hand, it has been used for kidney trouble, and in the Highlands[11] and Outer Hebrides[12] for colic. That heavy emphasis overall on righting and stimulating the system seems sharply at variance with a lingering reputation in the Outer Hebrides[13] for also staunching haemorrhages; but the plant was recommended as a wound healer by Classical writers, and a large quantity of its charred remains has been excavated from a Roman army hospital on the Rhine.[14]

Irish departures from service as a tonic are fewer by comparison. Louth[15] completes a predominantly Irish Sea focus of centaury's use for indigestion, 'Ulster'[16] has known it as a cough remedy, while in Wicklow[17] it has been rated excellent for the liver (perhaps the biliousness for which it has been valued by the Manx, in whose language it had a name translating as 'jaundice herb'[18]).

Gentianella campestris (Linnaeus)
Boerner
field gentian
northern and western Europe

Just as centaury stood in for 'gentian' (normally the eastern European species *Gentiana lutea* Linnaeus) in British Isles folk medicine, so in areas where centaury is absent the most widespread of the native *Gentianella* species, *G. campestris*, which tolerates colder climates, stood in for that in turn, its properties being very similar. Thus in Orkney, where it is common, it had a threefold value as a tonic, a remedy for gravel and a cure for jaundice,[19] while in Shetland it was used for digestive complaints.[20] Up in the Pennines bordering Cumbria, where centaury does not penetrate above the valleys, field gentian has similarly served as a digestive as well as being drunk 'to kill germs'.[21]

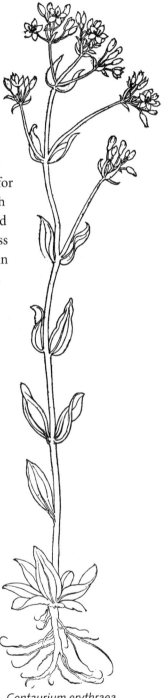

Centaurium erythraea,
centaury (Fuchs 1543, fig. 217)

APOCYNACEAE

Vinca major Linnaeus
greater periwinkle
southern Europe, North Africa;introduced into North America
and elsewhere

Vinca minor Linnaeus   PLATE 19
lesser periwinkle
Europe, western Asia; introduced into North America, Australasia
Alien plants which have run into the wilds from gardens and become well
naturalised in places, *Vinca major* and *V. minor* have acquired uses in folk
medicine to an extent that implies a lengthy history. Discovered in more recent
years to contain beneficial alkaloids, not only were they much recommended
in the herbals but in the hills of western Dorset they have acquired a name, 'St
Candida's Eyes', associating them with a medieval healer of local fame.[22]

A more widespread name, cutfinger, proclaims the healing properties
contained in the leaves, which when crushed or infused or included in an
ointment have been applied to minor cuts and sores of various kinds in
Devon,[23] Oxfordshire,[24] Cambridgeshire[25] and Lincolnshire,[26] to bruises and
persistent skin irritations in the Highlands,[27] to boils in Oxfordshire[28] and to
nosebleeds there, too, and in Devon.[29] The leaves also have a sedative effect
when chewed or otherwise consumed, making them valued in Devon for
nervous disorders, hysteria and to sufferers from nightmares[30] and for
toothache in Oxfordshire.[31] The roots, too, have been brought to bear on
colic in the Cambridgeshire Fens.[32] More esoterically, periwinkles even had
a reputation for keeping away cramp: in Somerset a decoction of the stems
was drunk to that end,[33] in Lincolnshire a piece of the plant was inserted
between the bedclothes and the mattress,[34] while in Devon the method was
to wind the stem around any part of the body.[35]

SOLANACEAE

Lycium barbarum Linnaeus
   L. halimifolium Miller
   Duke of Argyll's teaplant
   south-eastern Europe, western Asia; introduced into other
      temperate regions
There is a record from Warwickshire[36] of the stems of the sometimes natu-
ralised garden escape *Lycium barbarum* being used, as an alternative to those

of elder (*Sambucus nigra*), for the necklace placed round infants' necks when teething (for more on which see under henbane, *Hyoscyamus niger*).

Atropa belladonna Linnaeus
deadly nightshade
central and southern Europe, western Asia, North Africa;
    introduced into North America, New Zealand

(Name confusion suspected) The handful of records for folk uses allegedly of *Atropa belladonna* almost certainly belong to *Solanum dulcamara,* which so generally and confusingly shares its name among the non-botanical. The total lack of any convincing ones for the plant truly so called, by no means rare in the chalky areas of England, suggests that its notoriously ultra-poisonous character (three berries are sufficient to kill a child) firmly excluded it from the folk repertory. Though other poisonous species such as hemlock (*Conium maculatum*) were harnessed to some extent for healing purposes, this one alone would seem to have been accepted as prohibitively dangerous to handle or experiment with.

Hyoscyamus niger Linnaeus   PLATE 20
henbane
Europe, western Asia, North Africa; introduced into North America,
    Australasia

A mostly scarce plant of usually fleeting appearances after long periods of dormancy, *Hyoscyamus niger* has often been dismissed as wholly a relic in the British Isles of its past herbal use; but a good case can be made for considering it native on beaches, one of quite a number of species adapted to that open habitat as 'strand casuals'. 'Experience has shown that the wild seaside herb ... is more effective than the product of cultivation',[37] so it may even be distinct genetically. As one of the most ancient of herbs, traceable back in written records to the Babylonians and in prehistoric levels in Britain to the Early Neolithic, it is likely to have been prized in antiquity so highly as to form an exception to the general rule that in order to be utilised by humans a plant had to be plentiful, at least locally.

    Containing alkaloids which have a hypnotic as well as sedative effect, henbane's place in medicine was probably long subordinate to its value as a hallucinogen taken to induce trances and visions; though an archaeological find in Fife has been interpreted as indicative of that, conclusive evidence of such a use in Britain or Ireland is lacking.[38] The plant's name in Welsh has been interpreted as signifying an ability to prevent or cure faintness,[39] and a preparation once used in that country is said to have had a reputation for curing any mental trouble.[40] But the main function in folk medicine at least in more recent centuries has evidently been as a painkiller: relieving the pain of inflamed wounds and stomach-ache in Sussex,[41] but there and elsewhere (Kent (?),[42] Hertfordshire,[43] Norfolk[44]) toothache, too. A special practice in this last connection was the stringing of a necklace of beads cut from a henbane root round the neck of a teething infant. Though the only records traced of that are from Devon[45] and Sussex,[46] the dried berries of 'nightshade' have been used for the same purpose in Norfolk,[47] and other plants such as elder in Warwickshire and Gloucestershire have been drawn on for these necklaces, too; 'Verona root', made from imported orris (*Iris×germanica* Linnaeus or allied taxa), was even sold for them by herbalists, ready-made, at one period. What were regarded as the most potent parts of these plants and certain other members of the Solanaceae had the reputation of giving off fumes with a sedative effect. It was because of that effect that henbane was also given to women in childbirth, to bring relief in the form of 'twilight sleep', a practice on record from Wiltshire[48] but probably quite widespread.

It may have been primarily for this last reason that an infusion of the leaves has been given to children with whooping cough in Cavan, the county from which the only other Irish use traced, the drinking of the juice 'for the nerves', has been recorded as well.[49]

Solanum dulcamara Linnaeus
bittersweet, woody nightshade
Eurasia, North Africa; introduced into North America,
    New Zealand

Solanum dulcamara shares with other members of the Solanaceae alkaloids which affect the nervous system to a potentially dangerous degree, but instead of being used like henbane (*Hyoscyamus niger*) to treat mental disorders, its function in folk medicine in that particular direction appears to have been restricted to serving as a sedative to counter sleeplessness, as implied by one of its Gaelic names in Ireland[50] (and actually recorded as a use from Cavan[51]). In common with periwinkles (*Vinca*), the plant has a mildly narcotic property, and at one time in Cumberland schoolboys kept a stock of the twigs in their pockets and copied the tobacco chewing of their elders.[52]

The main use of this common plant, though, was for fingers inflamed by the cold. 'Divers countrie people doe use the berries bruised and laid to the finger that hath a felon thereon to cure it', wrote John Parkinson in the seventeenth century,[53] and in several English counties 'felon-wort' and 'felon-wood', names it shares with masterwort (*Peucedanum ostruthium*), have persisted in currency down to more recent years. In Essex,[54] Warwickshire[55] and Oxfordshire[56] the juice was mixed with lard to produce an ointment valued for chilblains—an allied complaint.

In Ireland a herb recorded in Limerick as 'guinea goul' and clearly this from the description has been used for cuts that have festered.[57] In the Isle of Man a decoction made from bittersweet was said to be effective in healing inward bruises[58]; boiled in a pint of beer, the plant has also enjoyed a reputation there as a strengthening tonic.[59] Each of these uses could be ascribed to its claimed ability to cleanse the system of impurities (hence its popularity in official medicine for skin diseases, rheumatism and gout), but how is its use in Kerry[60] for inducing blistering to be explained?

Datura stramonium Linnaeus   PLATE 21
thorn-apple
near-cosmopolitan weed

Like henbane (*Hyoscyamus niger*), *Datura stramonium* also appears unexpectedly after lying long dormant, especially in hot summers, and is no less dangerous for its violent action on the nervous system; it differs, though, in having no claim to be considered indigenous to the British Isles. It seems in fact to have been introduced from the East and reputedly owes much of its European dispersal to gypsies. The name *Datura* is of Sanskrit origin, and related species are popular in India as intoxicants.

Probably because East Anglia experiences the hottest temperatures in Britain it is from there that almost all the few records of the plant's use in folk medicine have come. The most interesting of these is an ointment made from boiling the juice in pork fat which was applied by a village herb woman in Norfolk c. 1920 to burns, scalds and inflammation in general[61]—exactly the same recipe as for a cure recommended more than three centuries earlier by John Gerard, who instanced the perfect healing it had achieved of a serious lightning burn suffered by a merchant's wife at Colchester in Essex.[62] It is also in Essex that the soporific fumes given off by the plant's juice (like that of henbane) have been harnessed as a pain-reliever, with vinegar added to make doubly sure.[63] Norfolk, too, is one county where the practice of smoking the dried leaves (or seeds) to relieve asthma, introduced into Britain by General Gent in 1802 and formerly widespread, has persisted at the folk level down to the twentieth century.[64]

CONVOLVULACEAE

Calystegia soldanella (Linnaeus) R. Brown
sea bindweed
coasts of west and southern Europe, Asia, North Africa, North and
  South America, Australasia

On the coasts of Sussex,[65] Hampshire[66] and the Isle of Wight,[67] *Calystegia soldanella* was known as scurvy-grass and either supplemented or stood in for *Cochlearia officinalis* in countering that once-common ailment. According to another author, 'the inhabitants of our coasts' (which from the context appears to refer to those of Norfolk) used to gather the young shoots and pickle these for employment as a gentle purge.[68]

Calystegia sepium (Linnaeus) R. Brown
hedge bindweed
Europe, western Asia, North Africa, North America, Australasia

The acrid roots of *Calystegia sepium* are much more violently purgative than those of *C. soldanella,* but despite their drastic action their use for that purpose in parts of the British Isles was for long not wholly displaced in remoter areas by its preferred relation, scammony (*C. scammonia* Linnaeus), imported from the Levant. In Northamptonshire 'the poor people' were still boiling the roots in ale as a purge as late as the 1830s.[69] However, the failure of folklore collectors to pick up mentions of that use of the plant and that it featured in herbals back to Dioscorides suggest that it originated in the written tradition.

There are nevertheless two records that seem likely to have had more spontaneous sources. One is as a wart cure in Leicestershire,[70] the other as a remedy for kidney trouble in Fermanagh—if it is indeed the plant known locally in the latter county as 'the tormentor' ('because it spreads its grip and chokes the plant').[71] In either case the species in question could equally well be the field bindweed, *Convolvulus arvensis* Linnaeus, which is known to be powerfully purgative, too, while the Fermanagh record might also belong to black-bindweed, *Fallopia convolvulus* (Linnaeus) A. Löve.

CUSCUTACEAE

Cuscuta europaea Linnaeus
greater dodder
Europe, western Asia, North Africa; introduced into North America,
  New Zealand

(Misinterpreted statement) A statement by Matthias de l'Obel,[72] that he had seen this species growing abundantly in Somerset and that it was effective as a diuretic, was misread by John Parkinson[73] as implying that that herbal use was a speciality of the region.

Cuscuta epithymum (Linnaeus) Linnaeus
dodder

Europe, western Asia; introduced into North America, South Africa, Australasia

'Hairweed', a name recorded for *Cuscuta epithymum* in three of the Eastern Counties of England, was added to nettle tea in the Fens of East Anglia and given to children whenever their mother detected signs of scurvy between their fingers.[74] The plant was recommended in herbals as a purge for 'ague' and the intention may have been to cleanse the system of the impurities suspected of being responsible.

MENYANTHACEAE

Menyanthes trifoliata Linnaeus
bogbean, *báchrán*

Europe, northern and central Asia, Morocco, North America

Wherever *Menyanthes trifoliata* occurs in any quantity, mainly in the boggy regions of the north and west of the British Isles, it has constituted one of the staples of the folk repertory and in some parts has been the most prized herb of all. Its intense bitterness has led it to be used as a substitute for hops in brewing or for adulterating beer, and it was probably in that connection that large quantities of the plant's pressed leaves and stems found round some of the ancient Irish raths are thought to have been deposited.[75] Whether or not that interpretation is correct, it is highly likely that bogbean was in favour for medicine as well at the same period.

Except in Wales the plant has predominantly served in Britain as a tonic, like the various imported bitters that have largely replaced it, while in the course of revitalising the system also resolving digestive problems (Cumbria,[76] Berwickshire,[77] Shetland,[78] Isle of Man[79]). As an 'astringent' it has banished headaches in the Outer Hebrides[80] and stopped loose bowels in Colonsay in the Inner Hebrides[81] and the Highlands,[82] while in the last[83] and in Shetland[84] to the north it has been rated a cure for jaundice—so much so in Shetland that it bore a name there from the Old Norse word for that affliction.[85]

A second cluster of ailments for which bogbean has been widely used is rheumatism and the like. Though Scottish records for that seem to be lacking and English ones limited—Sussex,[86] Kent (?),[87] Hertfordshire[88] and, as one of five ingredients in a mixture, the East Riding of Yorkshire[89]—in Wales it has been recorded from at least six of its counties[90] with a marked peak in Denbighshire,[91] and that total would rise to nine if one could be sure that by 'backache' people meant this, too. Confusingly, though, 'backache' is sometimes a synonym of kidney trouble—which is bogbean's other principal application in Wales, known from five counties there but apparently nowhere else in Britain.[92]

As it 'helps to open up the tubes', bogbean has been a natural choice in Lewis in the Outer Hebrides for asthma[93] and elsewhere in Scotland for persistent coughs (Argyllshire[94]) and pulmonary tuberculosis (the Highlands[95]), while in the nearby Isle of Man it has been favoured for fevers.[96] More exclu-

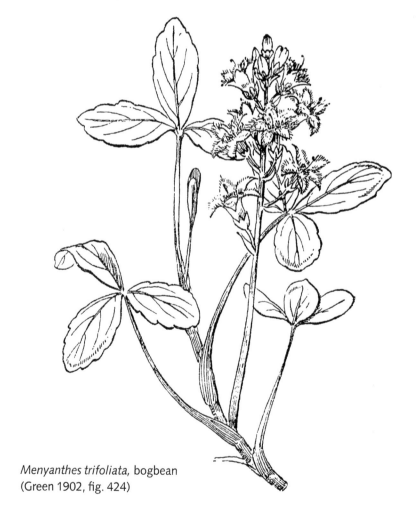

Menyanthes trifoliata, bogbean
(Green 1902, fig. 424)

sively Scottish has been the use of a decoction of the root for easing the pain of a stomach ulcer in the Highlands,[97] the plant's application as a poultice to the sores of scrofula in Orkney[98] and to those caused on the necks of fishermen in the Highlands by the friction of nets and ropes,[99] and a conviction in Lewis that the ribbed side of the leaf was good for drawing pus from a septic wound and the smooth side for healing it[100] (a property elsewhere ascribed to the leaves of other species, in particular, plantains).

The Irish pattern is broadly similar. Records of the use of bogbean, though, come largely from Ulster, showing a marked concentration in Donegal,[101] where in one area every household used to collect the roots in spring, 'when the blood gets out of order', and boil them with treacle and sulphur[102]; and as in Britain that reputation for cleansing the system has extended to the clearing up of boils and skin troubles (Londonderry,[103] Donegal,[104] Louth,[105] Clare,[106] Limerick[107]) and assisting the digestion (Antrim,[108] Louth[109]). Similarly, as an 'astringent' it has been valued for stomach upsets (Leitrim,[110] Roscommon,[111] Kerry[112]) though held to have the reverse effect in Tyrone[113] by *ending* constipation, while in Clare[114] and Cork[115] it is not clear in what way it assisted 'liver trouble' or how it cured jaundice in Wicklow.[116] One difference from England and especially Scotland, on the other hand, has been the wide valuing of bogbean juice for rheumatism and allied afflictions, the Irish records for which match the Welsh ones in the number of counties from which they have been traced—with an Ulster-tilted distribution in this case, too. More extremely, Ireland has a wider scatter of records than Wales of use for kidney trouble (Cavan,[117] Monaghan,[118] Clare,[119] Limerick,[120] Cork[121]) just as it greatly outstrips England and Wales in the extent to which the plant has been applied to the heavier kinds of coughs and colds (Donegal,[122] Cavan,[123] Louth,[124] Sligo,[125] Mayo[126]). But in heart disease (Mayo[127]) and its relation, dropsy (Louth[128]), Ireland's seeming lead is but a bare one.

Notes

1. Britten & Holland
2. Vickery 1995
3. Shaw, 50
4. Beith
5. Barbour
6. Taylor 1901, unpag.
7. Hodgson, 209
8. Beith

9. Moore 1898; Fargher
10. Williams MS
11. Grant
12. McDonald, 239; Carmichael, vi, 123
13. McDonald, 239; Carmichael, vi, 123
14. Majno
15. IFC S 657: 217, 248
16. Purdon

17. McClafferty
18. Moore 1898; Fargher
19. Spence
20. Jamieson
21. Duncan & Robson, 65
22. Duddridge
23. Baker, 52
24. Britten & Holland, 139
25. Porter 1969, 87; 1974, 46
26. Woodruffe-Peacock
27. Beith
28. Britten & Holland, 139; 'E.C.'
29. Lafont
30. Lafont
31. Baker, 52
32. Porter 1969, 79
33. Tongue
34. Woodruffe-Peacock; Rudkin, 202
35. Lafont
36. Bloom, 26
37. White, 444
38. Sherratt; Long et al.
39. Cameron
40. Trevelyan
41. A. Allen, 83
42. Pratt 1850–7
43. Ellis, 209
44. Wigby, 65
45. Wright, 248
46. A. Allen, 83
47. Taylor 1929, 127
48. Whitlock 1992, 109
49. Maloney
50. Moloney
51. Maloney
52. Hodgson, 222
53. Parkinson, 350
54. Hatfield, 27
55. Bloom, 25
56. 'E.C.'
57. IFC S 505: 117
58. Moore 1898
59. Fargher
60. IFC S 412: 98

61. Wigby, 65; Hatfield, 23
62. Gerard, 278
63. Hatfield, 40
64. Hatfield MS
65. Johnson 1633, 839
66. Johnson 1633, 839
67. Townsend, 218
68. Bryant, 63
69. Anon. (c. 1830), i, 60
70. Palmer 1985, 72
71. Glassie, 308
72. de l'Obel, 233
73. Parkinson, 11
74. Randell, 84
75. Sullivan, ccclxxiv
76. Wright, 239
77. Johnston 1829–31, i, 56
78. Jamieson
79. Quayle, 69
80. McDonald, 171; Shaw, 47
81. McNeill
82. Lightfoot, 1093; Hooker, 91; Grant
83. Beith
84. Beith
85. Tait
86. Arthur, 42
87. Pratt 1850–7
88. Ellis, 331
89. Vickery 1995
90. Vickery 1995; Williams MS
91. Williams MS
92. Williams MS
93. Beith
94. Fairweather
95. Beith; Murray, appendix, iv
96. Quayle, 69
97. Beith
98. Spence; Leask, 80
99. Beith
100. Beith
101. Hart 1898, 368; IFC S 1043: 71;
    1090: 282; 1098: 25, 130
102. McGlinchey, 84
103. Moore MS

104. IFC S 1121: 354
105. IFC S 657: 160
106. IFC S 617: 334
107. IFC S 484: 43
108. Vickery MSS
109. IFC S 657: 216
110. IFC S 190: 168, 176
111. IFC S 250: 273
112. IFC S 413: 227
113. *PLNN,* no. 11 (1990), 50
114. IFC S 617: 334
115. IFC S 385: 55
116. McClafferty

117. Maloney
118. IFC S 932: 239
119. IFC S 589: 62
120. IFC S 484: 41
121. IFC S 313: 213
122. IFC S 1090: 125
123. Maloney
124. IFC S 657: 216
125. IFC S 157: 254
126. IFC S 132: 98
127. IFC S 132: 37
128. IFC S 657: 216

CHAPTER 12

Comfrey, Vervain and Mints

Dicotyledonous flowering plants in the order Lamiales and families Boraginaceae (borages), Verbenaceae (vervains) and Lamiaceae (mints) are included in this chapter.

BORAGINACEAE

Lithospermum officinale Linnaeus
   common gromwell
   Europe, western Asia; introduced into North America
Identified with a herb recommended by Dioscorides as a cure for the stone, the hard-coated seeds of *Lithospermum officinale* became popular in that connection when plants supposed to reveal their utility through their form (the Doctrine of Signatures) were boosted in the herbals. There is a record of this use from the eastern Yorkshire moors dating from as late as 1897.[1]

In Ireland the plant was one of four herbs credited with that same virtue which went into a decoction drunk for gravel in several parts of the country half a century earlier.[2] While that, too, sounds like a legacy from written medicine, a record from Meath[3]—a region in which *Lithospermum officinale* was at one time locally abundant—of 'grumble seed', 'which grows along the Boyne River', being collected and boiled for kidney trouble may have more merit as a relic of the folk tradition.

A probable misidentification of this species as 'eyeseed' in Essex is discussed under wild clary (*Salvia verbenaca*).

Echium vulgare Linnaeus
viper's-bugloss
Europe, Asia Minor; introduced into North America, Australasia
An infusion of the leaves of *Echium vulgare* has been drunk in Somerset as a
cure for a headache.[4]

Pulmonaria officinalis Linnaeus   PLATE 22
lungwort
northern and central Europe, Caucasus; introduced into western
   Europe, North America
(Folk credentials questionable) Two members of the genus *Pulmonaria* are
accepted as native in England, but both are too limited in their range to have
been likely candidates for herbal use. That function has been served by the
introduced *P. officinalis,* which is very widely grown in gardens and often
naturalised on banks and in woods. Commonly dismissed as merely another
of the plants supposed to reveal their utility through their form (the Doctrine
of Signatures), the spots on its leaves supposedly having prompted its application to spots on the lungs, the plant does in fact contain active principles
which are claimed in alternative medicine circles to be genuinely beneficial
for respiratory complaints. Folk records of its use for pulmonary tuberculosis in Hampshire[5] and Norfolk[6] may thus not be the products of credulity, as
usually imagined—though the sources in these cases were more probably
cottage gardens than colonies of the plant growing wild. Alternatively, the
records may refer to the lichen *Lobaria pulmonaria,* which is sometimes called
'lungwort', too.

In Ireland, 'lungwort' was one of the names borne by mullein (*Verbascum thapsus*), to which Irish records can safely be referred.

Symphytum officinale Linnaeus
common comfrey
Europe, western Asia; introduced into North America, Australasia
Another of the chief stand-bys in the folk repertory, very widely known about
and still frequently used, *Symphytum officinale* is nevertheless a rarity, and
almost certainly not native, over most of the north and west of the British
Isles as well as in East Anglia. Two colour forms occur, one reddish, the other
white-flowered, each on the whole with different distributions. Populations
containing both are almost confined to the Thames Valley and to five of the
southernmost counties of England from Sussex to Devon.[7] Two of these, Sussex[8] and Dorset,[9] are also among the three counties (the third is Shropshire[10])

from which records have been traced of a presumably age-old belief that the reddish form must be used for healing men and the white one for healing women if success is to be assured (a gender distinction similar to that recorded for the two bryonies and several other 'paired' plants as well).

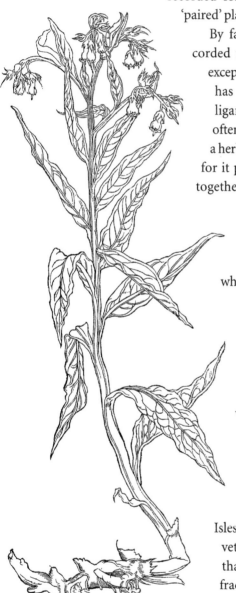

By far the commonest use of comfrey, recorded from most parts of the British Isles—except apparently the southern half of Wales—has been for treating injuries to limbs and ligaments, in particular, sprains (twice as often mentioned as fractures). Identified with a herb mentioned by Dioscorides, whose name for it passed into Latin as *Symphytum,* grow-together-plant, the plant is rich in allantoin, which promotes healing in connective tissues through the proliferation of new cells. Not for nothing was it widely known as 'knitbone', a name which still lingers on in places.

Various parts of the plant yield a strongly astringent oily juice, but for treating injuries the roots are most often preferred. The usual process is to clean, peel, pound or grate and boil these, in order to extract a thick paste which is then applied like plaster of Paris. Alternatively, the leaves and/or stem are heated and put on as a poultice. A third, much rarer method is to mix the juice with lard and rub the ointment in. Of 141 records traced from the British Isles as a whole for uses of comfrey for non-veterinary therapeutic purposes, no fewer than 60 are accounted for by sprains and fractures. But records for swellings of other kinds as well as for bruises and internal bleeding are perhaps logically combined with those, in which case 85, or well over half,

Symphytum officinale, common comfrey (Brunfels 1530, p. 76)

would fall into that category. The 56 records remaining can be classified for the most part into four broad groups: rheumatism and allied complaints (which the leaves have a reputation for relieving, though at the cost of large blisters); nasal and bronchial infections; boils; and wounds and cuts.

In Britain none of these four subsidiary categories of use seems to be on record from Scotland, where comfrey probably never grew wild in earlier times, though in the nearby Isle of Man a decoction of roots and stems has been drunk to get rid of phlegm[11] and the leaves bound on cuts to first draw foreign matter out and then heal them.[12] The English records traced for the application of the plant to colds and the like, however, are all from the southern half of the country (Devon,[13] Gloucestershire,[14] Norfolk[15]), though those for treating the rheumatism group (Devon,[16] Suffolk,[17] Caernarvonshire[18]) and for poulticing boils (Norfolk,[19] Shropshire,[20] Lancashire[21]) are more scattered, while the applying of an ointment made from the root to open wounds appears to be peculiarly East Anglian (Essex and Norfolk[22]). Apart from those, the only more minor use noted in Britain has been for leg ulcers (Norfolk,[23] Westmoreland[24]).

Ireland's speciality among the four subsidiary categories is applying the plant to wounds and cuts. Records have been picked up for that from seven counties there, all but two of them along the mid-western coast. The Irish records for treating colds and the like come from rather more counties than in England (Cavan,[25] Meath,[26] Sligo,[27] Wexford,[28] Kerry[29]) and the same is true of the poulticing of boils (Cavan,[30] Mayo,[31] Kilkenny,[32] Kerry[33]), but comfrey's use for rheumatism has been noted only from Sligo.[34] As so often, though, doubtless as a result of the more intensive investigation to which Ireland has been subjected, especially in the 1930s, that country has yielded a greater range of rare, minor applications: to toothache in Kilkenny,[35] kidney trouble in Tipperary[36] and warts and all manner of skin complaints in Limerick.[37] There is also an Irish record of the juice being rubbed into the face to improve the complexion[38]; like other astringent herbs this one had a role as a cosmetic as well, even if a tiny one apparently.

Symphytum tuberosum Linnaeus
tuberous comfrey
central and southern Europe, Asia Minor; introduced into North
America

There is a record of *Symphytum tuberosum* from Aberdeenshire, where *S. officinale* is much the scarcer of the two species, being valued for fractures, too.[39]

Anchusa arvensis (Linnaeus) M. Bieberstein
Lycopsis arvensis Linnaeus
bugloss
Europe, western Asia; introduced into North America
(Name confusion suspected) A herb described by Dioscorides under the name *Anchusa*, which means 'ox-tongue' in Greek, has been identified with various plants with rough and prickly leaves. The bugloss which occurs in light cultivated soils across much of the British Isles, *A. arvensis*, is a likely plant to have attracted herbal use, but the one or two records in the folk literature ascribed to that lack botanical authentication and could equally well belong to other species. In Ireland, the similar name *boglus* has also been applied too variously for any certainties.

Myosotis Linnaeus
forget-me-not
temperate regions of the northern and southern hemispheres
The name *Myosotis* in Latin translates as 'mouse-ear', a name which has generally been in herbal use for *Pilosella officinarum* (mouse-ear hawkweed), a favourite folk remedy for coughs. In view of that possible source of confusion and that only two records ascribed to a species of *Myosotis* have been traced in the folklore literature (Devon,[40] Kent[41]), and those both also of use for coughs (and other chest complaints in the former case), there must be some slight suspicion whether the identifications were correct. However, all the members of this genus are mucilaginous and astringent, like comfrey, and some at least have featured in official medicine, so the records can perhaps receive the benefit of the doubt.

Cynoglossum officinale Linnaeus
hound's-tongue
northern and central Europe, Asia; introduced into North America
Widespread in the south-eastern third of England, *Cynoglossum officinale* becomes essentially a maritime plant as it thins out northwards and westwards—as along the eastern coast of Ireland, where it is locally frequent. The one localised Irish record from within that range (Portrane, Co. Dublin[42]) seems likely to have involved the use of wild specimens; juice was rubbed on the arm rashes locally known as felons. Two other Irish records, however, are from counties in which the species is unknown outside gardens: in Monaghan it has been valued for coughs[43] and in Limerick its leaves have supplied a hot dressing for burns.[44] At one time it was also used in parts of Ireland by

'country herb-doctors' as a remedy for both external and internal cancers.[45] The plant certainly had a reputation in book medicine as a cure for skin troubles of various kinds, but a claim[46] that a name it has borne in Suffolk, 'scald-head', is a reference to that may be taking things too far.

VERBENACEAE

Verbena officinalis Linnaeus
vervain
Europe, western Asia, North Africa; introduced into North America, Australasia

For some unknown reason the not very conspicuous and rather scarce *Verbena officinalis* was credited with exceptional magico-religious potency, including as a divinatory, in parts of pre-Christian Europe. Belief in its powers seems to have survived into more recent times, especially strongly in Wales and the Isle of Man, leaving behind a legacy at least in the latter of ostensibly medicinal uses which are doubtless rooted in a reputation for countering adverse influences of all kinds. Some authors[47] have identified it as the plant known under the Manx name *yn lus*, 'the herb', but others hold that that correctly belongs to motherwort (*Leonurus cardiaca*), the 'gender twin' in the island of *V. officinalis* and known there as 'she-vervain'.[48]

There is nevertheless a sound phytochemical basis for some of the healing virtues attributed to vervain, for it contains a bitter principle, verbenaline, which has an action resembling that of quinine. For that reason the plant has been valued in the Isle of Man[49] for allaying fevers and in Gloucestershire[50] drunk as a strengthening tonic. A further internal use, also reported from Gloucestershire, has been as a vermifuge.[51] Probably more often, though, application has been external. 'Many country people', wrote John Quincy in 1718, 'pretend to get great feats with it in agues, by applying it to the wrist in the form of a cataplasm [i.e. plaster]; and also to cure gouty pains and swellings with it, used in the same manner.'[52] More recent such records are for wounds in Sussex,[53] sunburn in Norfolk[54] and as an eye lotion in Herefordshire.[55] Reportedly, the plant has also been used widely in England for sores.[56]

Ireland has produced the only certain mention (and that an unlocalised one[57]) of the wearing in a bag around the body of some portion of this plant as a remedy for scrofula, for which it was at one time held in particularly high repute; this may well have been the bag, though, that children were given to wear in Sussex to cure them of some unidentified sickness.[58] As vervain has no claim to be considered indigenous in Ireland, it is not surprising that only one other record of its use there has been traced: for allaying fever in Cavan.[59]

LAMIACEAE

Stachys officinalis (Linnaeus) Trevisan
   Betonica officinalis Linnaeus
   betony
   Europe, Caucasus, Algeria; introduced into North America

Like vervain, *Stachys officinalis,* too, seems to have owed much of its popularity as a medicinal herb to magico-religious associations underlying its use. It was early identified with a plant known to the Romans as *betonica* and described by Pliny the Elder as much in use by barbarian peoples as a nerve tonic and a cure for drunkenness and hangovers; no less questionably, a herb prominent in Anglo-Saxon lore was identified with it, too. To add to the confusion, another popular herb, common speedwell (*Veronica officinalis*), was known as *betonica Pauli* and, to judge from some of the purposes to which that species has been put according to the folk records, may have sometimes passed as betony as well. To the settlers in New England, betony on the other hand was a species of lousewort, *Pedicularis canadensis* Linnaeus, while in Ireland the name has been widely applied to bugle (*Ajuga reptans*).

Again like vervain, though, *Stachys officinalis* does possess some chemical potency: the roots are purgative and emetic, the leaves are reputed to act as an intoxicant, and alkaloids which the plant shares with yarrow give it the same wound-healing properties as that. Nevertheless, those virtues may not have been enough to warrant its being accorded such a high degree of reverence. Nor do they make it safe to assume that where 'betony' is mentioned in the folk records it is necessarily this species that is intended nor, for that matter, that it is the same plant in all cases. Those mentions all the same do show a reasonable consistency—and except for one ambiguous Irish one[60] are all from the southern half of Britain, the only part of the British Isles where *S. officinalis* is plentiful enough to have been able to meet any continuing herbal demand.

In only two counties (Wiltshire,[61] Sussex[62]) have records been traced of 'betony' in use for wounds. So highly was it valued in Sussex for this purpose, and even more for burns, that it gave rise to the saying there: 'Sell your coat and buy betony.'[63] Like other bitter 'astringents', though, the plant or plants bearing that name have principally served as a tonic, an infusion of the leaves being drunk as a tea. In Shropshire[64] that has been more specifically for purifying the blood, in Cumbria[65] for curing indigestion and in Somerset[66] for driving away a headache. Though household recipe books rank as folk records in the true sense only in part, a migraine remedy extracted c. 1800 from one in Cardiganshire is worthy of mention in that last connection: block the nostrils each day of the week with a mixture made from 'betony' leaves and primrose roots.[67] Finally, if it really was *Stachys officinalis* which existed in sufficient quantity in part of Kent for 'large bundles' to be hung up in cottages for winter use, the plant had a further use there as a drink for coughs and colds,[68] presumably because it cleared the nasal passages.

Stachys sylvatica Linnaeus
hedge woundwort
western and southern Europe, mountains of western and central
  Asia; introduced into North America, New Zealand

Stachys palustris Linnaeus
marsh woundwort
Europe, temperate Asia, North America; introduced into
  New Zealand

Stachys ×ambigua Smith
hybrid woundwort
'Woundwort' has probably always been applied interchangeably to both *Stachys sylvatica* and *S. palustris*, and to the hybrid between them, *S. ×ambigua*, as well. Though only botanists would normally be expected to distinguish hybrids, the one in this case occurs widely in some parts of Britain, especially the far north and west, in the absence of one or both parents even though it is normally—though by no means invariably—sterile. It is difficult to see how it could have attained an independent distribution which extends in the Hebrides to many remote parts without helping hands; elsewhere in the north of Scotland, for example, close observation does indeed leave the impression that in places it owes its origin to gardens instead of spontaneous crossing in the wild,[69] for noticeably more often than the parents it is found round houses and farmyards. Its presence in a cave in Rum has even led to the suggestion that it was introduced there and elsewhere in that region during the Bronze Age or later 'for medicinal or other purposes'.[70] The implication is that its hybrid character was recognised and that the plant was deliberately selected for propagation. That may have been for consumption as a vegetable—in the nineteenth century a Dr Joseph Houlton was awarded a medal

by the Society of Arts for demonstrating the palatability of the roots of *S. palustris*.[71] Hybrids that are more or less sterile tend to compensate for that with a greater profuseness in their vegetative parts than either parent species. Alternatively, or additionally, the plant may have been wanted as a medicine, in which case the belief may have been that the compensation for sterility was greater chemical potency.

It was presumably either the hybrid or *Stachys palustris* that was the 'all-heal' found by Martin Martin[72] in use in Lewis in the Outer Hebrides[150] as an ingredient in an ointment applied to green wounds. Wounds indeed appear always to have been the premier function of this herbal trio: the name borne by them collectively in Welsh translates as 'woundwort', it is the one use reported from the Highlands,[73] while John Gerard in his *Herball* cites a case from Kent that plainly counts as a folk one, too.[74] In places today the plants still continue to be prized for their remarkable healing power. The leaves have been used for poulticing boils and carbuncles in Essex and so bringing them to a head.[75]

In Ireland that reputation for curing wounds has similarly persisted here and there,[76] for example in Wicklow[77] and Galway.[78] The use of the leaves for dressed sores has also been reported from Westmeath.[79]

Ballota nigra Linnaeus
black horehound

Europe, south-western Asia, Morocco, Azores; introduced into
   North America, Australasia

In common with many other members of the mint family, *Ballota nigra* has had some use for colds, coughs, asthma and chest complaints. Except for Leicestershire[80]—where, puzzlingly, it was reportedly called 'lound's woundwort' (surely a corruption, or mishearing, of 'clown's woundwort', John Gerard's name for *Stachys palustris?*)—all the British records come from the Scottish Lowlands (Berwickshire,[81] Dumfriesshire,[82] Fife[83]), a distribution suggesting it has stood in there for some more warmth-demanding, less 'rough' alternative, perhaps white horehound (*Marrubium vulgare*). As *B. nigra* does not appear to occur in natural habitats anywhere in the British Isles except possibly the western Midlands (where it is represented by a distinct, woollier variety), its history as a folk herb is likely to have been a relatively short one, doubtless as a spill-over from book medicine.

The same remarks appertain to the only two Irish records traced (Londonderry,[84] Cavan[85]), for the same complaints as in Britain.

Leonurus cardiaca Linnaeus
motherwort
Europe; introduced into North America, New Zealand

A scarcely naturalised, cottage garden herb, reputedly introduced into Britain in the Middle Ages, *Leonurus cardiaca* features in folk medicine records apparently uniquely in the Isle of Man. There it has formed a 'gender pair' with vervain (*Verbena officinalis*),[86] regarded as the counterpart of that as a general protective against female ills, more particularly those associated with the womb and menstruation. It was grown in Manx gardens as a tonic at least to the 1940s.[87] Its similarity in appearance to that other long-venerated 'mother' plant, mugwort (*Artemisia vulgaris*), suggests that it may have become a stand-in for that.

Lamium album Linnaeus   PLATE 23
white dead-nettle, archangel
Europe, Himalaya, Japan; introduced into North America, New Zealand

Though so common and generally distributed in much of England, *Lamium album* appears to be unknown in natural habitats in the British Isles and has long lain under suspicion of having anciently been introduced, perhaps for food (it was at one time eaten extensively by peasants in Sweden). In Co. Dublin its distribution closely coincides with the known sites of early Norman settlements, while in parts of Wales an association with Roman way-stations has been postulated. It must be considered doubtful whether it was available for use anywhere in the British Isles prehistorically.

The few records suggest that the species has never enjoyed much popularity in the British Isles as a folk medicine. The ailments for which it has been used, moreover, are curiously diverse: skin complaints in Norfolk[88] and one region of north-western Eire[89] (where mixed with mutton suet it has been made into an ointment for treating eczema in adults), arthritis or sciatica in Norfolk[90] and Dumfriesshire,[91] bleeding and deep cuts in Somerset[92] and South Uist in the Outer Hebrides—and in this last also, sore feet and toothache.[93] None of these corresponds to uses for which the plant is recommended in at least some current books of herbal cures.

Lamium purpureum Linnaeus
red dead-nettle
Europe, western Asia; introduced into North America, Australasia

An infusion of *Lamium purpureum*, in a quart of wine, has been drunk in

Essex as a treatment for piles[94] (and elsewhere in East Anglia it features as a cure for certain diseases of poultry[95]).

In Ireland, on the other hand, a decoction of the roots has been taken in Meath to bring out the rash in cases of measles,[96] while in Kerry an infusion has been drunk for headaches.[97] As similar uses are on record for betony (*Stachys officinalis*), perhaps *Lamium purpureum* has served there merely as a stand-in for that.

Marrubium vulgare Linnaeus
white horehound
Europe, western and central Asia, North Africa, Macaronesia;
   introduced into North America, Australasia

Dubiously identified with herbs featured in Classical and Anglo-Saxon herbals, *Marrubium vulgare* has long been favoured in both book and folk medicine as a remedy for sore throats, hoarseness, colds, coughs of all kinds, bronchitis and asthma, for which there are records from many parts of Britain and particularly Ireland. However, the species is unknown as a macro-fossil from any pre-Roman site in the British Isles (or indeed from any pre-medieval one elsewhere in Europe) and it seems likely to have been a late addition to the folk repertory.

'Haryhound' was widely made into a beer and drunk as a spring tonic in East Anglia till the early twentieth century.[98] In the Fenland district of Cambridgeshire, expectant mothers used to drink an especially strong mixture of it with rue (*Ruta graveolens*, nowhere wild in the British Isles) if they wanted to delay a birth.[99] In Cumbria, by contrast, it has been valued for nosebleeds.[100]

That tonic of East Anglia has also been recorded from the opposite end of the British Isles, in the Aran Islands.[101] In other, unspecified parts of Ireland an infusion of the plant is said to have been a common remedy for earache or a headache,[102] while in Cavan a preparation has had the reputation of cleaning out the valves of the heart, and a tea has been drunk for rheumatism.[103]

Scutellaria galericulata Linnaeus
skullcap
Europe, northern and western Asia, Algeria, North America

(Folk credentials questionable) Prized in medieval herbalism for all disorders of the nervous system, the only alleged folk records of *Scutellaria galericulata* may in fact have come from that. Assertions that the plant continues 'in general use' in the Eastern Counties[104] have been found to be supported by a single localised record only from Norfolk,[105] where it has been used for insomnia.

Teucrium scorodonia Linnaeus
  wood sage, wild sage, mountain sage, heath sage
  southern, western and central Europe; introduced into North America
Mainly a plant of the acid soils of the north and west of the British Isles, *Teucrium scorodonia* seems to have featured as a folk herb only very marginally in England. A tea made from it in Hampshire has been drunk for swellings,

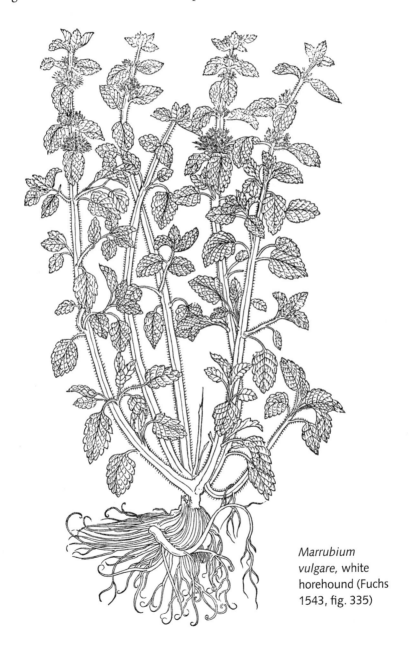

Marrubium vulgare, white horehound (Fuchs 1543, fig. 335)

'bad stomachs' and biliousness,[106] but more usually it has served to counter rheumatism, as in one district of Gloucestershire[107] and two counties in Wales (Pembrokeshire and Flintshire[108]). It has been used as a purifying tonic in Wiltshire,[109] Merionethshire[110] and the Isle of Man.[111] Like other members of the Lamiaceae, this species has the production of sweating as its most obvious property and the majority of its recorded applications reflect that. Though those records come principally from Ireland, they include the easing of 'a sore head' (presumably a headache) with a plaster made from the plant in the Highlands.[112] But that can hardly be why wood sage has been used for shingles in Caernarvonshire,[113] St Vitus' dance in Denbighshire,[114] jaundice in Orkney (as reflected in the plant's name there in Old Norse)[115] and dysentery in the Isle of Man.[116]

Though Ireland has echoed that limited use for rheumatism (Cork[117] and, assuming 'mountain sedge' was a mishearing for this, Mayo[118]), it is as a cure for colds and coughs, including those of tuberculosis, that the plant has predominantly featured there ('Ulster',[119] Mayo,[120] Co. Dublin,[121] Wicklow[122] and other unspecified areas of the country[123]). That it also has a relaxing effect could explain a subsidiary popularity in Ireland for such varied troubles as colic, gripe, indigestion,[124] palpitations[125] and—in Cork—sprains[126] and 'a pain near the heart'.[127]

Particularly striking is the extent to which wood sage has been employed in combination with other herbs. The Welsh cure for shingles already mentioned, for example, also involves navelwort and greater stitchwort[128]; as a cure for tuberculosis in Wicklow it has been mixed with thyme and honeysuckle[129]; in Wexford it has shared with equal parts of chickweed the role of poulticing boils and ulcers[130]; while in Mayo it was merely one of eight ingredients in a juice taken for coughing after a fever.[131] Was this because it was typically seen as fulfilling a supporting role, in need of a boost from some other source if it was to overcome the more deep-seated complaints? Yet some people do seem to have had great faith in its effectiveness even if utilised alone: according to one Mayo informant, indeed, it 'can cure every disease'.[132]

Teucrium scordium Linnaeus
water germander
southern, western and central Europe, western Asia

Locally abundant in the Cambridgeshire Fens until the eighteenth century, as 'English treacle' *Teucrium scordium* was said by John Ray to have been in use by women 'very frequently' two centuries earlier in a decoction to suppress menstruation.[133] Smelling powerfully like garlic, it was also used 'by the peasantry' as a vermicide, according to a later source.[134] In both cases, though, it is left ambiguous whether it was specifically Cambridgeshire that was referred to. No other mentions of the plant have been traced in the folklore literature of Britain.

Ajuga reptans Linnaeus
bugle
Europe, south-western Asia, North Africa; introduced into North
America, New Zealand

There is one British record, from Sussex,[135] of the ostensibly folk use of *Ajuga reptans* for wounds, a purpose for which it was anciently valued on account of its considerable astringency.

Two Irish records add support to that. In the early nineteenth century, country people in Londonderry are said to have applied the juice to bruises as those were at the stage of turning black.[136] And in Sligo—if, as seems likely, *glas-na-coille* was a mishearing of *glasnair choille* (the name in Irish)—it supplied till much later a cure for whitlows reckoned infallible.[137]

Nepeta cataria Linnaeus
cat-mint
Europe, western and central Asia; introduced into North America,
South Africa

(Confusion suspected) A herb boiled in Meath to drive out a cold by inducing sweating has been recorded as *Nepeta cataria*[138]; however, no other mention of the species in the folklore literature has been traced, and as it is a rarish plant in Ireland and not accepted as indigenous there, there must be an element of doubt. Possibly it was a mishearing of 'calamint' (*Clinopodium ascendens*), another herb used for colds and said to have been formerly drunk as a tea in parts of Ireland.[139]

Glechoma hederacea Linnaeus
ground-ivy, robin-run-in-the-hedge
Europe, north and western Asia; introduced into North America,
New Zealand

'Women of our northern parts, especially about Wales and Cheshire', wrote John Gerard in his *Herball*,[140] put pieces of *Glechoma hederacea* in their ale to clear the head of 'rheumatic humour flowing from the brain'—hence its names of 'ale-hoof' or 'tun-hoof'. By the time John Ray wrote, nearly a century later,[141] that custom had gradually disappeared, following the arrival of hops (*Humulus lupulus*); he accepted, however, that the herb had the power to clear the brain, usually within twenty-four hours. Many subsequent authors have attested to its action on the mucous membranes, which have caused it to be extensively prescribed and used for cleansing the system as a whole as well as, more specifically, as an expectorant or inhalant for colds, coughs and respiratory complaints in general. Records of its folk use for this last purpose

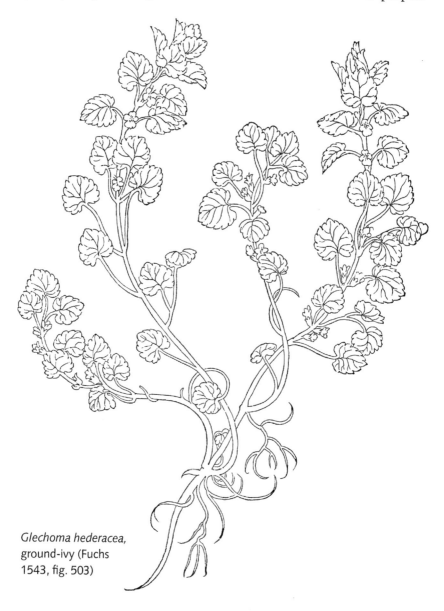

Glechoma hederacea,
ground-ivy (Fuchs
1543, fig. 503)

are very widely spread but especially frequent from the 'Celtic' west. A natural follow-on from the reputation for clearing the head has been to bring that property to bear on deafness (reported from Lincolnshire[142]) and, of course, headaches, too. The method of administering it for the latter is not mentioned in the one unlocalised Irish record,[143] but in the case of a seventeenth-century one from Staffordshire the juice was put up the nostrils,[144] while in the Highlands the dried leaves have been made into a snuff.[145] Predictably, the eyes have been seen to benefit, too. The deriving of an eye lotion from the plant evidently goes back a very long way, for it features among the recipes of the physicians of Myddvai in thirteenth-century Carmarthenshire; more recent records come from Dorset[146] and Warwickshire.[147]

Ground-ivy's more broadly cleansing action has caused its second most widespread use, as a purifying tonic. Whereas its records as a cold cure show a preponderantly 'Celtic' distribution, by contrast they come noticeably much more from the southern half of England: Devon,[148] Dorset,[149] Wiltshire,[150] Berkshire and Oxfordshire,[151] Kent[152] and Warwickshire.[153] In this last area, the plant was boiled with the young shoots of nettles to produce a very bitter drink known as 'gill tea', which children were made to drink on nine successive days every spring. Like other purifying herbs, this one has been credited, too, with clearing up skin complaints of a variety of kinds—in Devon[154] and Gloucestershire[155] as far as Britain is concerned.

The plant further enjoyed a reputation, if a more minor one, for healing externally. In Cornwall, wounds and lesser cuts have been bound with its fresh leaves, a secondary function of which has been to draw out thorns and splinters.[156] It has been valued for wounds in Caernarvonshire,[157] too, and for adder bites in the Highlands.[158] And no doubt its claimed success with lard as an ointment for corns in Suffolk[159] belongs in this category, too.

Ireland's share of these lesser uses extends from clearing up skin complaints (Westmeath,[160] Limerick,[161] Cork[162]), flushing out the kidneys (Kilkenny,[163] Tipperary[164]), stimulating menstruation in cases of chlorosis ('Ulster'[165]), healing sores and blisters (Louth[166]) and making ulcers disappear (Westmeath,[167] Wexford[168]).

Prunella vulgaris Linnaeus

self-heal; *ceannbhan beg*, heart's-ease (Ireland)

Europe, temperate Asia, North Africa; introduced into North
America, Australasia

An Irish herb *par excellence*—despite being common over most of the British

Isles—*Prunella vulgaris* has had three principal but distinct functions in folk medicine: to staunch bleeding, to ease respiratory complaints and to treat heart trouble. For the first of those the plant was once highly valued in official medicine as well, but by the eighteenth century it largely fell into disuse and has lingered on only in country areas: the Weald of Kent (where charcoal burners applied it to cuts and bruises as recently as World War II[169]), Suffolk,[170]

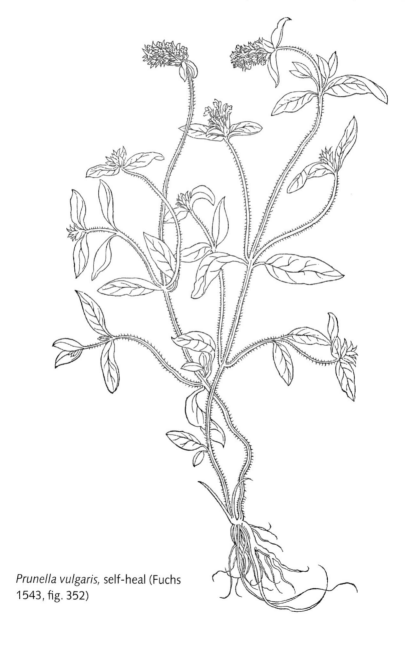

Prunella vulgaris, self-heal (Fuchs 1543, fig. 352)

Gloucestershire[171] and the Highlands[172] as far as Britain is concerned. The second function, as a treatment for colds and respiratory problems, was reportedly popular c. 1700 in several parts of Wales[173] and is on record more recently from two remote areas where dying usages are likely to linger longest: the Pennines of Westmoreland[174] and the island of Colonsay in the Inner Hebrides.[175] (Elsewhere in the Hebrides a tea made from self-heal and tansy (*Tanacetum vulgare*) was once drunk for cooling the blood.[176]) For the third main function of the plant, however, no records at all from Britain have been traced.

Ireland seems to have had little interest in self-heal's ability to staunch bleeding, at any rate in more recent times, and the three counties from which that action is recorded (Londonderry,[177] Co. Dublin,[178] Cork[179]) are suspiciously ones containing large centres of population, suggesting a late arrival. One of John Ray's correspondents, a physician in Kilkenny accustomed to that use of the plant elsewhere, was surprised to find that Irish herb doctors instead gave it frequently, boiled in a posset, 'in all sorts of common continual fevers, some also in intermittent ones'.[180] It has persisted as a cure for ailments of that type in at least Donegal,[181] Cavan,[182] the Aran Islands[183] and Wicklow,[184] but it is in the more particular guise of a remedy for easing tubercular coughs that it features in the later records, with a marked concentration—and striking frequency—in the counties of the centre: Kildare (especially),[185] Laois,[186] Carlow[187] and Offaly.[188] If this is the plant known there as 'pusey', it is on record for that from Fermanagh, too.[189] There was a saying in those parts that you could tell whether a person had this fever-like illness, known there under the name *mionnérach*, by rubbing the plant in the hand and seeing if a froth developed.

The third main function of the plant, as a heart remedy, appears to have been exclusively Irish, recorded especially along the western coast (Donegal,[190] Sligo,[191] Clare Island off Mayo,[192] Limerick[193]) but also farther east (Cavan,[194] Kildare[195]). In that capacity it has variously borne the names of *cailleach's tea*[196] and *ceann de dohosaig*.[197] A presumably related use, in some unspecified part of Eire,[198] has been for a sudden stroke (or *poc*).

That medicinal uses of self-heal in Ireland have acquired some accretions of special ritual strengthens the impression that the history of the plant in that country is especially deep-rooted. Not surprisingly, therefore, it has attracted some further applications there of a more marginal kind: in Kildare[199] and Wicklow[200] to rid children of worms, in Londonderry[201] and Wexford[202] as a treatment for piles, in Meath[203] as a cure for eczema, in Carlow[204] as a remedy for 'a pain in the back' (renal colic?) and in Cavan[205] for 'weak blood'.

Clinopodium ascendens (Jordan) Sampaio
Calamintha ascendens Jordan, *Calamintha sylvatica* subsp. *ascendens*
(Jordan) P. W. Ball
common calamint
western and southern Europe, North Africa; introduced into
North America

(Folk credentials questionable) There is one vague statement[206] that the aromatic *Clinopodium ascendens* was in frequent use as a herbal tea in parts of Ireland in the early nineteenth century, leaving it unclear whether that was for medicinal purposes (it has been drunk for colds quite widely elsewhere). The species is accepted as a native of that country, occurring there in some quantity in limestone districts, so it is a likely one to have been exploited.

Origanum vulgare Linnaeus
marjoram
Europe, northern and western Asia, North Africa; introduced into
North America, New Zealand

Though the native version, *Origanum vulgare*, of this well-known pot-herb is locally common in the British Isles on chalk and limestone and its varied medicinal virtues have been much publicised in the literature, folk records of its use are curiously almost wanting. In Kent (?) it was at one time gathered in large quantities in autumn. Some was made into a tea for drinking immediately as a prophylactic and the rest hung up in bunches to dry for winter use.[207] On the Isle of Portland in Dorset it has the reputation of relieving headaches[208] and in 'Ulster' a decoction has been drunk to counter indigestion and acidity.[209] Otherwise it appears to have been essentially a remedy for horses. That pennyroyal (*Mentha pulegium*) was widely known as 'organ', presumably a corruption of *Origanum*, suggests that the latter largely took its place at least in English folk medicine.

Thymus Linnaeus
thyme
northern Eurasia; introduced into North America

Like so many other members of the mint family, *Thymus* has been one of many possible alternatives used for treating coughs and respiratory ailments (including tuberculosis). British records for this usage come from Devon,[210] Somerset,[211] Suffolk[212] and the Highlands.[213] The most important reason for drinking thyme tea, though, has been to calm the nerves: the plant is a well-known sedative. Once drunk almost universally in remote parts of Scotland,

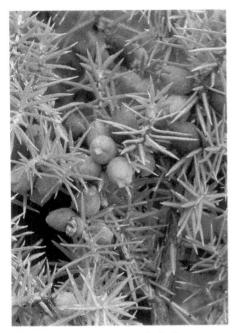

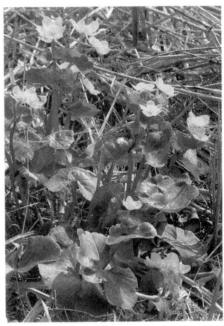

Plate 1. *Juniperus communis*, juniper
(Cupressaceae)

Plate 2. *Caltha palustris*, marsh-marigold
(Ranunculaceae)

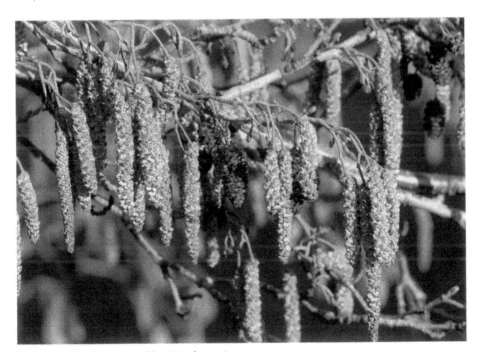

Plate 3. *Alnus glutinosa*, alder (Betulaceae)

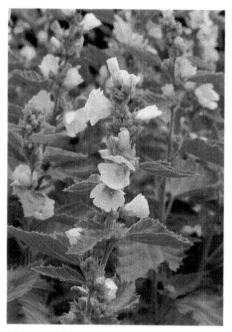

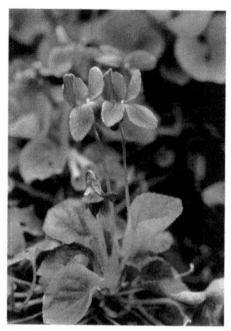

Plate 4. *Althaea officinalis*, marsh-mallow (Malvaceae)

Plate 5. *Viola odorata*, sweet violet (Violaceae)

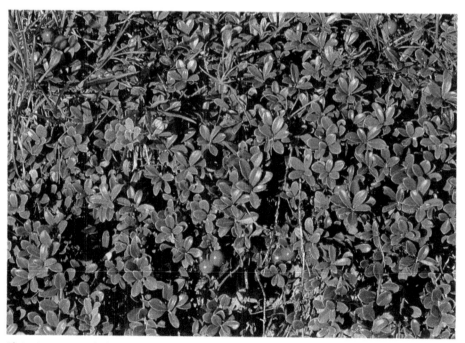

Plate 6. *Arctostaphylos uva-ursi*, bearberry (Ericaceae)

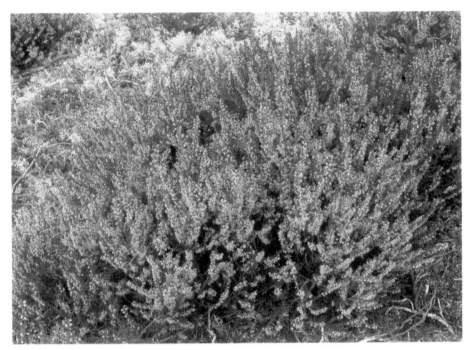

Plate 7. *Calluna vulgaris*, heather (Ericaceae)

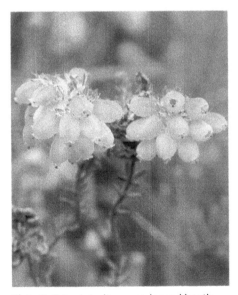

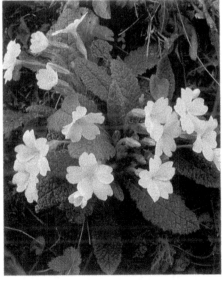

Plate 8. *Erica tetralix*, cross-leaved heath
(Ericaceae)

Plate 9. *Primula vulgaris*, primrose
(Primulaceae)

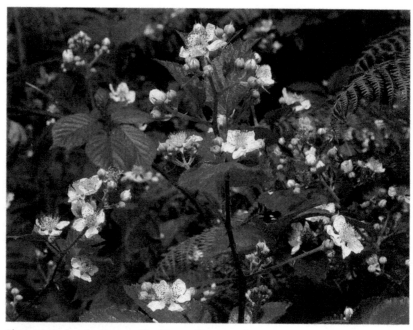

Plate 10. *Rubus fruticosus*, blackberry (Rosaceae)

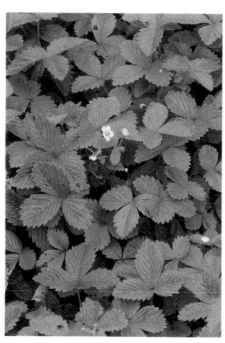

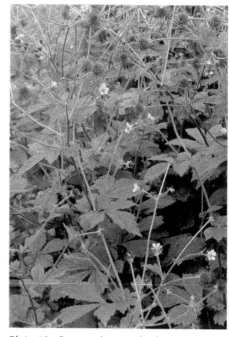

Plate 11. *Fragaria vesca*, wild strawberry (Rosaceae)

Plate 12. *Geum urbanum*, herb-Bennet (Rosaceae)

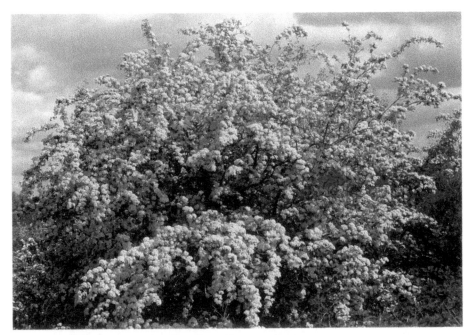

Plate 13. *Crataegus monogyna* , hawthorn (Rosaceae)

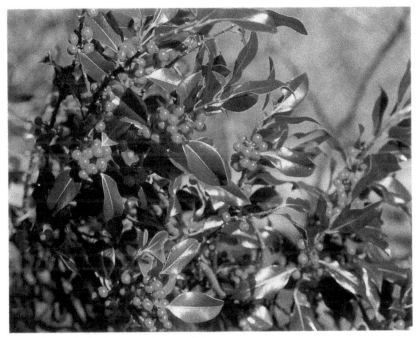

Plate 14. *Ilex aquifolium,* holly (Aquifoliaceae)

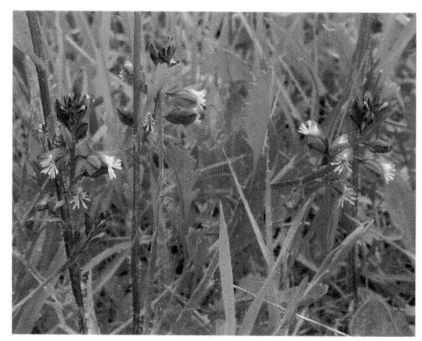

Plate 15. *Polygala vulgaris*, common milkwort (Polygalaceae)

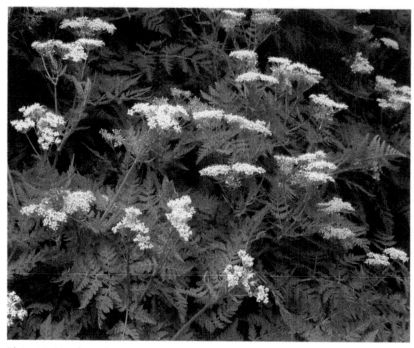

Plate 16. *Myrrhis odorata*, sweet cicely (Apiaceae)

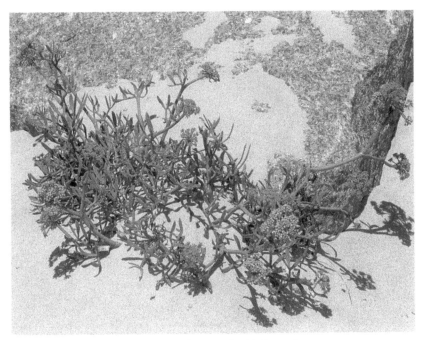

Plate 17. *Crithmum maritimum,* rock samphire (Apiaceae)

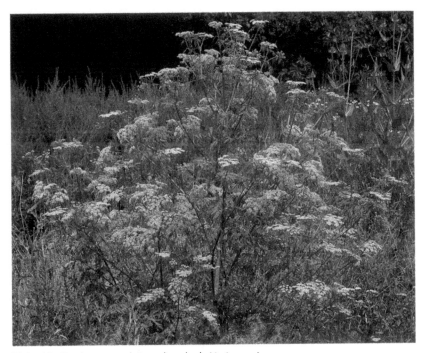

Plate 18. *Conium maculatum,* hemlock (Apiaceae)

231

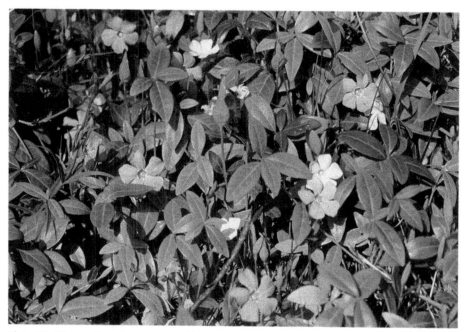

Plate 19. *Vinca minor*, lesser periwinkle (Apocynaceae)

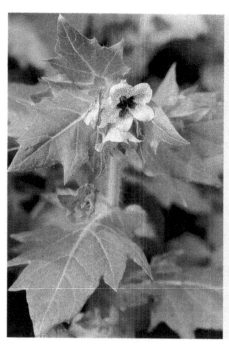

Plate 20. *Hyoscyamus niger*, henbane (Solanaceae)

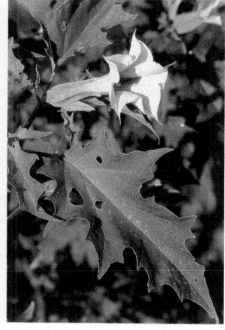

Plate 21. *Datura stramonium*, thorn-apple (Solanaceae)

232

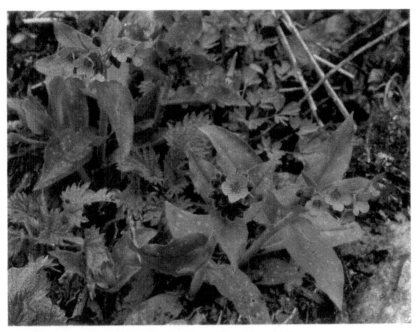

Plate 22. *Pulmonaria officinalis,* lungwort (Boraginaceae)

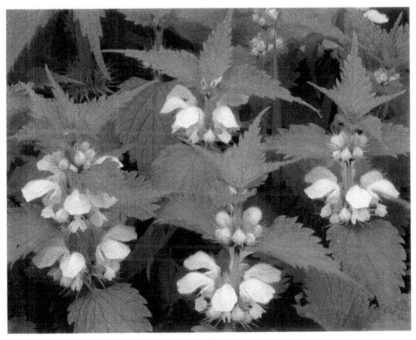

Plate 23. *Lamium album,* white dead-nettle (Lamiaceae)

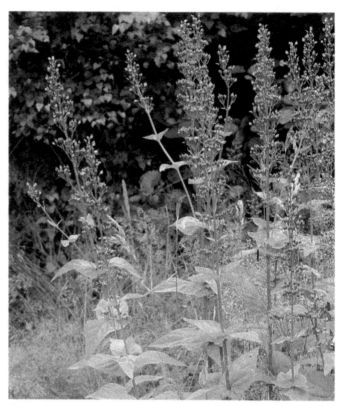

Plate 24. *Scrophularia nodosa*, common figwort
(Scrophulariaceae)

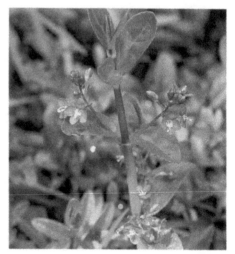

Plate 25. *Veronica beccabunga*, brooklime
(Scrophulariaceae)

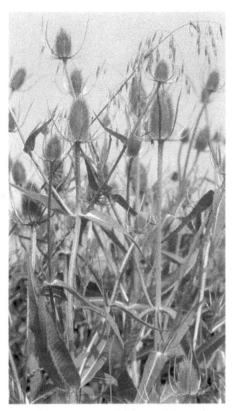

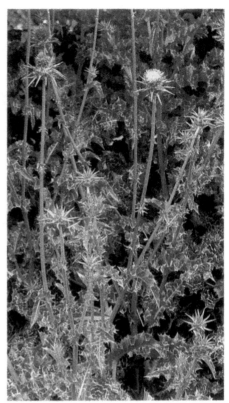

Plate 26. *Dipsacus fullonum*, wild teasel (Dipsacaceae)

Plate 27. *Silybum marianum*, milk thistle (Asteraceae)

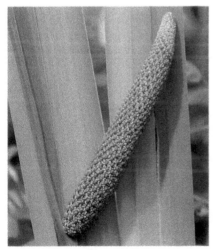

Plate 28. *Acorus calamus*, sweet flag (Araceae)

235

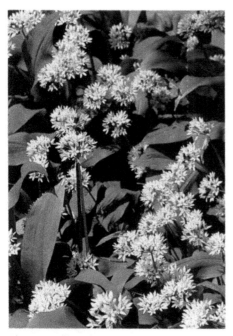

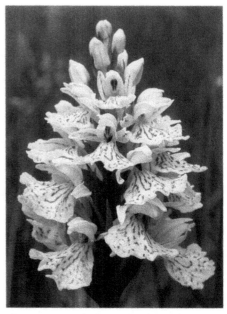

Plate 29. *Allium ursinum*, ramsons (Liliaceae)

Plate 30. *Dactylorhiza maculata* subsp. *ericetorum*, heath spotted-orchid (Orchidaceae)

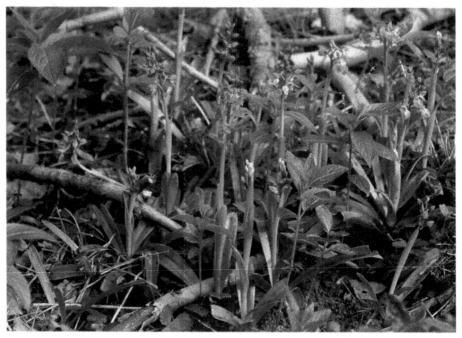

Plate 31. *Orchis mascula*, early-purple orchid (Orchidaceae)

236

both there[214] and in Suffolk[215] that infusion also had the supposed extra virtue of preventing bad dreams. But whereas in Suffolk it has additionally been a specific for headache,[216] in Wiltshire it has been looked upon as a wart cure, boiled in urine with pepper and nitre,[217] while from Cumbria there is a record of a mixed bunch of nettle, dock and thyme leaves being applied to lumbago as a counter-irritant switch.[218]

The Irish uses are similar but records of them noticeably less widespread, with a marked concentration in the south-east: in Wexford[219] the infusion has been drunk *both* to counter respiratory troubles *and* as a sedative to calm the nerves or induce deeper sleep, though in Wicklow[220] a tuberculosis cure has taken the form of an infusion mixed with honeysuckle and wild sage instead. In Limerick, headaches were banished by sniffing the plant plucked fresh.[221]

Mentha Linnaeus
mint
Old World temperate regions

Mentha aquatica Linnaeus
water mint
Europe, south-western Asia, North and South Africa, Madeira;
    introduced into North America

Mentha ×piperita Linnaeus
peppermint
horticultural

Mentha spicata Linnaeus
spearmint
horticultural

Except for pennyroyal (*Mentha pulegium*), the members of the genus *Mentha,* if distinguished at all in the folk literature, have borne their vernacular names interchangeably and have been used medicinally for such a broadly similar range of ailments that it is appropriate to discuss them together. Most records probably relate to the native water mint (*M. aquatica*), the common species of wet places. That is widely known also as 'water peppermint' or 'wild peppermint', names rarely relating to the true peppermint (*M. ×piperita*), which is a garden hybrid, originating in England in the seventeenth century. Though spearmint (*M. spicata*) is probably always distinguished correctly, only two folk records of that have been found, while the solitary one for 'horse mint' cannot confidently be ascribed to any of the species or hybrids now recognised by taxonomists. Until grown as pot-herbs, some of which have crept out of gardens and become naturalised in the wild, 'mint' doubtless denoted a single wild entity for all practical purposes.

Like so many other members of the family Lamiaceae, mint has found its principal use in countering colds and coughs—though, curiously, the British records for that are all from the southern half of England: Dorset,[222] Wiltshire,[223] Warwickshire,[224] Suffolk,[225] and Norfolk.[226] A secondary focus has been on the digestive system, as a cure for constipation, stomach-ache or inflammation of the appendix (Kent,[227] Norfolk[228]), perhaps also the 'stomach trouble' reported from Gloucestershire[229] and even the 'heart complaints' for which 'horse mint' has been commended in Lincolnshire[230] if those are 'heartburn' at least in part. But 'a pain in the side after jaundice', recorded from the Highlands,[231] must belong in a separate category, as clearly does a tradition persisting in rural Somerset[232] and the mining communities of Fife[233] of relieving 'curdled milk' in nursing mothers by applying a hot 'peppermint' or spearmint compress to the breasts. The same applies to rubbing the gums with the leaves to ease the pain of toothache in Wiltshire.[234]

Ireland's uses have been similar, but the two leading ones in Britain have exchanged their places there: indigestion and stomach pain have been the main troubles remedied (Cavan,[235] Limerick,[236] Cork[237] and unlocalised records[238]) whereas the only cold cure traced is a record from Co. Dublin—where it was eaten raw[239]—and the only cough cure is represented by a spearmint syrup made with water-cress and honeysuckle for whooping cough in Cork.[240] In the last county a decoction has also been drunk for headaches,[241] while deafness has been treated there by squeezing the juice from nine plants and pouring a thimbleful into the relevant ear.[242] Other Irish applications have been to jaundice in Limerick,[243] measles in Cavan[244] and nettle stings (as a counter-irritant) in Co. Dublin.[245] In some unspecified part of the country a bunch tied to the wrist or worn elsewhere about the person has also been held to ward off infection.[246]

Mentha pulegium Linnaeus

pennyroyal (pennyroyal of North America is a quite different plant,
Hedeoma pulegioides (Linnaeus) Persoon), organ, hop marjoram
central and southern Europe, North Africa, Macaronesia; introduced
into North and South America, Australasia

The name pennyroyal is a corrupted translation of the Latin *pulegium regium*, under which the herbals propagated the belief that *Mentha pulegium* was the plant recommended by Classical writers as a flea repellent. In deference to that, posies of the plant were at one time frequently kept in cottages in Devon[247] and no doubt elsewhere. The Classical authors, however, also praised this plant as useful to 'bring away the afterbirth' and pennyroyal has consequently enjoyed a secondary, apparently much more widespread reputation as an abortifacient—and the plant does indeed harbour a toxic chemical, pulegone. Though records of its use for that purpose predictably feature but rarely in the folk literature and the handful that have been traced are mostly from the east of England (Essex,[248] Cambridgeshire,[249] Norfolk,[250] Lancashire,[251] Yorkshire[252]), there is considerable evidence to suggest that it has been one of the most popular solutions for unwanted pregnancies down through the years and continued in currency more or less down to the present. An associated use, more freely reported, has been for menstrual obstruction (Dorset,[253] Suffolk,[254] Norfolk,[255] Lancashire[256]).

In its non-clandestine roles, however, pennyroyal has principally served as just another mint, sharing with so many other members of the Lamiaceae an obvious ability to clear the nasal and bronchial passages. In that capacity it has evidently been preferred to the wild marjoram (*Origanum vulgare*), which has a similar scent, and usurped its Latin name *Origanum* in the corrupted forms of 'organy' and 'organ(s)'. Under the last name a tea made from it has been drunk very extensively in Cornwall[257] and particularly Devon[258] at least since the seventeenth century,[259] either as a refreshing pick-me-up or, mixed with honey, for colds and the like. It was traditionally taken out to har-

Mentha pulegium, pennyroyal (Brunfels 1530, p. 227)

vesters in the fields and also used by sailors to sweeten their drinking water when at sea.[260] Beyond this south-western headquarters its recorded use for these particular purposes has extended to Wiltshire,[261] Wexford[262] and (in an infusion with bramble roots) the Highlands.[263] In Gloucestershire[264] also it has been drunk to cure flatulence, and in Wales, as *coludd-lys*, to open the bowels.[265]

Miscellaneous uses, unrelated to any of the foregoing, have been for cramp in Devon[266] and, mixed with barley-meal, as a dressing on burns in the Isle of Man.[267] The sole Irish one is as a corn cure in Wexford.[268]

Though now a scarce plant, only in the New Forest to be found in quantity still, pennyroyal was allegedly once much more plentiful in lowland England. Requiring short turf, it was characteristic of village greens and ponds frequented by farm geese, both habitats much exposed to modern changes. A marked association of the older records with the wide verges of old roads that may have been ancient trackways has been noted.

Salvia verbenaca Linnaeus
S. horminoides Pourret
  wild clary
  southern and western Europe, Algeria; introduced into North
    America, Australasia

The seeds of some *Salvia* species have a seed coat which, when soaked in water or melted by the warmth and moisture of the eyeball, becomes jelly-like and adheres to any foreign body, enabling it to be extracted with the minimum of pain. 'Clary' is allegedly a corruption of 'clear-eye'.

Though other foreign or cultivated species were normally recommended in official medicine for this purpose, the native English *Salvia verbenaca* attracted some use for it as well, under the name 'eyeseed'. There are definite records of that from Oxfordshire and Denbighshire[269] and a more doubtful one from Lincolnshire[270]; it also seems more likely than gromwell (as claimed[271]) to be the 'eyeseed' used in Essex, in precisely the same way.

An infusion of the plant formerly drunk as a tea in Berwickshire has provoked the suggestion that it was anciently grown there (and elsewhere?) medicinally.[272] If so, perhaps that was for sprains, for which a plant known as 'eyeseeds' and queried as this species, was at one time used in the Louth district of Lincolnshire.[273]

Notes

1. Barbour
2. Moore MS
3. IFC S 630: 39
4. Tongue
5. Wright, 241
6. Taylor 1929
7. Perring
8. Payne, 92 footnote
9. *Folk-lore Record*, 6 (1888), 116
10. Burne, 190; Wright, 243
11. Quayle, 69; Fargher
12. Killip, 135
13. Briggs 1880
14. Ibbott, 11
15. Hatfield, 30
16. Vickery MSS
17. Hatfield, appendix
18. Vickery MSS
19. Hatfield MS
20. Hayward
21. Hatfield MS
22. Hatfield, 33
23. Hatfield, 52
24. Vickery MSS
25. Maloney
26. IFC S 710: 48
27. IFC S 157: 295, 314
28. Barbour
29. IFC S 475: 207
30. Maloney
31. Vickery MSS
32. IFC S 850: 113
33. Logan, 61
34. IFC S 170: 197
35. IFC S 850: 113
36. IFC S 550: 288
37. IFC S 505: 117
38. Logan, 77
39. Murray
40. Lafont
41. Pratt 1850–7
42. Colgan 1904, 309
43. IFC S 931: 303

44. IFC S 524: 8
45. Wood-Martin, 185
46. Grigson
47. e.g. Roeder; Moore 1898
48. Garrad 1976 and in litt.
49. Moore 1898
50. Roberts
51. Roberts
52. Quincy, 133
53. A. Allen, 185
54. Hatfield, 50
55. Vickery MSS
56. Wright, 247
57. Moloney
58. Latham, 38
59. Maloney
60. Moore MS
61. Whitlock 1992, 103
62. A. Allen, 185
63. Whitlock 1992, 103
64. Hayward, 230
65. Newman & Wilson
66. Tongue
67. Jones 1996, 89
68. Pratt 1850–7
69. R. C. Palmer, in litt.
70. Harrison
71. Kirby, 60
72. Martin, 94
73. Cameron
74. Gerard, 852
75. Hatfield MS
76. Moloney
77. McClafferty
78. IFC S 21: 11
79. IFC S 736: 191
80. Bethell
81. Johnston 1853, 162
82. CECTL MSS
83. Simpkins, 133
84. Moore MS
85. Maloney
86. Larch S. Garrad, in litt.

87. *North Western Naturalist*, 18 (1944), 168
88. Hatfield MS
89. Logan, 73
90. Hatfield MS
91. CECTL MSS
92. Tongue
93. Shaw, 48, 49
94. Hatfield, 45
95. Hatfield, appendix
96. IFC S 717: 352
97. IFC S 413: 228
98. Randell, 87; Hatfield, 55
99. Porter 1969, 10
100. Newman & Wilson
101. Ó hEithir
102. Wilson
103. Maloney
104. Newman 1945; 1948, 150
105. Hatfield MS
106. Beddington & Christy, 212
107. Riddelsdell et al., 398
108. Williams MS
109. Macpherson MS
110. Williams MS
111. Fargher
112. Carmichael, vi, 114
113. Williams MS
114. Vickery 1995, 404
115. Spence; Leask, 71
116. Moore 1898
117. IFC S 386: 118
118. IFC S 138: 466
119. Purdon
120. Colgan 1911; IFC S 93: 32; 132: 97
121. Egan
122. McClafferty
123. Wood-Martin, 177; Wilson
124. Moloney; Ó Súilleabháin, 310
125. Wood-Martin, 177
126. IFC S 287: 67
127. IFC S 286: 56
128. Williams MS
129. McClafferty
130. IFC S 897: 238
131. IFC S 132: 97
132. IFC S 133: 339
133. Ray 1670, 67
134. Johnson 1862, 205
135. A. Allen, 185
136. Moore MS
137. IFC S 170: 256
138. Farrelly MS
139. Farrelly MS
140. Gerard, 707
141. Ray 1670, 161
142. Woodruffe-Peacock
143. Wilson
144. Ray 1690, 281
145. Beith
146. Dacombe
147. *PLNN*, no. 32 (1993), 147
148. Lafont
149. Dacombe
150. Macpherson MS
151. Vickery 1995
152. Pratt 1850–7
153. Wright, 239
154. Lafont
155. Britten & Holland
156. Deane & Shaw
157. Williams MS
158. MacFarlane
159. Hatfield, 53
160. IFC S 736: 170
161. IFC S 524: 83
162. IFC S 385: 55
163. IFC S 850: 114
164. Vickery MSS
165. Barbour
166. IFC S 672: 259
167. IFC S 736: 137
168. IFC S 897: 236
169. Mabey, 317
170. Jobson 1967, 60
171. Hopkins, 80
172. Beith
173. Lankester, 372

174. Duncan & Robson, 69
175. McNeill
176. Swire, 76
177. Moore MS
178. IFC S 795: 124
179. IFC S 386: 118
180. Lankester, 372
181. IFC S 1090: 241, 274
182. Maloney
183. Ó hEithir (as *Eriophorum*)
184. McClafferty
185. IFC S 781: 3, 11, 51, 79, 108
186. IFC S 837: 56, 130
187. IFC S 907: 414
188. IFC S 800: 53
189. Glassie, 308
190. Hart 1898, 377, 379; Vickery MSS
191. IFC S 170: 258
192. Colgan 1911
193. IFC S 484: 41
194. IFC S 969: 225
195. IFC S 771: 241
196. Moloney
197. Vickery MSS
198. Ó Súilleabháin, 314
199. *Journal of the County Kildare Archaeological Society*, 16 (1983–4), 379
200. McClafferty (as *Eriophorum*); IFC S 908: 98
201. Moore MS
202. IFC S 888: 108
203. IFC S 710: 49
204. IFC S 907: 414, 415
205. Maloney
206. Moore MS
207. Pratt 1850–7
208. Vickery MSS
209. Egan
210. Vickery MSS
211. Tongue
212. Chamberlain 1981, 257
213. MacFarlane
214. Cameron; Beith

215. Jobson 1959, 32
216. Jobson 1959, 32
217. Whitlock 1976, 164
218. *PLNN*, no. 54 (1998), 261
219. IFC S 897: 239
220. McClafferty
221. IFC S 524: 30
222. Dacombe
223. Whitlock 1976, 167
224. Vickery MSS
225. Kightly, 222; *Folk-lore*, 35 (1924), 356
226. Hatfield, 8, 30
227. Vickery MSS
228. Hatfield, 72, 88
229. Knight, 182
230. Woodruffe-Peacock
231. Beith
232. Tongue
233. Simpkins, 411
234. Macpherson MS
235. Maloney
236. IFC S 504: 136
237. IFC S 287: 180
238. Wood-Martin, 220; Sargent
239. IFC S 787: 282
240. IFC S 385: 286
241. IFC S 287: 67
242. IFC S 287: 180
243. IFC S 512: 407, 523
244. Maloney
245. IFC S 787: 336
246. Sargent
247. Lafont
248. Hatfield, 20
249. Porter 1969, 10
250. Hatfield, 17
251. Vickery 1995
252. Vickery 1995
253. Dacombe
254. Jobson 1959, 144
255. Hatfield MS
256. Vickery 1995
257. Davey; Wright, 241

258. Briggs 1880; Wright, 241; Lafont
259. Parkinson, 30
260. Lafont
261. Macpherson MS
262. IFC S 897: 263
263. Beith
264. Vickery 1995
265. Cameron
266. Lafont
267. Fargher; Garrad 1984
268. IFC S 897: 81
269. *Gardeners' Chronicle* (1871: I), 45, 106
270. Britten & Holland, 172
271. Gepp, 45
272. Johnston 1853, 159
273. Woodruffe-Peacock

CHAPTER 13

Plantains, Figworts, Foxglove and Speedwells

Dicotyledonous flowering plants in the orders (and families) Callitrichales (Callitrichaceae, water-starworts), Plantaginales (Plantaginaceae, plantains) and Scrophulariales (Oleaceae, the ash family; Scrophulariaceae, figworts; Orobanchaceae, broomrapes; Lentibulariaceae, bladderworts) are included in this chapter.

CALLITRICHACEAE

Callitriche stagnalis Scopoli
common water-starwort
Europe, North Africa, North America; introduced into Australasia
A plant identified botanically as *Callitriche stagnalis* was found to be an ingredient, along with chamomile and ragwort, in plasters used to promote the formation of pus in wounds in the island of Colonsay in the Inner Hebrides in the late nineteenth century.[1] Possibly it had been used in mistake for some similar-looking herb.

PLANTAGINACEAE

Plantago coronopus Linnaeus
buck's-horn plantain
western and central Europe, western Asia, North Africa, Azores;
    introduced into North America, Australasia
Though *Plantago coronopus* has shared in the Isle of Man[2] the reputation of the genus more generally for staunching cuts and wounds, as *P. maritima* Linnaeus has in Cork,[3] it at one time acquired very special fame as an antidote

to the bites of rabid dogs and resulting hydrophobia, under the name 'star-of-the-earth'. Though the recorded uses of the latter seem to have been veterinary, it could well have been used when humans were bitten, too.

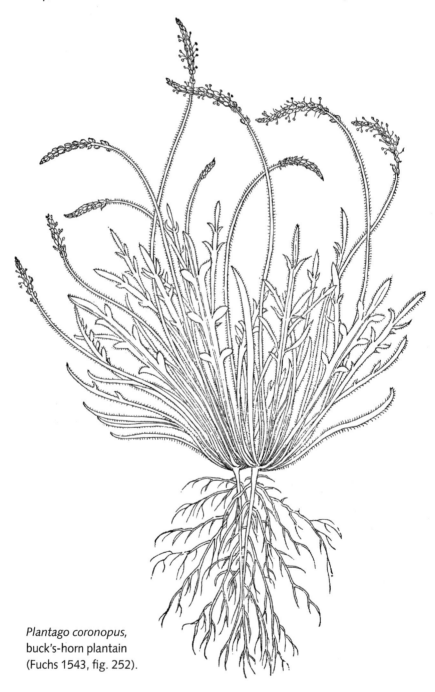

Plantago coronopus,
buck's-horn plantain
(Fuchs 1543, fig. 252).

Plantago lanceolata Linnaeus
ribwort plantain, rib-grass, *slánlus,* St Patrick's leaf
Europe, northern and central Asia; cosmopolitan weed

Plantago major Linnaeus
greater plantain, St Patrick's leaf
Europe, northern and central Asia;
   cosmopolitan weed

The commonest species of plantain in the British
Isles, both for the most part followers of human
activity but probably indigenous in marshes
(*Plantago major*) and in sea-cliff sward (*P. lanceolata*), these two have naturally been the normal choices for the purpose for which this genus
is renowned in many parts of the world (including Sikkim and Peru): the ability to stop bleeding from an external injury in a matter of minutes. Usually it is found sufficient for just a fresh
leaf to be crushed (or chewed) for enough of the
healing chemicals to be released, but to treat
severer haemorrhages the whole plant has sometimes been boiled; alternatively, an ointment
has been produced and applied. The two species seem to have been used throughout
the British Isles for this primary purpose,
and interchangeably.

In Britain that famed effectiveness
has led the leaves to be applied as
well to rashes (Somerset[4]) and
soreness from any rubbing (South
Uist in the Hebrides[5] and elsewhere
in Scotland[6]), piles (Devon[7]) and
burns (Devon,[8] Shetland[9]). Credited with antiseptic properties[10] and
the ability to prevent festering, they
have been valued further for treating
varicose veins (Montgomeryshire[11]) and
for drawing the pus out of an infected
wound or swelling (Gloucestershire,[12]

Plantago major, greater plantain
(Brunfels 1530, p. 23)

the Inner[13] and Outer Hebrides,[14] Orkney[15]). A reputation for also alleviating pain has encouraged a use for all kinds of stings, too, mostly in southern England (Devon,[16] Dorset,[17] Somerset,[18] Kent (?),[19] Bedfordshire,[20] the Fens of East Anglia[21]) but in the Highlands[22] as well. A still further use, recorded from Denbighshire,[23] is as a tonic, mixed with yarrow and nettles.

Ireland is distinctive for the wide presence there (Longford,[24] Leitrim,[25] Mayo,[26] Tipperary[27]) of a belief—common to several other plants—that one side of the leaf does the drawing out of septic matter from a wound and the other the healing, a belief recorded apparently only from the Outer Hebrides[28] in Britain. More exclusively Irish has been drinking plantain juice for a cough (Monaghan,[29] Mayo,[30] Laois[31]). While the two countries have yielded similar numbers of similarly scattered records for applying the leaves to burns (Monaghan,[32] Limerick,[33] Tipperary[34]) and to drawing pus out of boils, wounds or swellings (Donegal,[35] Laois,[36] Tipperary[37]), Ireland seems to have found other uses for the leaves unknown, or at any rate untraced, in Britain: lumps and swellings (Monaghan,[38] Clare-Galway borderland[39]), pimples (Laois[40]), chapped hands or legs (Limerick,[41] Tipperary[42]), corns (Longford[43]), warts (Westmeath[44]), headaches (Meath,[45] Cavan[46]) and gout (Cavan[47]). The sole records for some internal uses are Irish, too: drinking the boiled juice for liver trouble (Cavan[48]) or jaundice (Laois[49]) and putting it into the milk of children that are delicate (Tipperary[50]). Even 'sore eyes' have had their share of attention (Galway,[51] Limerick[52]) though it is unclear—as also in the case of a record from the Highlands[53]—whether that meant styes or merely the result of straining.

OLEACEAE

Fraxinus excelsior Linnaeus
ash

Europe, western Asia, North Africa; introduced into North America, New Zealand

Another tree traditionally believed to exude special power from its every part, *Fraxinus excelsior* has been valued for one healing purpose at least which seems to betray a magico-religious origin: as an antidote for the bites of venomous snakes. That this is based on superstition rather than anything else is shown by the fact that the cure, or the power to avert such bites in the first place, is attributed to the wearing of a collar woven out of ash twigs or to the carrying of an 'ash-stick'. Records of its use in those ways for people and/or dogs have been traced from Cornwall,[54] Devon,[55] Dorset,[56] 'Wales'[57] and Galloway[58]—all areas where adders occur in particular numbers. In Moray[59] in the north of Scotland, soaking the affected limb in a preparation of the leaves and buds was a more down-to-earth alternative. That that belief is not only ancient but was once Europe-wide is shown by its presence in the Norse sagas as well as the writings of Pliny the Elder.

Though healing powers attributed to any plant with a magical aura are *ipso facto* suspect, it is nevertheless possible that some chemical property of the sap does have a genuinely beneficial effect. Before the advent of quinine (from *Cinchona* spp.), the bark was popular in learned medicine for allaying fevers, and although no reflection of that particular use has been found in the folk records, they do contain other applications that are clearly cognate. One is a cure for earache (or deafness or tinnitus or even a headache), recorded from Sussex[60] and a chain of Irish counties, which involves heating a twig or young sapling in the fire, catching on a spoon the liquid that emerges and putting that hot into the ear, normally on cotton wool (or presumably a puffball before that product was invented). The sap has been similarly extracted to put on warts in Devon[61] and Leicestershire[62] or on an aching tooth in the Highlands.[63]

Apart from the buds, which are a slimming remedy in Gloucestershire,[64] and the seeds, reputedly an aphrodisiac in Devon,[65] it is the leaves that have otherwise been used. Reputed to purge, these have been valued in Gloucestershire for eliminating 'gravel'.[66]

It is in Ireland, though, that the leaves have been pre-eminently valued herbally: boiled or laid on fresh, they have been a remedy for rheumatism and its allies (Roscommon,[67] Meath,[68] Co. Dublin,[69] Laois,[70] Wexford,[71] Waterford,[72] Cork,[73] Kerry[74]) or for gout (Cavan,[75] Cork[76]). More compact, and more intriguing, is the distribution pattern displayed by the records for the earache cure described above. All those traced come from the eastern province of Leinster (Westmeath,[77] Co. Dublin,[78] Kildare,[79] Offaly,[80] Wicklow,[81] Wexford[82]) and thus perhaps have a Norse origin as the explanation. Ireland's greater valuing of the tree is further shown by a wider range of minor uses recorded for it: for ringworm in Down[83] and Antrim[84] (by enveloping the affected part in the smoke from smouldering twigs), for heartburn in Meath[85] and for burns in Kilkenny (by boiling the bark in linseed oil).[86] Even England's application to warts has echoes in Westmeath[87] and Co. Dublin.[88]

Ligustrum vulgare Linnaeus

privet

western, central and southern Europe, North Africa; introduced
into North America, New Zealand

A decoction of the berries of *Ligustrum vulgare*, which contain a potentially dangerous glycoside, has been recorded in more recent years as a home remedy for mumps in Wiltshire.[89]

In unspecified parts of Ireland, though, a similar decoction is said to have enjoyed great popularity for earache, while an infusion has been drunk for sore throats.[90] In Kildare, on the other hand, anyone following advice to chew the leaves to heal a sore lip has been carefully warned against swallowing the juice.[91]

All the records leave it unclear whether the native *Ligustrum vulgare* or the cultivated *L. ovalifolium* Hasskarl is the species resorted to. They could be expected to be more numerous, and from earlier periods, had the former been used.

SCROPHULARIACEAE

Verbascum thapsus Linnaeus

great mullein; Mary's candle (Ireland)

Europe, temperate Asia; introduced into North America, Australasia

The favourite remedy for pulmonary tuberculosis in Ireland throughout recorded history and doubtless long before, known from virtually every part of that country, has been to boil the woolly leaves of *Verbascum thapsus* in milk, strain the thick, mucilaginous liquid produced by that and then drink it warm, twice daily.[92] So valued has this plant been there both for that and for coughs and colds more generally, sore throats, catarrh, bronchitis and asthma that it was formerly often grown in cottage gardens, sometimes on a considerable scale. Advertisements were placed in newspapers, offering it for sale, and it was available even in the best chemists' shops in Dublin.

Though species of *Verbascum* have been used for lung and chest complaints over much of Europe at least since Classical times, very curiously that heavy Irish use is not matched in the records from elsewhere in the British Isles. Such English ones as have been traced are all from the south-east (Sussex,[93] Buckinghamshire,[94] Norfolk[95] and the Eastern Counties more generally[96]) and it would appear not even to have been a member at all of the Welsh or Scottish folk repertories.

In so far as great mullein has had additional, minor uses, the records are again Irish almost wholly. In unspecified parts of Ulster a decoction has been taken for diarrhoea and, mixed with other herbs, for cramp and for liver and kidney ailments, while a leaf roasted between dock leaves and moistened with spittle has been a treatment for boils.[97] The leaves have also predictably found favour as a poultice: in parts of Ireland for 'running sores',[98] in Meath for bee stings[99] and in Westmeath for goitre.[100] In Kerry, though, it was the water in which the plant had been boiled that was rubbed into the body to ease doctor-resistant 'pains' (a word most often denoting rheumatism in the rural areas of Ireland).[101]

Verbascum lychnitis
Linnaeus
white mullein
southern half of Europe,
western Siberia,
Morocco; intro-
duced into North
America

(Name confusion suspected) If the plant known under the name 'white mullein' in Wiltshire is correctly taken to be *Verbascum lychnitis*, its juice has been used there as a wart cure.[102] However, there are no certain botanical records for it from that county and perhaps the white leaves of *V. thapsus* have made that 'white mullein' locally.

Verbascum thapsus, great mullein
(Fuchs 1543, fig. 485)

Scrophularia nodosa Linnaeus   PLATE 24
common figwort, rose noble, brown(s)wort; *fothrom* (Irish)

Europe, temperate western and central Asia, allied species in North
  America; introduced into New Zealand

Like great mullein (*Verbascum thapsus*), the far less conspicuous *Scrophularia nodosa*, with a rank smell and bitter-tasting leaves (as William Withering noted), has been outstandingly and preponderantly an Irish herb. Known
in Ireland as 'queen of herbs', the consort of the foxglove (*Digitalis purpurea*),
it was a plant of ancient veneration there, its usual name in Gaelic, *fothrom*,
being a corruption of *faoi trom*, 'under elder': just as mistletoe partook of
the magical properties of the oak by growing on that, so this was believed to
have special power through thriving in the shade of that other sacred tree. Just
like mistletoe, too, it was supposed to lose power if allowed to touch the
ground once picked.

A name borne by any of the figworts in Devon, 'poor man's salve',[103] indicates one way in which these plants, and more specially *Scrophularia nodosa*,
were used: the roots, which in *S. nodosa* are swollen and knobby, were ground
into a powder and mixed with lard to produce an ointment applied to piles
and skin troubles of all kinds. More often, though, the roots or leaves, or sometimes the berries or seeds, were boiled and the liquid drunk—either as the
standard kind of tonic held to clear the blood of impurities, including boils
and rashes (Donegal,[104] Monaghan,[105] Cavan,[106] Co. Dublin,[107] Tipperary[108]),
or as yet one further cure for bronchial ailments, sore throats, coughs and
consumption (Donegal,[109] Cavan,[110] Meath,[111] Waterford[112]). In Kilkenny,[113]
on the other hand, sore throats were rubbed with the ointment and perhaps
that is also how goitre in Waterford[114] has been treated with the plant.

Alternatively, one of the leaves might be applied as a poultice: to sprains
or other swellings in Donegal,[115] Londonderry[116] and Leitrim[117] (particularly extensively in the latter two), to burns in Leitrim[118] and Mayo,[119] to
wounds and cuts in Mayo[120] and, mixed with moss and herb-Robert, in
Wicklow.[121] For poulticing erysipelas in Donegal, however, it was not a leaf
but the ground-up root that was used as one of several ingredients.[122]

We are not told which part of the plant went into a herbal cocktail drunk
at one time in Ulster for the liver and kidneys,[123] nor which has been
employed in Donegal for liver trouble[124] nor in Cavan for stomach ailments[125]; nor can we be sure what the 'pains' were for which it was valued in
Waterford 'long ago'[126] unless they belonged to that 'any class of sudden pains'
for which a leaf or a stem was dipped in Easter water in Kilkenny[127] and then

rubbed on the part of the body affected. Frustrating in a different way is the failure to specify in which part of Ireland the plant has been used for a sudden stroke[128] or believed to have the yet further property of producing a copious flow of the menses[129] (though that was presumably the basis for the practice in Londonderry of giving rose noble to cows to help clear the afterbirth[130]).

British use of this herb has been very slight by comparison and apparently restricted to the leaves alone: for poulticing skin eruptions, abscesses or ulcers in Devon[131] and wounds in Surrey—as testified by the name 'cut finger leaves' recorded for it there.[132] And it was presumably through its employment for such purposes that the plant earned a name in Welsh that translates as 'good leaf'.[133]

Scrophularia auriculata Linnaeus

S. aquatica of authors

water figwort, water betony

western and southern Europe, north-western Africa, Azores;
    introduced into New Zealand

Though in English counties as far apart as Sussex, Oxfordshire, Leicestershire and Yorkshire[134] *Scrophularia auriculata* has suggestively had the supposedly all-healing betony as one of its local names, it seems doubtful whether it was consistently distinguished for herbal purposes from *S. nodosa*. In Ireland, at any rate, both have passed as 'rose noble',[135] and although in Cornwall[136] and Devon[137] there is a long tradition of singling out *S. auriculata* as a dressing for ulcers (and in Devon for cuts as well), ulcers are one of the ailments for which *S. nodosa* has been recorded in use in that same corner of the country[138]— though maybe uncritically. On the other hand it is expressly the leaves of 'water bitney' that have been sought out in Oxfordshire, a county in which both species are present in quantity, for tying round festering fingers.[139] In the Cambridgeshire Fens, again it was leaves of 'water bitney'—'from the river'— that were used to poultice sore heels and chapped and gathered toes.[140] It thus seems possible that in England, in contrast to Ireland, it was *S. auriculata* that on the whole was the primary recipient of folk attention.

Linaria vulgaris Miller

common toadflax

Europe, western Asia; introduced into North America, Australasia

Only two folk records of *Linaria vulgaris* have been traced, both from southern England: in Sussex it has served as a wart plant[141] and in Gloucestershire it has been mixed with yarrow leaves in a poultice to ease pain, staunch bleeding and induce sleep.[142] Though frequent to common over much of the British Isles at least since the time of William Turner, it tends to occupy only late-created habitats and has the suspect look of a slow-spreading invader from the Continent. That so conspicuous and easily distinguished a plant scarcely features as a folk herb in the British Isles, even though long established in official medicine, adds strength to that suspicion.

Digitalis purpurea Linnaeus
foxglove, fairy fingers, fairy thimble, throatwort, floppy dock;
  lus mór (Irish and Scots Gaelic)
  western Europe, Morocco; introduced into North America,
  Australasia and elsewhere

The story of William Withering's testing of the therapeutic value of the old folk herb *Digitalis purpurea* and its subsequent adoption by official medicine has been recounted many times, particularly in more recent years. Not only was it a landmark in the gradual reawakening to the possible genuineness of many long-derided country remedies, but Withering's ten years of patient experimenting with the plant's properties and his pioneering development of the technique of dose titration have earned him acclaim as the founder of clinical pharmacology. The story, however, often underplays the extent to which species of foxglove had already been recommended for various purposes by earlier writers, including the authors of the most widely read English herbals (though not of the Classical texts[143]). Medieval Irish monks are even known to have valued the plant as a diuretic to cure dropsy, the particular action which caught Withering's attention in 1775,[144] when he was introduced to an old family recipe handed down from that of a Shropshire herb woman and, thanks to his recently acquired expertise as a field botanist, identified which of the score or so ingredients in that 'cocktail' was producing the effect in question. Withering's interest was confined strictly to the plant's diuretic action and its ability to slow the pulse rate, the latter which eventually brought it into general use for treating heart failure. It is now known that about a dozen different glycosides are present in *Digitalis* species but that the content of them varies through the year and in different parts of the plant, the root having the least.

Considering how well known its violent and even fatal action was, it is surprising that foxglove has been used as extensively as it has been in both the written and unwritten traditions, and for a considerable range of ailments. In Scotland the older legal records contain numerous cases of children's deaths caused by drinking an infusion of the plant,[145] and it had a reputation in English villages for causing alarming illnesses if recklessly used for treating colds.[146] In Orkney the observation that foxgloves proved deadly poisonous to geese caused them to be shunned for human remedies entirely.[147]

In Ireland, too, the generality of folk practitioners avoided prescribing the plant for internal use,[148] at any rate latterly (by which time its dangers had probably become more widely known).

Heart troubles feature in the folk records as the single most widespread use, if the British and Irish ones are combined. While it is possible that this usage partly antedates the publicity given to the treatment for that complaint

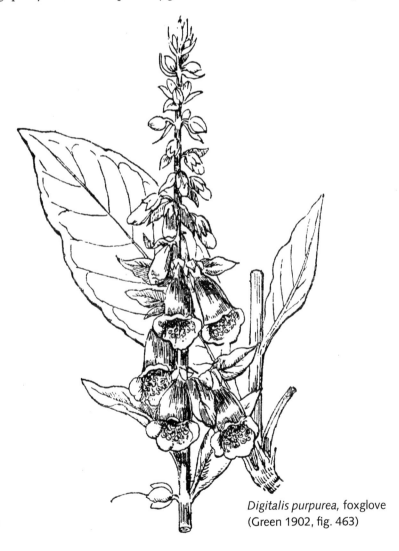

Digitalis purpurea, foxglove
(Green 1902, fig. 463)

stemming from Withering's work, a post-Withering acquisition from learned medicine seems more probable. The very scattered distribution of the folk records traced, in Britain and Ireland alike, lends support to that (just Devon,[149] Shropshire[150] and the Scottish lowlands[151] as far as the British ones are concerned). As a diuretic, though, valued for dropsy or gravel, the plant's credentials as a folk medicine of much longer standing are more convincing, with British records from Oxfordshire,[152] Shropshire,[153] Yorkshire[154] and the Highlands.[155]

In the later herbals, foxglove is recommended as a remedy for tuberculosis pre-eminently, but of its use for that in folk medicine only a single record (an Irish one) has been discovered. The herbals also make much mention of its value for the tubercular condition of the glands known as scrofula, but folk records of that, too, are no less conspicuous by their absence. Instead, the plant seems to have served for the most part as an all-purpose salve: for bruises, especially when festering, in the Isle of Man,[156] to bring boils to a head there, too,[157] and in the Highlands[158] for skin complaints of various kinds as well as in the Isle of Man[159] and Devon,[160] for cuts and wounds in Montgomeryshire,[161] for lumps and swellings in Inverness-shire[162] and for burns and scalds in Eriskay in the Outer Hebrides.[163] In Gloucestershire within living memory, large foxglove leaves have been placed on the breasts to dry up milk at weaning.[164]

A further quite widespread use—though much less in evidence in Britain (Kent (?),[165] Fife[166])—has been for colds, sore throats and fevers. This was the standard function of foxglove tea, though a broth sometimes took the place of that. Some of the sore throats, however, may really have been diphtheria, cases of which in Inverness-shire are known to have been treated with a hot poultice (made from the pulped roots) placed on the neck—a treatment reserved there, too, for 'bad knees' (presumably rheumatism).[167] In the days when fever victims were assailed with purges and emetics a decoction of the foxglove, notorious for the violence of its effects, was found in use for this purpose in the Somerset Levels in the sixteenth century by Matthias de l'Obel [168] and still persisted in that county and Devon nearly three centuries later.[169] To remove pains following a fever, the inhabitants of Skye also at one time found a foxglove poultice useful.[170] But it was presumably because it was seen as dangerous to expose children to its properties too directly that the preferred treatment for those suffering from scarlet fever, at least in Shropshire, was for them to wear the leaves in their shoes for a year.[171]

The compounds which this plant contains not only affect the heart but can powerfully influence the nervous system, too. In Derbyshire, according to

Withering's son, women 'of the poorer class' used to drink large amounts of foxglove tea as a cheap form of intoxication.[172]

A herb so patently poisonous has predictably been deployed against pests as well. In the Forest of Dean in Gloucestershire the practice has survived of boiling the plant to produce a disinfectant wash for the walls of houses, to rid them of insects and the like.[173]

Ireland has shared about the same set of uses in varying degrees. While the plant features in the records more widely there as a remedy for heart trouble, apart from Sligo[174] and Cavan[175] the counties concerned form a noticeable cluster along the eastern coast (Co. Dublin,[176] Wicklow,[177] Wexford[178]), possibly indicative of post-Withering intrusion by learned medicine. As one general practitioner with an experience stretching back many years in the region just south-west of the border never encountered any use for this purpose at all,[179] it may be that those records from Sligo and Cavan are merely recent intrusions, too. Even for use as a diuretic, the sole Irish record traced is from 'Ulster' (unlocalised but probably one or more rural areas[180]), which is one further reason for considering the knowledge of, or at any rate valuing, of these particular actions of the plants to be of no great age in this country.

In Ireland, too, as in Britain, the foxglove has failed to make headway against alternative remedies for tuberculosis (the sole record traced of use for that is a Limerick one[181]), and it is either as an all-purpose salve or as a cough cure that it seems to have featured almost exclusively. In the first of those roles it has been applied to skin complaints in Donegal[182] and Limerick,[183] wounds in Cork,[184] lumps and swellings in Carlow[185] and Wexford,[186] sprains in Kilkenny,[187] burns in Limerick,[188] old ulcers in Londonderry[189] and festering stone-bruises in Donegal.[190] In the second role, as a tea, the plant has outdone Britain, with records from twice as many counties (Monaghan,[191] Mayo,[192] Limerick,[193] Wexford[194]). But only Limerick, once again, has produced an instance of its use as a repellent: pieces of foxglove were there at one time strewn around to kill rats and mice.[195]

Veronica serpyllifolia Linnaeus
thyme-leaved speedwell
Europe, temperate Asia, North Africa, Macaronesia; introduced into
North and South America, New Zealand

(Misidentification suspected) According to one far from reliable source,[196] *Veronica serpyllifolia* is the herb known in Gaelic as *luibh a treatha* and the classic Irish remedy for whooping cough. Confusion with the similarly small-leaved *V. officinalis* seems probable.

Veronica officinalis Linnaeus
heath speedwell
Europe, Asia Minor, Azores, Australia (?), eastern North America;
introduced into New Zealand

John Gerard in his *Herball*[197] described and figured *Veronica officinalis* as the herb long esteemed in Wales for great healing virtues under the name 'fluellen'. That identification may or may not have been correct, but he immediately confused matters by extending that name to the two British species of *Kickxia* (to which it has mainly been applied in books since) and to other members of the genus *Veronica* as well. If he *had* been correct, one would expect numerous Welsh folk uses of this species to have persisted in the folk records down to recent times. However, only a single mention of any speedwell valued there medicinally has been met with: as a cure for piles and impetigo, in some unstated part of the country and without indication of the species.[198]

Although *Veronica officinalis*, as the specific name implies, was the speedwell focused on by official medicine as the possessor of a range of healing properties (and its folk use in Romania for treating stomach ulcers appears to have had its efficacy confirmed as well founded by experiments[199]), it features too rarely in the Scottish and Irish folk records—and seemingly not at all in those for England—to be accepted as a wholly convincing member of the unwritten tradition in the British Isles, as opposed to being a late requisition from book-based lore. That a tea made from this species has been drunk for gouty and rheumatic complaints in Angus[200] is suspiciously similar to a recommendation that appears in books. It is hard to believe that it was really the plant intended by Martin Martin as *betonica Pauli* (a name for *V. officinalis* in the herbals) which he reported accompanied goldenrod and St John's-wort in an ointment made in Skye for treating fractures,[201] for such a use seems at odds with the other claimed virtues of this species.

The Irish evidence is only a little better. That the plant has been employed for colds in one district of Donegal stands safely on the authority of an experienced botanist[202]; in the adjoining county of Londonderry, however, another botanist found the country people mistook germander speedwell for this species, using that for asthma and lung complaints.[203] Another Irish source claims *Veronica* species in general have been used in (unspecified) parts of the country for coughs from chest troubles of all kinds[204]—and *V. officinalis* is the one which in Germany has enjoyed a reputation for pulmonary tuberculosis. But that it was once used in Ireland by nursing mothers for sore nipples is an assertion based merely on a translation of a Gaelic name identified with this species.[205]

Veronica chamaedrys Linnaeus
  germander speedwell, cat's-eye,
    bird's-eye
  Europe, northern and western Asia;
    introduced into North America,
    New Zealand

Veronica chamaedrys has been so particularly mentioned in the folk records as a remedy for two ailments almost exclusively that it seems safe to assume that 'speedwell' is intended for this in instances where just that name is given in either of those connections.

One of those ailments is tired or strained eyes. The records traced of the use of a lotion for that are all from the southern half of England: Cornwall,[206] Somerset,[207] Suffolk[208] and Norfolk.[209] In some areas, this use was apparently so deeply entrenched that the plant was known as 'eyebright',[210] a name normally borne by *Euphrasia* species (with which speedwell was combined in the decoction recorded from Somerset[211]).

In sharp contrast, the records of use for the other ailment, jaundice, are Irish exclusively: Cavan,[212] Longford,[213] Offaly,[214] Wicklow,[215] Tipperary,[216] Limerick[217] and Kerry[218] —mostly around the fringes of the central plain. The leaves and stems in these cases were boiled and the resulting liquid drunk, with milk and sugar sometimes added. According to one Kerry informant, after drinking this twice daily the jaundice will disappear after the ninth day; but if the yellow colour of the skin turns to black, the cure has no effect.[219]

If this was 'cat-eye', the plant has performed the further service in Limerick, pounded and boiled in milk, of healing the 'falling sickness', i.e. epilepsy.[220]

Veronica chamaedrys,
germander speedwell
(Fuchs 1543, fig. 501)

Veronica beccabunga Linnaeus   PLATE 25
brooklime
Europe, temperate Asia, North Africa; introduced into North America
Mainly Irish as a folk herb, *Veronica beccabunga* has shared with *V. officinalis*
a reputation for easing colds and coughs (Wicklow,[221] Limerick,[222] Clare[223])
or as an expectorant (the Belfast area[224]), but in other ways its use has displayed a pattern markedly different from other speedwells. Valued as a
diuretic, it has treated kidney and urinary troubles in 'Ulster',[225] Wicklow[226]
and Clare,[227] while it has served as a 'spring juice' for cleansing the system of
impurities and curing scurvy in Clare[228] and Cork[229] and been applied to
wounds in Londonderry.[230] But the famous eighteenth-century doctress of
Macroom in Co. Cork, Mrs Elizabeth Pearson, whose renowned cure for
scrofula based on this plant made her such a fortune that she was able to buy
a house in the most fashionable part of London,[231] would appear to have
been alone in the folk community in prescribing it for that.

Outside Ireland the use for colds seems to have been reported solely from
the Isle of Man,[232] but the very few British records are, curiously, almost all
either unlocalised or unattributable to a county with certainty. The plant has
been valued for healing 'bad legs' (leg ulcers produced by scurvy?) in Hampshire[233] and perhaps also in Devon,[234] applied to fresh wounds in, probably,
Norfolk,[235] and in at least some part of the country people are said to have
placed the bruised leaves on burns.[236]

Melampyrum pratense Linnaeus
cow-wheat
Europe, western Asia
(Name ambiguity) Conceivably *Melampyrum pratense* was the plant known
as 'golden wheat' recorded as boiled in Cavan for kidney ailments.[237]

Euphrasia officinalis Linnaeus, in the broad sense
eyebright
northern temperate zone; introduced into New Zealand
Euphrasia officinalis seems a unique instance of a well-known and widely
used herb which has apparently been valued in folk medicine for one purpose
only: to remedy eye troubles (of just about every kind short of blindness).
That the mildly astringent juice does act at least as a comforting lotion
appears well attested, though physicians learned to advise against its use
because of its danger if that was done to excess. An ancient remedy, recorded
from much of Europe and almost every part of the British Isles, it normally

took the form of application to the eyes direct, but in Shropshire it has long been customary to trust to the drinking of a tea made from the plant to achieve the same purpose.[238]

Though 'eyebright' has been recorded as a jaundice cure in Cavan,[239] the record in question probably arose through the sharing of that name by ger-

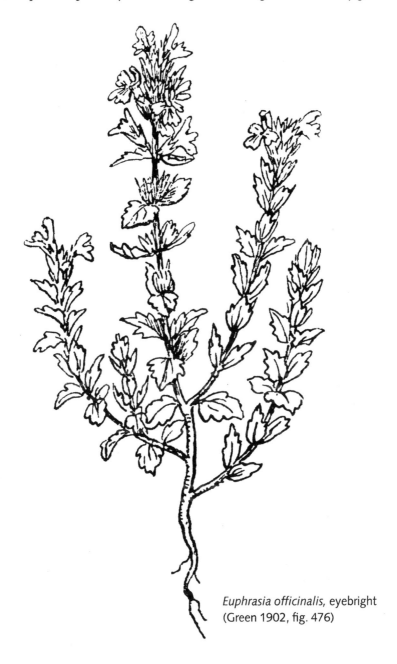

Euphrasia officinalis, eyebright
(Green 1902, fig. 476)

mander speedwell (*Veronica chamaedrys*), a known jaundice herb (including in that county.)

Pedicularis palustris Linnaeus
marsh lousewort, red rattle
northern and central Europe, Caucasus, North America
In the second half of the eighteenth century the Rev. Dr John Walker visited Jura in the course of a fact-finding survey of the Hebrides. A remarkable number of its inhabitants, he found, were crippled for life by a disease allegedly caused by a reddish worm, about an inch in length, which lodged under the skin of the knees or the ankles, causing intense pain. The affliction was known in Gaelic as the *fillan* (under which name cases were recorded from elsewhere in the Hebrides and western Highlands by other early authors). The only known cure as far as he could ascertain was derived from the root of a local plant: pounded and mixed with the marrow of beef bones or goat tallow, this was applied on a hot poultice to the part affected. An experienced botanist who became professor of natural history at Edinburgh University, Walker identified the plant as *Pedicularis palustris*,[240] which is now known to contain a glycoside poisonous to insects. Thomas Pennant, who had had a session with Walker three years before his second Scottish tour in 1772, asked further about the worm when he, too, visited Jura. Pennant was able to add that it was 'small as a thread', caused redness and moved quickly from one part of the body to another; the only cure mentioned to him, however, was a poultice of cheese and honey.[241]

The only other record traced of the plant's use in the British Isles is also from the Highlands, where its flowers are said to have been used to procure a cosmetic.[242]

OROBANCHACEAE

Lathraea squamaria Linnaeus
toothwort
Europe, western Asia
According to John Gerard, country women in England in his day called *Lathraea squamaria* 'lungwort' and used it against 'the cough' (presumably pulmonary tuberculosis) and other lung troubles.[243] No other record has been traced of the plant's presence in folk medicine in either Britain or Ireland.

LENTIBULARIACEAE

Pinguicula vulgaris Linnaeus
common butterwort, bog violet
Europe, northern Asia, Morocco, North America

Repeatedly referred to in the literature, from the eighteenth century onwards, as a folk medicine in use for cattle, the butter-like juice of *Pinguicula vulgaris* had its uses for human afflictions as well. According to John Parkinson, 'the country people that live where it groweth' applied it to hands chapped by the wind ('felons'), while in Wales the poorer sorts of people made it not only into a syrup with which to purge themselves and their children, but also mixed it with butter to produce an ointment rated excellent for obstructions of the liver.[244] Similarly there is a nineteenth-century record, apparently from Kent,[245] of the use of the juice for skin irritations caused by the wind, also of the crushed leaves as a village remedy for bruises. More recently still, an infusion has been drunk in the uplands of Westmoreland in the belief that this helps to procure a smoother skin.[246] Unexpectedly, though this is a widespread plant of bogs, it does not seem to have featured as a folk medicine, at any rate for people, in either Ireland or Scotland.

Notes

1. McNeill
2. Moore 1898
3. Sargent
4. Tongue
5. Shaw, 49
6. Britten & Holland
7. Lafont
8. Lafont
9. Tait
10. Lafont
11. Evans 1940
12. Palmer 1994, 122
13. McNeill
14. Goodrich-Freer, 205
15. Spence; Leask, 75
16. Lafont
17. Vickery MSS
18. Tongue
19. Pratt 1850–7
20. Vickery MSS
21. Randell, 87
22. Beith
23. Williams MS
24. Vickery 1995
25. IFC S 226: 484
26. IFC S 133: 94
27. IFC S 550: 274; 572: 90
28. Goodrich-Freer, 205
29. IFC S 932: 240, 312
30. IFC S 132: 97
31. IFC S 837: 128
32. IFC S 932: 217
33. IFC S 498: 383
34. IFC S 572: 90
35. IFC S 1043: 269
36. IFC S 837: 122
37. IFC S 550: 274
38. IFC S 932: 311

39. Gregory
40. IFC S 837: 125
41. IFC S 484: 219
42. IFC S 572: 69
43. IFC S 752: 223
44. IFC S 736: 190
45. IFC S 690: 114
46. Maloney
47. Maloney
48. Maloney
49. IFC S 857: 118
50. IFC S 571: 208; 572: 298
51. IFC S 22: 509
52. IFC S 485: 237
53. Pennant 1776, ii, 42
54. Spooner, 195
55. Bray, i, 95: Gordon, 184; Lafont
56. Vickery 1995
57. Mabey, 328
58. MacKerlie, 305
59. Pennant 1771, 290
60. Arthur, 42
61. Lafont
62. Dyer 1889, 295
63. Pennant 1776, ii, 43
64. Gibbs
65. Lafont
66. Gibbs
67. IFC S 250: 35
68. IFC S 690: 41
69. IFC S 787: 37
70. IFC S 825: 94
71. IFC S 897: 82
72. IFC S 654: 89
73. IFC S 385: 54
74. IFC S 476: 91
75. Maloney
76. IFC S 385: 54
77. IFC S 736: 22, 24, 171; 746: 554
78. IFC S 787: 216, 219
79. IFC S 771: 149
80. *PLNN*, no. 4 (1988), 14
81. McClafferty
82. IFC S 888: 232
83. Ulster Folk and Transport Museum
    (ex Vickery MSS)
84. Vickery 1995
85. IFC S 689: 103
86. IFC S 862: 376
87. IFC S 737: 405
88. IFC S 787: 215
89. Macpherson MS
90. Wilson
91. IFC S 775: 83
92. Quinlan 1883a
93. A. Allen, 46
94. *Hardwicke's Science-gossip* (1866),
    83
95. Bardswell; Hatfield, 30
96. Newman 1945, 356
97. Egan
98. Moloney
99. Farrelly MS
100. IFC S 737: 480
101. IFC S 413: 205
102. Whitlock 1976, 164
103. Britten & Holland
104. IFC S 1098: 130
105. IFC S 932: 241, 312; 960: 212, 282
106. Maloney
107. IFC S 786: 181, 204; 787: 53, etc.
108. Barbour
109. IFC S 1098: 130
110. Maloney
111. IFC S 710: 42
112. IFC S 654: 242
113. IFC S 850: 166
114. IFC S 654: 290
115. Hart 1898, 385
116. Hart 1898, 385
117. IFC S 190: 167–71
118. IFC S 190: 112
119. IFC S 93: 528
120. IFC S 93: 528
121. IFC S 914: 549
122. McGlinchey, 83
123. Egan
124. IFC S 1098: 130

125. Maloney
126. IFC S 655: 356
127. IFC S 849: 315
128. Ó Súilleabháin, 314
129. Purdon
130. Moore MS
131. Lafont
132. Britten & Holland
133. Johnson 1862
134. Britten & Holland; *PLNN,* no. 56
     (1998), 269
135. Hart 1898, 385
136. Couch, 174; Davey, 325
137. *PLNN,* no. 2 (1988), 3
138. Lafont
139. *PLNN,* no. 2 (1998), 3
140. Marshall 1967, 221
141. A. Allen, 178
142. Ibbott, 64
143. Groves & Bisset
144. Withering 1785
145. Dalyell, 113
146. Pratt 1857, 24
147. Leask, 79
148. Moloney
149. Vickery MSS
150. Hayward
151. Simpson, 159
152. Withering 1785, 9–10
153. Withering 1785, 9–10
154. Withering 1785, 9–10
155. Polson, 32; Beith
156. Fargher
157. Fargher
158. Polson, 32; Beith
159. Fargher; Polson, 34; Beith
160. Lafont
161. Davies 1938
162. Polson, 32; Beith
163. McDonald, 171
164. Hatfield MS
165. Pratt 1857, 24
166. Simpkins, 133
167. Beith

168. de l'Obel, 308
169. Bray, i, 317
170. Martin, 224
171. Vickery 1995
172. Withering 1830
173. Hopkins, 52; Palmer 1994, 122
174. IFC S 157: 253
175. Maloney
176. IFC S 787: 281
177. IFC S 913: 64
178. IFC S 898: 87
179. Logan, 28
180. Egan
181. IFC S 485: 191
182. IFC S 1098: 64
183. IFC S 504: 135
184. IFC S 1128: 26
185. IFC S 907: 176
186. IFC S 897: 234
187. IFC S 850: 114
188. IFC S 491: 255
189. Moore MS
190. McGlinchey, 84
191. IFC S 932: 311
192. IFC S 138: 314
193. IFC S 498: 128
194. IFC S 888: 294
195. IFC S 483: 256
196. Moloney
197. Gerard, 504
198. Jones 1930, 143
199. *Journal of Ethnopharmacology,* 13
     (1985), 157–63
200. Gardiner
201. Martin, 230
202. Hart 1898, 370
203. Moore MS
204. Moloney
205. Moloney
206. Macpherson MS
207. Tongue
208. Chamberlain 1981, 217
209. Hatfield MS
210. Friend 1883–4, ii, 363

211. Tongue
212. IFC S 993: 19
213. *PLNN,* no. 22 (1991), 101
214. IFC S 290: 159
215. McClafferty
216. IFC S 530: 300b
217. IFC S 489: 91; 491: 255; 524: 255
218. IFC S 412: 97; 413: 228
219. IFC S 413: 228
220. IFC S 512: 446
221. Ó Cléirigh
222. IFC S 483: 84
223. IFC S 601: 183
224. Barbour
225. Egan
226. IFC S 921: 90
227. IFC S 617: 334
228. IFC S 617: 334
229. IFC S 385: 56
230. Moore MS
231. 'Ó Clara', 35
232. Fargher
233. Yonge, 226
234. Friend 1882
235. Bryant, 117
236. Johnson 1862
237. Maloney
238. Hayward
239. Maloney
240. McKay, 116, 238
241. Pennant 1774, 215
242. Cameron
243. Gerard, 1388
244. Parkinson, 534
245. Pratt 1850–7
246. Freethy, 128

CHAPTER 14

Bedstraws, Valerian and Scabious

Dicotyledonous flowering plants in the orders (and families) Rubiales (Rubiaceae, bedstraws) and Dipsacales (Caprifoliaceae, honeysuckles; Valerianaceae, valerians; Dipsacaceae, teasels) are included in this chapter.

RUBIACEAE

Galium odoratum (Linnaeus) Scopoli
Asperula odorata Linnaeus
woodruff
Europe, Siberia, North Africa; introduced into North America
Bruising the fresh leaves of *Galium odoratum* and applying them to wounds and cuts was a very common practice of country people in seventeenth-century England[1] and was recorded in use in Norfolk as late as 1911.[2] Otherwise woodruff seems to have featured in folk medicine only as a tea made from the dried leaves and drunk for feverish colds and lung infections—and only in the Highlands, where that function was reflected in its name in Gaelic.[3]

Galium palustre Linnaeus, in the broad sense
marsh bedstraw
Europe, western Asia, North Africa, North America
A plant of muddy streams known as *gairgean* (or *geirgein*) in either South Uist or Eriskay of the Outer Hebrides, of which a preparation has been applied there externally for dropsy, has been identified as *Galium palustre*.[4]

Galium verum Linnaeus
lady's bedstraw
Europe, western Asia; introduced into North America
Though common over much of the British Isles and a herb much in favour in other European countries, especially for its ability to staunch bleeding, *Galium verum* appears to have had no place in folk *medicine* in Britain and Ireland except as a veterinary one. However, its use persists in Berkshire,[5] if not elsewhere, as a deterrent of moths, dried and placed in drawers.

Galium saxatile Linnaeus
heath bedstraw
western and central Europe, Newfoundland
The name *llysiau'r eyr*, shingles plant, reported from Cardiganshire and attributed to woodruff (*Galium odoratum*) in the University of Wales dictionary of the Welsh language, *Geiriadur Prifysgol Cymru*, has been conclusively established as *G. saxatile*: two informants, in Denbighshire and Anglesey, respectively, still using it today for shingles, pointed it out, thus enabling the identification to be clinched by the National Museum of Wales.[6]

    Galium saxatile also features in an Isle of Man list as a remedy used there for nosebleeds,[7] which suggests that it shares the styptic property of lady's bedstraw; alternatively, the record may have been referred to the wrong species.

Galium aparine Linnaeus
cleavers, goosegrass, Robin-run-in-the-hedge, catchweed
Europe, northern and western Asia; introduced into North America
   and elsewhere
The very common *Galium aparine*, largely scorned by learned medicine over the years, has enjoyed an impressively diverse and widely scattered number of uses in its folk counterpart, though none with any particular pre-eminence or marked geographical clustering. Principally it has served as a spring tonic, either on its own or mixed with nettles and/or other plants, with the traditional reputation of herbal tonics of cleansing the system of impurities (Essex,[8] Norfolk,[9] Montgomeryshire[10]) and for skin complaints such as psoriasis (Norfolk[11]). A special use which may belong in that same category is to counteract scurvy. After a Dublin hospital physician had published a note in the *British Medical Journal* in 1883 reporting the beneficial effects of mullein for tuberculosis patients, he received letters from 'several parts' of the British Isles recommending him to test on his patients similarly the claims made for goosegrass as a cure for chronic ulcers.[12] It is unclear whether that knowledge

was derived from the herbals (in which the plant was recommended for this purpose) or folk sources; if the latter, disappointingly little evidence of those has proved traceable, records of that use having been located only from Devon,[13] Norfolk[14] and somewhere in Ulster.[15]

The next most widely reported applications in Britain are for colds (Devon,[16] Dorset (?),[17] Berwickshire[18]) and cuts and wounds (Essex,[19] Nor-

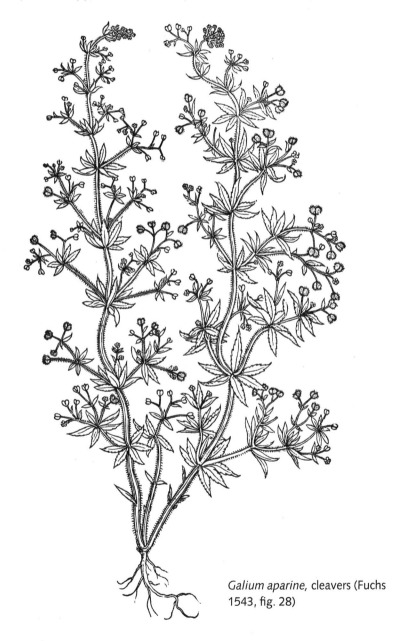

Galium aparine, cleavers (Fuchs 1543, fig. 28)

folk[20]), the second of which in 'some English country districts' unspecified has extended to drinking the juice mixed with wine as a remedy for the bites of adders.[21] Single records only have been met with of applications to cancerous tumours (Devon[22]), boils (Somerset[23]), rheumatism (Essex[24]) and warts (South Riding of Yorkshire[25]).

Ireland's uses have been largely different but even more diverse. While tumours have similarly been among those (Londonderry[26] and some part of the country unspecified[27]), unlike Britain it has produced records for burns (Westmeath,[28] Wicklow[29]), whooping cough (unlocalised[30]), swellings (Wicklow[31]), inflammation of the bowels in children (Donegal[32]), stomach-ache (Limerick[33]) and 'softening the joints' (Tipperary[34]). Though this plant has had a reputation in learned medicine as a diuretic, the sole hint of that traced in the folk record is its mixing with crane's-bill (*Geranium* sp.) in a preparation drunk for kidney trouble in Kerry.[35]

So lengthy a tail of miscellaneous uses with an apparently very restricted distribution is normally characteristic of herbs with a much more salient presence in the folk records. It may be that this species was once much more prominent in that repertory but lost that place over the centuries to other plants whose effectiveness was more readily apparent. An alternative explanation could lie in its strictly seasonal character as a remedy, for it is effective for healing only in the spring; other reputed cures would therefore have had to be resorted to at other seasons.

CAPRIFOLIACEAE

Sambucus nigra Linnaeus
elder
Europe, western Asia, North Africa, Azores; introduced into
    North America
Sambucus nigra rivals only docks, nettles and dandelions in prominence and diversity of use as a folk herb. Some of that it may owe to its former magico-religious status as a tree redolent of special powers, but it does also seem to possess some genuine therapeutic effects.

Of the total of 159 records traced, just under half are accounted for by the four leading uses. Much the commonest of these, with 32 records, is for colds and respiratory troubles (the liquid from the boiled flowers induces sweating and the berries are rich in vitamin C); but whereas that is found mostly in the southern half of England, the 14 records for burns or scalds and the 12 for swellings and inflammation are preponderantly Irish. The 16 for skin sores and related complaints such as erysipelas and ringworm on the other hand exhibit no particular geographical pattern, and the same is true of cuts (8), rheumatism (7), warts (7), boils (6) and use as a cosmetic (6).

The lesser uses are intriguingly diverse but have been much the same in Britain and Ireland. Britain's uses have included treatment for insect bites and stings (Somerset,[36] Norfolk,[37] Isle of Man[38]), nettle stings (Devon,[39]

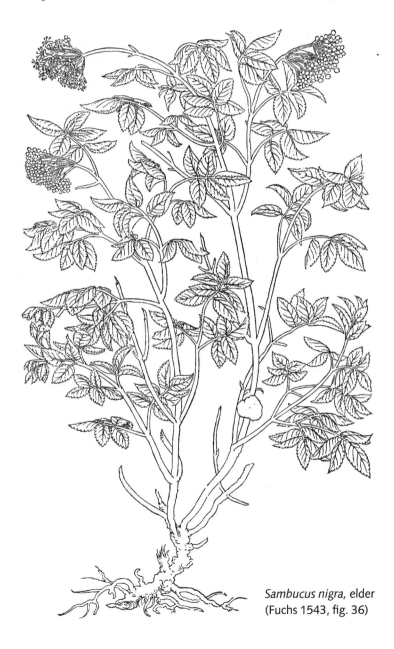

Sambucus nigra, elder
(Fuchs 1543, fig. 36)

Somerset[40]), dropsy and kidney trouble (Cambridgeshire,[41] Berwickshire,[42] Fife[43]), toothache (Devon,[44] 'South Wales',[45] Gloucestershire[46]), gout (Norfolk,[47] Cumbria[48]), sprains (Gloucestershire,[49] Berwickshire[50]), eye troubles (Hampshire,[51] Orkney[52]), constipation (Devon,[53] the Highlands[54]), jaundice (Herefordshire[55]), measles (Suffolk[56]), tonsillitis (Devon[57]) and piles (Sussex[58]). A wine made from the flowers has also been widely drunk as prophylaxis in Gloucestershire and Buckinghamshire, and in the former's Forest of Dean is remembered as a cure-all which was taken for a day or two before calling a medical practitioner—for if it failed to clear up the trouble in question, then it could only be that something serious was afoot.[59]

Ireland has yielded records from up to three counties for all the above ailments in the list above except insect bites, sprains, constipation, measles, tonsillitis and piles. Epilepsy (Cavan,[60] Cork[61]) and indigestion (Sligo,[62] Carlow[63]) are the only two noted that are additional.

Sambucus ebulus Linnaeus
dwarf elder
central and southern Europe, western Asia; introduced into North
  America, Madeira

(Folk credentials questionable) Much rarer than *Sambucus nigra* and reputedly with similar but stronger properties, *S. ebulus* does not appear to set good seed in the British Isles, depending for its persistence on adventitious shoots. It presumably therefore owes its presence where it occurs in the British Isles to deliberate introduction, though it is possible that it was fertile at some hotter period in the past. The name danewort long applied to it in many places and an apparent association with prehistoric sites have occasioned frequent suggestions in the literature that it was brought across from the European mainland by one or more waves of early invaders for some specific utilitarian purpose. According to John Parkinson,[64] though, it owes that name merely to its strong purging effect: those who took it medicinally were spoken of as 'troubled with the Danes'. Certainly it was a herb well known to the Romans and the Anglo-Saxons and consequently recommended in herbals.

Curiously, although the populations of the plant in Berkshire are on record as having been heavily raided by herb collectors early in the nineteenth century (on account of its popularity for treating dropsy),[65] the only records traced of actual folk uses are from remote areas where it must always have been extremely scarce or even non-existent in the wild. In Aberdeenshire it was noted by James Robertson on his 1768 tour as in use for plasters for dispelling tumours,[66] and in Londonderry—the sole Irish record—it was allegedly sometimes employed for dropsy and rheumatic pains in the early nineteenth century.[67] All the evidence seems to indicate that this was late, book-derived medicine.

Viburnum lantana Linnaeus
wayfaring-tree
central and southern Europe, northern Asia Minor, north-western
    Africa; introduced into North America

There is one Suffolk record of the leaves of *Viburnum lantana* being used for making 'an excellent gargle'.[68]

Lonicera periclymenum Linnaeus
honeysuckle
western and central Europe, Morocco; introduced into
    North America

In a somewhat ambiguous statement, probably rightly interpreted by a later author[69] as referring to 'the common people' of England, John Parkinson[70] poured scorn on a deep-rooted practice of employing the leaves and flowers of *Lonicera periclymenum* for gargles and for lotions for inflammations of the mouth or 'the privy parts of men and women'. By these he clearly meant that fungus infection known as thrush, which most characteristically attacks the lining of the mouth and tongue, especially in infants, or the vagina, especially in pregnancy. And this is in fact the ailment which features in the folk records as the one for which honeysuckle has, by a small margin, been most widely used—though those records are Irish exclusively (from Sligo,[71] the Aran Islands,[72] Wicklow[73] and Wexford,[74] on the assumption that 'sore mouth' in two of those counties refers to this; on the other hand 'a cold broken out on the lips', recorded from Monaghan,[75] sounds more like herpes).

Some of the other uses recorded in Ireland echo those of the elder tree: jaundice in Cavan[76] and (especially) Leitrim,[77] consumption or whooping cough—mixed with other herbs—in Wicklow[78] and Cork,[79] burns in Louth[80] and erysipelas in Donegal.[81]

The many fewer British records are partly for similar complaints: asthma and/or bronchitis in Norfolk[82] and the Highlands[83] is clearly similar to the Irish remedy for coughs, and an infusion drunk to cure a headache in those same two areas[84] is no doubt cognate; but the same cannot be said of the emergency remedy for adder bites in Devon,[85] the cure for stings in Hampshire[86] or the wash for removing freckles or soothing sunburn known from the Highlands.[87]

Lonicera caprifolium Linnaeus
goat-leaf honeysuckle
central and southern Europe, Asia Minor; introduced into western
Europe, North America

In parts of southern Devon the blossoms of the non-native *Lonicera capri-folium* have been drunk as an infusion for asthma,[88] evidently as an alternative to those of *L. periclymenum*. But they are more likely to have been obtained from gardens than from naturalised bushes.

VALERIANACEAE

Valeriana officinalis Linnaeus
valerian
most of Europe, temperate Asia; introduced into North America

Though the roots of the common valerian, *Valeriana officinalis,* have been valued as the source of a nerve relaxant since ancient times and an extract has become fashionable in alternative medicine as a sedative, no undoubted folk records of the plant's use for that purpose have been traced. Nor does William Withering's[89] recommendation of it as a laxative find any reflection in them either—other than for cows in the Hebrides.[90] Similarly, its reputation today of reducing the ill effects of alcohol appears to have no parallel in folk medicine.

As a folk herb, *Valeriana officinalis* has principally fulfilled two quite other functions in the British Isles: as yet another tonic to stimulate and cleanse the system (Suffolk,[91] Gloucestershire[92]) and to staunch bleeding from wounds and other cuts (Sussex[93]) or heal a festering finger (Wiltshire,[94] Gloucestershire[95]). In Wiltshire the marsh valerian, *V. dioica* Linnaeus, has also been recorded as bearing the name cut-finger-leaf, but doubtless the two species have passed as one and the same in the eyes of country people. A slight variant of that name borne in Hampshire[96] by a plant whose leaves have been used there for binding wounds has been attributed, however, rightly or wrongly, to the garden valerian or 'setwall', *V. pyrenaica* Linnaeus. That attribution may have been influenced by the passage John Gerard has about 'set-wall' in his *Herball*[97]:

The dry roote . . . is put into counterpoisons and medicines preservative against the pestilence . . . ; whereupon it hath beene had (and is to this day among the poore people of our northerne parts) in such veneration among them, that no brothes, pottage, or physicall meates are worth anything, if setwall were not at one end: whereupon some woman poet or other hath made these verses:

They that will have their heale
Must put setwall in their keale.

It is used in slight cuts, wounds, and small hurts.

Valeriana pyrenaica lingers on as a naturalised plant in northern country areas, and it seems likely that following its introduction into the British Isles it partly displaced *V. officinalis* as a wound plant.

One or two minor uses of *Valeriana officinalis* have been recorded in Britain in addition: for indigestion in Skye and South Uist in the Inner Hebrides[98] and for barrenness in the Highlands.[99] Though said to have been held in high repute in Wales at one time for its healing as well as magical powers,[100] no more specific Welsh records have been traced. Maybe that was one of 'the countries of this land' that Parkinson had in mind in reporting that this plant was generally called 'the poor man's remedy'; a decoction of its root drunk if cold after sweating, troubled with colic or wind or 'otherwise distempered', or its leaves bruised and applied to a cut or to draw out a thorn or splinter.[101]

Irish records are far fewer and have been traced only from the north: in Donegal[102] and Londonderry[103] for cleansing the system and in Londonderry as a wound plant—both as in Britain—but in Cavan[104] for such unrelated purposes as sore eyes, liver trouble and tuberculosis.

DIPSACACEAE

Dipsacus fullonum Linnaeus   PLATE 26
  wild teasel
  Europe, south-western Asia, North Africa, Canary Islands
  According to a deep-seated folk belief going back at least to Pliny the Elder, the rain-water or dew collecting in the natural cup between the connate leaves of *Dipsacus fullonum* (known as the 'bath of Venus' or the 'lip of Venus') had certain healing properties. Sundew and lady's-mantle, similarly endowed with droplets of moisture of mysterious origin, were treated with special respect for much the same reason. Teasel's version of 'holy water' was thought particularly beneficial when used as an eye lotion (Somerset,[105] Sussex,[106] Denbighshire[107]) but it is also recorded as used in Wales for ridding the complexion of freckles.[108]

The heads of the plant were formerly in demand as well in 'various parts of England'[109] (and sold in London in Covent Garden market[110]) as a certain cure for the ague. Three, five or seven—note the magical odd numbers—of the thin 'worms' found in these in the autumn were sealed up in a quill or a bag and worn against the pit of the stomach or some other part of the person. More mundane than those two uses was boiling the root and applying it to abscesses (in Suffolk[111]) or to warts (in Wiltshire[112]). The absence of records from Scotland or Ireland is noteworthy.

Knautia arvensis (Linnaeus) Coulter
Scabiosa arvensis Linnaeus
   field scabious
   Europe, western Siberia

Two records of the use of 'scabious' in Essex, as an infusion for rheumatism[113] and as a decoction sat over to cure piles,[114] seem more likely to belong to *Knautia arvensis* than *Succisa pratensis* on distributional grounds.

Succisa pratensis Moench
Scabiosa succisa Linnaeus
   devil's-bit scabious
   Europe, western Siberia, North Africa

A common plant of the acid soils of the west of the British Isles, *Succisa pratensis* has been widely valued there for the properties of its root. At least part of this use may have been magico-religious, for the peculiarly truncated shape of the root is supposed to have suggested the notion that this was the product of some malign influence (hence the vernacular name), for which reason it was recommended for the scaly eruptions known as 'devils' bites'. It was still in use precisely for those in the Rossendale Valley in south-eastern Lancashire well into the nineteenth century,[115] doubtless by those who took the herbals as gospel.

It is tempting to ascribe to that same superstition the reserving of this plant in Somerset specifically for bites by dogs—but in fact it has a seemingly well-founded reputation as an antiseptic. The wound caused by those bites was bathed with water in which devil's-bit had been steeped, then covered with the leaves to check the bleeding and initiate healing.[116] The plant has accordingly been favoured for sores of all kinds, of which British examples include sore throats[117] and bruises[118] in the Isle of Man and, if the use for scurvy reported from there is correctly interpreted, scorbutic sores in Shetland.[119] 'The itch', which this plant has relieved in the Highlands,[120] must surely have been scabies (hence 'scabious'), too. If devil's-bit also has an aspirin-like effect, that could explain its use for rheumatism in the Isle of Man[121] and for toothache in the Highlands,[122] afflictions which were perhaps among the 'all manner of ailments' this plant is said to have been employed against in Cornwall.[123]

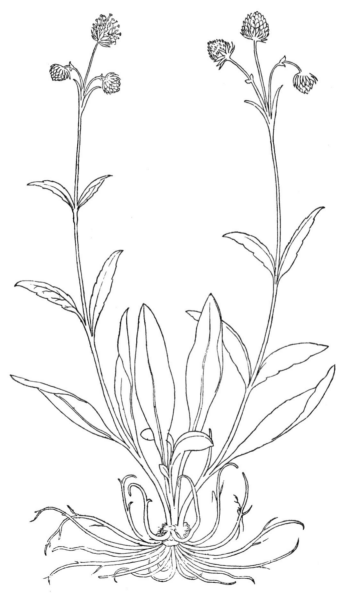

Succisa pratensis, devil's-bit scabious (Fuchs 1543, fig. 408)

The Irish uses have shared the same dominant theme: 'sores such as boils' in Mayo[124] and—assuming this was *meena madar*, 'a nice little blue flower'—running sores on the Clare-Galway border.[125] If the 'evil' it helped to assuage in Sligo[126] was a reference to the king's evil, i.e. scrofula (tuberculosis of the glands), then that belongs in that category, too.

Notes

1. Parkinson, 563
2. Bardswell
3. Cameron; Beith
4. McDonald, 134; Goodrich-Freer, 206
5. Vickery 1995
6. Williams MS
7. Fargher
8. Hatfield, 56
9. Harland; Hatfield 56, 87
10. Evans 1940
11. Hatfield, 88
12. Quinlan 1883b
13. Lafont
14. Hatfield, 77, 88
15. Hatfield MS
16. Lafont
17. Quelch, 64
18. Johnston 1853
19. Hatfield, 33, 88
20. Hatfield, appendix
21. Hole, 12
22. Lafont
23. Tongue
24. Newman & Wilson
25. CECTL MSS
26. Hart 1898, 384
27. Moloney
28. IFC S 747: 187
29. McClafferty
30. Wright, 252; Ó hEithir MS
31. IFC S 914: 322
32. Hart 1898, 379
33. IFC S 482: 357
34. IFC S 550: 282
35. IFC S 412: 96
36. Tongue
37. Hatfield MS
38. Moore 1898
39. Vickery MSS; Lafont
40. Tongue
41. Porter 1969, 80
42. Johnston 1853
43. Vickery MSS
44. Lafont
45. Trevelyan, 315
46. Gibbs, 57
47. Wigby, 65; Hatfield, appendix
48. Freethy, 79
49. Vickery MSS
50. Johnston 1853
51. Yonge, 218
52. Leask, 72
53. Lafont
54. Beith
55. Leather, 80
56. *Folk-lore*, 35 (1924), 356; Jobson 1959, 144
57. Lafont
58. Vickery 1995
59. *PLNN*, no. 37 (1994), 181–2
60. Maloney
61. IFC S 385: 55
62. IFC S 170: 256
63. IFC S 907: 208
64. Parkinson, 210
65. Lousley
66. Henderson & Dickson, 155
67. Moore MS
68. Chamberlain 1981, 253

69. Deering, 46
70. Parkinson, 1461
71. IFC S 170: 256
72. Ó hEithir
73. McClafferty
74. IFC S 876: 240
75. IFC S 932: 240
76. IFC S 800: 122; 992: 29
77. IFC S 190: 167, 168, 170
78. McClafferty
79. IFC S 385: 286
80. IFC S 672: 210
81. McGlinchey, 83
82. Hatfield, appendix
83. Beith
84. Hatfield, 39; Beith
85. Lafont
86. Eyre, 75
87. Beith
88. Lafont
89. Withering 1787–92, 21
90. McDonald, 248
91. Chamberlain 1981, 203
92. Palmer 1994, 122
93. Vickery 1995
94. Dartnell & Goddard, 39
95. Vickery 1995; Wright, 246
96. Wright, 243
97. Gerard, 919
98. McDonald, 248

99. Carmichael, iv, 203
100. Trevelyan
101. Parkinson, 124
102. Hart 1898, 380
103. Moore MS
104. Maloney
105. Vickery 1995
106. Latham, 45
107. Mabey, 353
108. Trevelyan
109. Dyer 1880, 21
110. Cullum MS
111. Jobson 1959, 144
112. Whitlock 1976, 164
113. Newman & Wilson
114. Hatfield, 43, appendix
115. *Notes and Queries,* ser. 9, 4 (1899),
      98
116. Tongue
117. Paton
118. Moore 1898
119. Jamieson
120. Beith
121. Fargher
122. Pennant 1776, ii, 43
123. Deane & Shaw
124. IFC S 138: 465
125. Gregory
126. IFC S 171: 53

CHAPTER 15

Daisies

Dicotyledonous flowering plants in the order Asterales and family Asteraceae (thistles, daisies and the like) are included in this chapter.

ASTERACEAE

Carlina vulgaris Linnaeus
carline thistle
Europe, Asia Minor, Siberia; introduced into North America
In Limerick a preparation from *Carlina vulgaris* has been rubbed into the skin for a disease described as spreading over the body.[1]

Arctium Linnaeus
burdock, cockle; crádán (Ireland); *meac-an-dogh* (Highlands and Western Isles); *bollan-dhoo* (Manx)
Europe, Caucasus, North Africa; introduced into North America, Australasia
Arctium is another example of a well-known and widely popular herb— strictly speaking herbs, for more than one species is involved—with one principal use and an impressive diversity of other subsidiary ones as well. That principal one, mainly via a decoction of the roots, has been and still is as a forceful cleanser of the system and consequent eliminator of boils and skin complaints. In that it resembles sarsaparilla, the tropical drug to which burdock was even rated superior by some eighteenth-century physicians, according to William Withering. Unexpectedly, though—if the records traced accurately reflect its distribution—that use has been restricted in Britain just to extreme south-western England (Cornwall,[2] Devon[3]) and parts of Scotland

(Berwickshire,[4] Colonsay in the Inner Hebrides[5]) together with the Isle of Man,[6] a pattern suggestive of overspills from Ireland, where the use has been markedly widespread (see below). Though it might be supposed that cleansing the system has extended to treating rheumatic complaints, as has been the case with some other herbs, the very different distribution of records for those (Montgomeryshire,[7] Suffolk,[8] East Riding of Yorkshire [9]) lends no support to such an assumption. Nor is there any apparent connection, similarly,

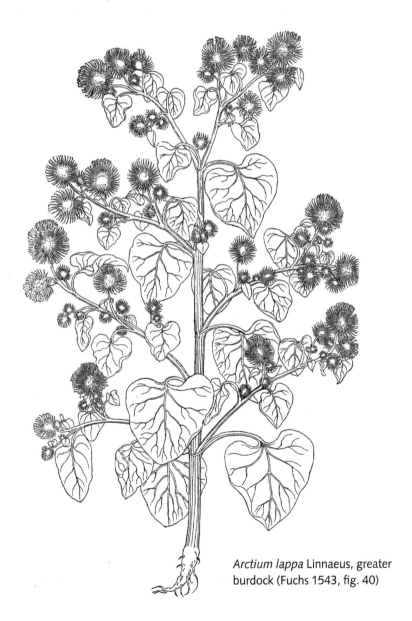

Arctium lappa Linnaeus, greater burdock (Fuchs 1543, fig. 40)

between any of the other uses of burdock recorded from Britain: for jaundice (South Uist in the Outer Hebrides[10]), urinary complaints (Berwickshire[11]), inflammatory tumours ('much in use amongst the country people' for those, according to John Quincy in 1718[12]), allaying nervousness (Isle of Man[13]) and, by application of a poultice of the bruised leaves to the soles of the feet, such other conditions as epilepsy, hysteria and convulsions (the 'west of England'[14] and other (?) unspecified rural areas[15]).

   In Ireland the plant's predominance as a cleansing herb has been particularly pronounced, with a bunching of records in Leinster. Otherwise, as in Britain, its applications have been very various and some of them different ones: for instance, for burns (Meath,[16] Wicklow[17]), cuts (Cavan[18]), flatulence (Donegal[19]) and to poultice boils (Sligo[20]). An ancient Irish remedy for scrofula,[21] the glandular swellings it has more recently been deployed against,[22] may be the same as Quincy's inflammatory tumours, however. And Ireland has shared with Britain that same special cure for convulsions (Louth[23]) as well as the uses for nervousness (Meath[24]), jaundice (Donegal[25]), rheumatism (Londonderry,[26] Cavan,[27] Limerick[28]), colds and respiratory trouble (Cavan,[29] Mayo[30]) and, as a powerful diuretic, dropsy and kidney and urinary complaints (Ulster,[31] Cavan,[32] Wicklow[33]).

Cirsium arvense (Linnaeus) Scopoli
creeping thistle
Eurasia, North Africa; introduced into North America, Australasia

Silybum marianum (Linnaeus) Gaertner   PLATE 27
milk thistle, blessed thistle, lady's thistle, speckled thistle
southern Europe, south-western Asia, North Africa; introduced into
   western and central Europe, North and South America, Australasia
Because of the vagueness with which the name thistle has been applied in folk medicine, it is difficult in most cases to be at all sure to which particular species any one record relates. Any valued for a milky juice applied as a wart cure (sometimes known as 'milk thistle', 'soft thistle' or 'soft white thistle') is almost certainly one of the sow-thistles (*Sonchus* spp.), and all records for that use are therefore listed under that genus. One or more other kinds seem to have been well known as a specific for whooping cough, boiled in new milk, just in one tight group of counties in the north-eastern corner of what is now the Irish Republic: Cavan,[34] Monaghan[35] and above all Louth.[36] Though recorded under some names which could refer to various species, such as 'larger kind of thistle', 'white thistle', 'crisp thistle' and 'bracket thistle',

others—'blessed thistle', 'lady's thistle' and 'speckled thistle'—are indicative of *Silybum marianum*, even though that is quite rare in Ireland and certainly introduced. If that identification is correct, possibly the sole source of it for herbal medicine was cottage gardens, in which case these records do not rightly belong in this book. 'Blessed thistle' has also been used for loss of appetite in Meath.[37] That name originally referred in learned medicine to the southern European *Cnicus benedictus* Linnaeus, also known as 'holy this-tle', which was recommended in herbals for colds. That could account for a record from Cavan[38] of 'holly thistle' as a cure for those.

That leaves a residue of records which may belong to one or more of the very common wild, purple-flowered thistles such as *Cirsium arvense* and *C. vulgare* (Savi) Tenore. The 'Scotch thistle' or 'bull thistle' still employed for kidney infection in Donegal[39] is presumably one of those. But the identity of the species employed as a wound plant in Co. Dublin[40] and Limerick[41] is quite uncertain, and the same applies to the one whose tops, mixed with plan-tain and sorrel, have yielded a juice drunk for tuberculosis in Kildare.[42]

Whatever their identity, records for true thistles thus seem to be Irish almost exclusively. The sole exception is a thistle tea drunk in the Highlands to dispel depression.[43]

Serratula tinctoria Linnaeus
saw-wort
northern and central Europe, Siberia, Algeria; introduced into
    North America
There is just one record, from Sussex, for *Serratula tinctoria* as a wound plant.[44] The species is still locally frequent in that county and thus plentiful enough to be utilised herbally.

Centaurea cyanus Linnaeus
cornflower, bluebottle
south-eastern Europe; introduced into the rest of Europe, south-
    western Asia, North Africa, North America, Australasia
There is an apparently long-standing East Anglian tradition of collecting the heads of the once common cornfield weed *Centaurea cyanus*, bruising and distilling them in water, and dropping the liquid into the eyes, to cure them of inflammation or merely clear those of the elderly enough to make wearing glasses unnecessary (hence 'break spectacles water'). There is a recipe to this effect in a late seventeenth-century Suffolk household book which has sur-vived in a Norwich church.[45] The practice is referred to rather grudgingly by

John Gerard[46] and, though mentioned in at least one later herbal, seems more likely to have been a folk use adopted by official medicine than *vice versa*. Lending support to that is a twentieth-century Essex record of boiling the flowers with chamomile heads and applying the mixture as a compress to tired eyes.[47]

Centaurea nigra Linnaeus
common knapweed, hardheads; blackheads, blackbuttons
(Ireland)
western Europe; introduced into North America, Australasia

As a medicinal herb almost exclusively Irish, the common *Centaurea nigra* has been used in that country principally for jaundice and liver trouble (Ulster,[48] Cavan,[49] Offaly,[50] Laois,[51] Wicklow[52]), the decoction of its roots in milk rivalling dandelion as a treatment for that. That it has also been valued as a cleansing tonic is suggested by its reputation for removing boils in Limerick[53] and—significantly, if drunk in a mixture with burdock—for curing scurvy in Wicklow.[54] On the Clare-Galway border the same preparation has been drunk for 'pains in the bones' (presumably rheumatism or osteoarthritis),[55] while in Donegal a much-favoured remedy locally for 'the decline' (presumably tuberculosis) was seven stalks of this, seven of 'fairy lint' (purging flax, *Linum catharticum*) and seven of maidenhair, pounded together and mixed with seven noggins of water drawn from a place where three streams meet[56]; it may well also be the 'buttonweed' of which an infusion has been drunk in Kerry for asthma.[57] It is possible that more Irish records are hidden within the numerous ones for plantain, for both that and knapweed have been known as 'blackheads' in Co. Dublin,[58] Donegal[59] and no doubt other counties, too.

The only British use recorded that is certainly the same as any of the Irish ones is a reputation for boils in Montgomeryshire[60]; this plant may, how-

Centaurea nigra, common knapweed (Green 1902, fig. 354)

ever, be the 'horse knaps' that has found favour for rheumatism in Furness.[61] Peculiar to Essex, apparently, is an infusion drunk as a digestive.[62] In the Isle of Man the one-time name *lus-y-cramman-dhoo* hints at a medicinal use but what that was has never been ascertained.[63]

Lapsana communis Linnaeus
nipplewort
Europe, western and central Asia, North Africa; introduced into
North America, Australasia

Under Gaelic names translating as 'good leaf' and 'breast leaf', *Lapsana communis* has had the special function in the Highlands of allaying the soreness of the nipples of nursing mothers[64] (a function alleged to have been performed in Ireland by heath speedwell, *Veronica officinalis*[65]). This may also have been the purpose left undisclosed—on grounds of delicacy?—by the mid-nineteenth-century author who knew the plant featured at that time in village medicine in 'parts of England'.[66] Yet the fact that John Parkinson was led to coin the name nipplewort only on learning of its use for this same particular purpose in Prussia[67] seems to suggest that it had no vernacular name in English before that, which suggests in turn that the use may merely have been a late infiltration into the folk repertory of Britain.

That in Ireland *Lapsana communis* has apparently been recorded only as an application to cuts, bruises or burns (Wexford,[68] Tipperary[69]) could be evidence in support of that possibility. On the other hand, a use for the breast may well not have been revealed to the male or child enquirers responsible for most of the Irish folk records.

Hypochaeris maculata Linnaeus
spotted cat's-ear
northern and central Europe

In one district in the Yorkshire Pennines in the eighteenth century, *Hypochaeris maculata* was believed a cure for 'tetters' and other skin complaints—because of its spotted leaves, it has been (perhaps fancifully) suggested.[70]

Sonchus arvensis Linnaeus
perennial sow-thistle
Europe, western Asia; introduced into other continents

Sonchus asper (Linnaeus) Hill
prickly sow-thistle
cosmopolitan

Sonchus oleraceus Linnaeus
smooth sow-thistle
cosmopolitan

Sonchus arvensis, S. asper and *S. oleraceus,* three common weeds of cultivation, have doubtless not been differentiated in folk medicine, the only record of herbal use attributable to one of them specifically being the result of a Lincolnshire user pointing out *S. arvensis* to a botanist.[71] Probably all three share much the same properties, in particular the white juice that has given rise to the names 'milkweed', 'milkwort' and 'milk thistle' in England and Ireland alike and been widely applied to warts in both countries. In Wales, however, where the plants' association with pigs seems to have been particularly strong, with even a magical tinge, they are said to have been reserved for applying to

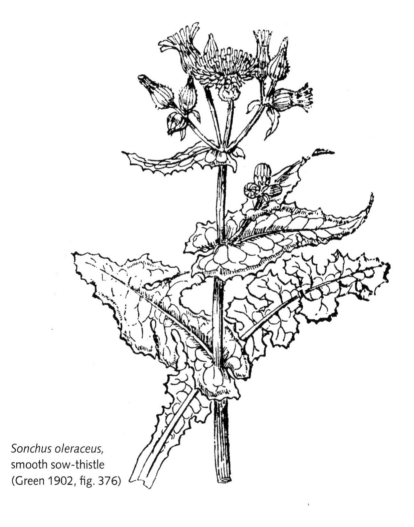

Sonchus oleraceus,
smooth sow-thistle
(Green 1902, fig. 376)

a gash made by the hoof or teeth of a hog.[72] Also, to the seventeenth-century English antiquarian John Aubrey we owe an unlocalised record of the use of the heads for relieving cramp.[73]

The Irish records have yielded only one additional use: for burns in Westmeath.[74]

Mycelis muralis (Linnaeus) Dumortier
wall lettuce
Europe, Asia Minor, north-western Africa; introduced into North
America, New Zealand
According to the Dublin botanist Caleb Threlkeld, writing in 1726, 'the poor people' in Ireland boiled *Mycelis muralis* in a posset to take against fevers.

Taraxacum officinale Weber, in the broad sense
dandelion
Eurasia; introduced into North America, Australasia
Vying with elder and nettles as the wild plant drawn on most widely and heavily in the British Isles for folk medicine, dandelion also rivals the docks in the extent to which it is used and known for one purpose in particular: in this case for promoting the flow of urine and thus assisting kidney and associated troubles in general. Renowned all over Europe for that diuretic effect, *Taraxacum officinale* features in the folk records too near-universally for logging of those in terms of individual counties to serve any useful purpose.

Even with that group of ailments set aside, there still remain 333 British and Irish records traced for dandelion's numerous other uses. Chief among those, by a big margin, accounting for almost exactly one-quarter of that total, is the plant's application to warts, a practice known from most parts of both countries. After that in popularity of use come coughs, colds and respiratory troubles (55 records). All the remaining leading uses are mainly or wholly Irish except for the plant's service as a tonic to 'cleanse the blood' and purge the system of skin complaints and boils; the combined total of 38 records for that include several from southern English counties and parts of Scotland. Britain's share of the large number of minor applications is also markedly smaller than Ireland's. These include indigestion in Dorset[75] and Essex,[76] corns in Devon,[77] stings in Somerset,[78] scarlet fever in Leicestershire,[79] lip cancer in Norfolk,[80] ulcers in Argyllshire[81] and internal pains in general in the Highlands.[82]

Ireland's use of the dandelion has been markedly more diverse than Britain's. The two countries' combined total of 55 records for coughs, colds ·

and respiratory troubles includes a large number for 'consumption', all 25 for the last of these Irish. If the British and Irish records for application to liver trouble (24) and jaundice (22) are added together, those constitute the fourth largest ailment overall—and the majority of them are Irish. So are most of those for use as a cleansing tonic (38 records jointly), for stomach pains or upsets (24) and for rheumatism (19). Heart trouble, however, seems an exclusively Irish affliction as far as the use of dandelion is concerned, and the 21 records are noticeably numerous along the western coast from Leitrim to Limerick. Finally, in the long 'tail' of much more minor applications, normal in the case of most widely used folk herbs, Ireland appears to have had a monopoly with regard to cuts (Cavan,[83] Wicklow,[84] Limerick,[85] Kerry[86]), nervousness (Cavan,[87] Wicklow,[88] Limerick[89]), thrush (Co. Dublin,[90] Carlow,[91] Limerick[92]), sprains and swellings (Kildare,[93] Limerick[94]), weak or broken bones (Limerick,[95] Kerry[96]), headaches (Cavan,[97] Limerick[98]), diabetes (Kilkenny[99]), sore eyes (Roscommon[100]), external cancers (Carlow[101]), anaemia (specific record untraced[102]) and—the ultimate cure—'every disease' (Tipperary[103]). Rather curiously, the only ones with Irish records to complement British ones are for indigestion (Donegal,[104] Carlow[105]) and corns (Co. Dublin[106]). Uniquely Irish also is the wide reputation dandelions are said to have once enjoyed in parts of the country for easing toothache, allegedly because their much-toothed leaves were held to be a signature.[107] Another belief associated with the leaves, recorded from Limerick, was that to be effective as a tonic those with a white vein had to be eaten by a man and those with a red one by a woman.[108]

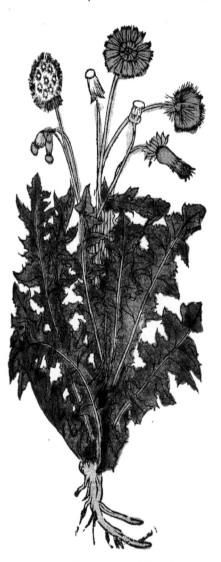

Taraxacum officinale, dandelion (Bock 1556, p. 100)

Pilosella officinarum F. W. Schultz & Schultz 'Bipontinus'
Hieracium pilosella Linnaeus
mouse-ear hawkweed
temperate and subarctic Europe, western Asia; introduced into
North America, New Zealand
Usually known simply as 'mouse-ear' and a cause of the misattribution of
records to mouse-ear chickweed (*Cerastium* spp.) or forget-me-not (the
generic name of which, *Myosotis*, has the same meaning), *Pilosella offici-*

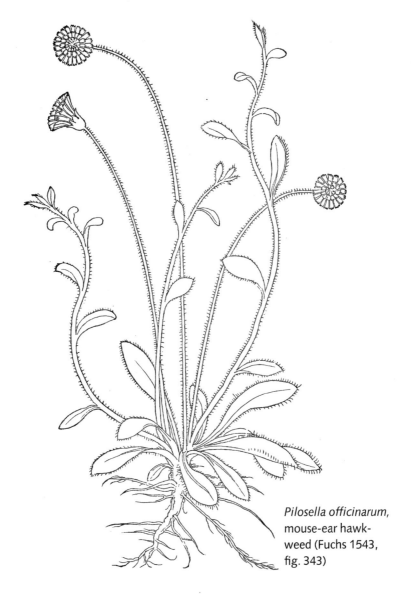

*Pilosella officinarum,
mouse-ear hawk-
weed (Fuchs 1543,
fig. 343)*

narum has been a widely favoured herb for coughs, especially whooping cough, and throat infections in parts of England (Hampshire,[109] Kent,[110] Suffolk,[111] Staffordshire[112]) and the Isle of Man.[113] A specially Manx herb, it has been used in that island, too, as a diuretic[114] as well as to 'draw' splinters and promote 'healing pus'.[115] The name 'felon herb' recorded in Cornwall[116] hints at one further use.

Almost all those have been Irish uses also: for whooping cough in Meath[117] and Limerick,[118] for urinary trouble in Roscommon,[119] Westmeath[120] and Wicklow,[121] and as a salve for burns (Wicklow[122]), whitlows (Meath[123]) and other sores (Cavan[124]).

The concentration of records in the Isle of Man and the Irish counties on either side of Dublin may possibly have some significance.

Hieracium Linnaeus
hawkweed
mainly arctic, alpine and temperate regions of the northern
hemisphere; introduced into New Zealand

As *Pilosella officinarum* seems to have been known in general as 'mouse-ear', without the addition of 'hawkweed' so favoured by book authors, it can probably be safely taken that the plant recorded under the latter name as in use in 'Ireland' (part unspecified) as a jaundice remedy[125] was one or more of the numerous asexual microspecies of *Hieracium*. That the complaint is not among the folk uses traced for mouse-ear adds strength to that assumption.

Filago vulgaris Lamarck
F. germanica Linnaeus, not Hudson
common cudweed
central and southern Europe, western Asia, North Africa, Canary
Islands; introduced into North America, New Zealand

Anaphalis margaritacea (Linnaeus) Bentham
American cudweed, pearly everlasting
North America; introduced into Europe

Under the name *Centunculus* (a generic name long used by botanists for the minuscule plant now called *Anagallis minima* (Linnaeus) E. H. L. Krause), William Turner described a herb 'thought to be good for chafinge of anye man's flesh with goynge or rydinge', for which reason it was known in his native Northumberland, he wrote, as 'Chaf[e]weed' and in Yorkshire as 'cudweed'.[126] Though some authors[127] have argued that he must have been referring to heath cudweed (*Gnaphalium sylvaticum* Linnaeus), as he separately

CHAPTER 15 Daisies **291**

mentioned the species now known as *Filago vulgaris* under a different name, others[128] have assumed he meant the latter nonetheless. Matters have not been helped by the fact that John Gerard[129] chose to illustrate what he called 'English cudweede' with a figure of what is unambiguously *G. sylvaticum*—though it is apparent from the text that he understood by 'cudweed' and 'chaffweed' various *Filago* and *Gnaphalium* species in just a vague, collective sense.[130]

Fortunately, Matthias de l'Obel in 1576 was a model of clarity by comparison: his figure is undoubtedly *Filago vulgaris*, which he says the common people in the west of England pound, steep in oil and boil for use on spots, bruises, cuts and lacerations.[131] By the west of England he doubtless meant the neighbourhood of Bristol, where he practised medicine on first arriving as an immigrant, and *Gnaphalium sylvaticum* is much too scarce in that part of the country to have served as a herbal source.

Though the use of the plant appears to have died out in England a century or so after de l'Obel wrote (John Parkinson in 1640 merely paraphrases his words), *Filago vulgaris* has borne a name in Manx, *lus ny croshey*, which has been interpreted as implying a herbal application of some (unknown) kind.[132] At the same time 'cudweed' can be short for the American cudweed or pearly everlasting, *Anaphalis margaritacea*, a garden plant which is on record as smoked like tobacco for a cough or headache in Suffolk.[133] This was probably the 'cudweed' reported from Wexford in the 1930s as a whooping-cough cure.[134]

Antennaria dioica (Linnaeus) Gaertner
  mountain everlasting, cat's-ear, cat's-foot
  northern and central Europe, northern and western Asia,
    North America
'A plant that grows wild named cat's-ear' when chewed and mixed with cobwebs has been used in Clare for staunching bleeding from cuts.[135] *Antennaria dioica* has a reputation as astringent and styptic, and happens to occur particularly frequently in the calcareous turf of the Burren for which that county is botanically renowned.

Inula helenium Linnaeus
  elecampane, wild parsnip, horseheal, scabwort
  central Asia; introduced into Europe, western Asia, Japan, North
    America, New Zealand
Inula helenium falls into the same category as greater celandine (*Chelidonium majus*): an ancient herb largely fallen into disuse but lingering on stub-

bornly in semi-wild conditions. Probably a native of central Asia, it was much valued by the Romans and the Anglo-Saxons and, serving for food as well as medicine, was evidently a favourite subsistence plant of early Christian times, as in Ireland it is found on some of the islets off the coasts as well as on and around ancient monastic sites more generally. Its ability to survive grazing by sheep probably accounts for this remarkable persistence.

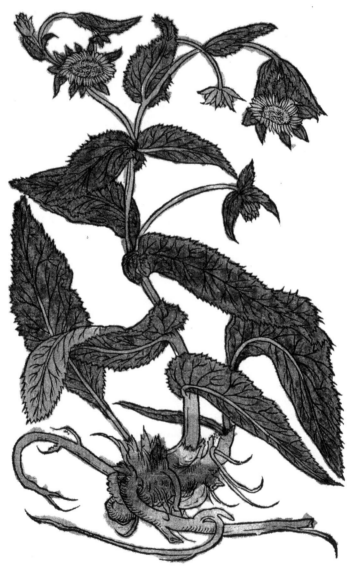

Inula helenium, elecampane (Bock 1556, p. 65)

A veterinary medicine as much as a human one, the plant's roots contain a white starchy powder extracted by boiling, which has been drunk in particular for lung and chest complaints, pulmonary tuberculosis, whooping cough and asthma (Norfolk,[136] Orkney[137] and the Isle of Man[138] as far as Britain is concerned). Wounds (in Sussex[139]) and toothache (in Cheshire[140]) are further ailments for which there are British records.

In Ireland the lung and chest application has similarly been the main one (Cavan,[141] Wexford[142] and doubtless—as the cough cure obtained from *meacan uilian* or 'wild parsnip'—Clare[143] and Limerick,[144] too).

Pulicaria dysenterica (Linnaeus) Bernhardi
common fleabane
Europe, Asia Minor, North Africa; introduced into New Zealand
(Folk credentials questionable) A plant of the herbals, hopefully identified by their authors with one celebrated in Classical times for insecticidal properties, *Pulicaria dysenterica* enjoyed a vogue for that purpose in what seem to have been relatively sophisticated circles and the only two allegedly folk records sound suspiciously like hand-downs from book learning. In Devon it was recommended to be gathered and dried for burning every morning in rooms to rid them of flies,[145] and in Sussex it was one of four strewing herbs principally employed to keep away fleas.[145a] That those records are both from southernmost England, despite the plant's wide distribution elsewhere in the British Isles, supports the impression that it was at best a marginal interloper as far as the folk tradition was concerned. Tansy, mugwort and the wormwoods have amply served the same purpose instead.

Solidago virgaurea Linnaeus
goldenrod
Eurasia; introduced into New Zealand
In learned medicine long popular as a wound herb, *Solidago virgaurea* has lingered on in use for that purpose in Sussex,[146] the East Riding of Yorkshire[147] and the Hebrides.[148] Martin Martin, to whom we owe our knowledge of its survival in the last-named, recorded it as an ingredient in two different ointments, one combined with 'all-heal' (*Stachys* spp.?) and applied to wounds in Lewis in the Outer Hebrides, the other smeared in Skye on fractures at the stage of healing when splints could be removed.[149]

In Ireland, however, the ailments for which this common plant has been recorded in use are very different from those, so much so as to suggest that not only was it never a wound herb there (perhaps purple-loosestrife,

Lythrum salicaria, took its place?) but the treatment of wounds may never have been one of its functions in the British Isles folk repertory in its pristine state. In Cavan,[150] where herbal uses are known with particular completeness, only heart trouble, stomach upsets and kidney problems feature in the records. Stomach upsets are the function of the plant in Cork,[151] too. In Louth, on the other hand, its leaves have been boiled as a remedy for colds,[152] and it may be because that use extended to pulmonary tuberculosis that an ˂ infusion was drunk in Londonderry for the spitting of blood.[153] In other parts of Ulster, though, its reputation, and that a well-known one, was merely for curing flatulence.[154]

Bellis perennis Linnaeus
daisy

Europe, western Asia; introduced into North America, Australasia

Considering its near-ubiquity, it is striking that *Bellis perennis* has featured as a folk herb only to a limited extent. Though William Turner knew it in his native Northumberland as 'banwort', 'because it helpeth bones to knyt againe'[155] (a statement repeated by Caleb Threlkeld who, though raised in Cumberland, was probably merely parroting Turner), no further mention of that use has been discovered. Instead, as far as Britain is concerned, its functions subsequently seem to have been limited to serving as an ointment— either alone or combined with other herbs—for burns (Hampshire[156]) or cuts and bruises (the Highlands and Western Isles[157]), or as an infusion made from the flower-heads drunk for coughs and colds (Wiltshire[158]) or eye troubles (the Highlands[159]). But simply eating the flower-heads, for curing boils (Devon,[160] Dorset[161]) or toothache (Cumbria[162]), sounds like a procedure based on magic rather than on any supposed chemical influence: two of them sufficed for toothache, but at least in Dorset seven or nine, those magic-laden numbers, were required to heal a boil and had to be picked from plants growing close enough to be covered with one foot.

The plant is also on record in Ireland as an ointment for burns and as an eye lotion but in both cases much more widely: from at least six counties, but entirely different ones in the case of each and with no apparent geographical patterns. As a cure for coughs and colds, however, records have been noted only from Cavan[163] and Mayo,[164] though it has been used in Roscommon[165] for headaches. A treatment for boils is known from Wexford but of a down-to-earth kind, involving boiling pieces with soap and sugar in a tin until the mixture turns black.[166] Cavan similarly appears to have been unique in finding a use for stomach and/or liver complaints.[167] It is especially in applying this plant to skin troubles, though, that Ireland differs most from Britain. Broadly classifiable under that head are records for ringworm from Leitrim,[168] whitlows[169] and chilblains[170] from Meath, 'blasts' (facial swellings) from Carlow[171] and erysipelas from Donegal.[172]

Tanacetum vulgare Linnaeus
tansy
Europe, Siberia; introduced into North
   America, Australasia

Though convincingly a native of beaches and riversides in other parts of north-western Europe, *Tanacetum vulgare* may owe its presence in the British Isles wholly to human influence and perhaps in large part to former cultivation for herbal purposes. Significantly, its Gaelic name, recorded as early as 1698 from Skye, translates as 'French herb'. With properties similar to wormwood, its primary use through the centuries and over much of Europe has been as a repellent: either drunk as an infusion to purge the system of intestinal worms (for which its effectiveness is well attested) or strewn about in the fresh state to keep away any noxious insects and even mice. Records of the former practice in Britain have been traced from Lincolnshire,[173] Skye[174] and Orkney,[175] and of the latter from South Wales,[176] the East Riding of Yorkshire,[177] Berwickshire[178] and the Highlands[179]— in other words, curiously, their known distributions do not overlap. In the days when it was believed that infections were transmitted by inhaling them, some of Orkney's inhabitants so trusted in the plant's effectiveness that they made a habit of

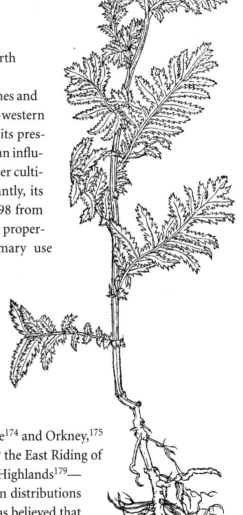

Tanacetum vulgare, tansy
(Brunfels 1530, p. 250)

carrying a piece of it between their upper lip and their nose.[180] Similarly, to keep at bay the influence of the 'miasma' arising from the ground that was supposed to give rise to ague, country folk in Hampshire[181] and Sussex[182] took the precaution of lining their boots with pieces of the plant.

A toxic oil powerful enough to rid the system of worms and other parasites would have commended itself as an abortifacient, too, if taken in a quantity large enough, and the plant is on record as used for that purpose in Wiltshire,[183] Gloucestershire[184] and the Cambridgeshire Fens.[185] In all three of those, however, it also had a reputation for aiding conception, presumably because of a separate relaxing effect. Such an effect could explain the drinking of tansy tea to counter palpitations in Gloucestershire,[186] rheumatism and indigestion in Essex[187] and period pains in Norfolk.[188] In the 'nórth of England' where an alternative was to apply a hot compress of the plant to the seat of any rheumatic pain, drinking that tea three times a day was held to clear the system of any tendency to gout[189]; it was as an antidote to gout that the plant was once much used in Scotland also[190] (though possibly on the recommendation of John Gerard's *Herball*, as a decoction of the root).

Ireland's uses seem to have been broadly similar but more thinly spread. As a vermicidal purge it has featured in Londonderry[191] and Louth[192] (and for veterinary purposes in further counties, too); in 'Ulster', where it was extensively grown in cottage gardens, it was valued as an emmenagogue of much power[193] as well as for indigestion and pains in the joints, these last relieved by being bathed with the product of boiling the leaves in salted water[194]; in the Aran Islands the juice has been drunk for fevers[195] and in some unspecified parts the plant is said to have shared that northern British popularity for gout.[196] Cavan is alone idiosyncratic in having yielded records as a jaundice cure and as an application to cuts.[197] That tansy is predominantly a herb of Ulster may be evidence for its having been introduced primarily from Scotland.

Seriphidium maritimum (Linnaeus) Poljakov
Artemisia maritima Linnaeus
   sea wormwood
   Europe, south-western and central Asia
Though *Seriphidium maritimum* has properties similar to the two *Artemisia* species (of which more below), its effects were found to be weaker and so led to its recommendation by village doctresses in preference to its inland counterpart for ridding children of worms.[198] Apothecaries also gave it priority

over the commoner plant because its less bitter taste gave it more 'consumer appeal'.[199] Once collected along the Sussex coast[200] on a commercial scale, the name 'savin', by which some people knew it, suggests that, by borrowing that from juniper, the 'deleterious purposes too generally known' for which that collecting was said to take place[201] may have been as an abortifacient at least in part. In the south of Scotland, though, it was to treat fevers and consumption that the peasants apparently primarily favoured it: Lanarkshire and Galloway folk tales tell of its being recommended by mermaids,[202] as if to underline that only the maritime plant would do. Another use, reported from Essex, was to rub one's forehead with a handful of it to cure a headache.[203]

Artemisia vulgaris Linnaeus
mugwort, muggons

northern temperate zone

A common component of the tundra vegetation that clothed the British Isles at the termination of the Ice Age, *Artemisia vulgaris* has lingered on in other parts of northern Europe as a member of the natural vegetation of the drift lines at or above the level of high-water spring tides (like tansy). In Britain and Ireland, however, it appears in modern times to have been confined exclusively to man-made habitats, especially dry waste ground, on which it is common throughout the lowlands. Like other nitrophiles, it may have acquired this weed status even as early as Mesolithic times and is likely to have been available for exploitation for several millennia at least. The medico-magical potency with which this visually unprepossessing plant has been credited through much of Eurasia and the strikingly similar beliefs associated with it in different regions of that landmass indeed suggest that it may be one of the oldest herbs known to mankind.[204] Sacred to thunder gods, its power to ward off evil influences was believed to be greatest on Midsummer Eve, the time of year when light and heat were rated their most intense. In that role it has rivalled, and probably preceded, St John's-wort and attained a particularly exalted status in the Isle of Man, where the custom was revived c. 1924 of wearing a sprig of it on Tynwald Day, when the island's ancient parliament is traditionally convened for an open-air proclamation of each year's new laws.

Why, though, did it attract such an extraordinarily widespread and tenacious faith in its efficacy? It is only slightly aromatic and its flowers are inconspicuous. It is, however, narcotic and was probably once a favourite divinatory, a use which is known to have persisted into more recent times in East

Prussia. The practice of smoking the dried leaves as a substitute for tobacco, general among country lads in Berkshire till late in the nineteenth century (under the name 'docko'[205]), may well be a relic of that, for unlike colt's-foot it appears to have had no medical justifications attached to it. As the plant shares with tansy and the wormwoods vermicidal properties, that it may have been used like them to purge the system of internal parasites is another possibility. If so, however, those two rivals must have usurped such former popularity as it may have enjoyed for that, for no mentions of such an application have been found. (An eighteenth-century record from Moray of its use as a purge, boiled in whey,[206] does not indicate the purpose of the purging.) And though 'mugwort' means midge-herb, it seems to have been rated much inferior to those others for keeping away insects, too—records of its serving that function have been traced from Devon,[207] Sussex[208] and Berwickshire[209] alone.

A further well-attested property of the plant is its ability to restore menstrual flow, ease delivery and cleanse the womb, for which functions it was once highly valued by midwives and nurses. Not for nothing is the genus named after the Greek goddess Artemis, the patron of maternity and childbirth, for since ancient times mugwort has been the female plant above all others, the *mater herbarum* or *herba matrum*. It may indeed be on account of the similarity of its leaves that motherwort (*Leonurus cardiaca*) acquired, through misidentification, a comparable degree of respect in the Isle of Man under the name 'she-vervain'. Though long valued in official medicine in cases of difficult parturition, mugwort features in the folk records in this and allied connections much less than expected but has probably suffered, like abortifacients in general, from a degree of reticence on the part of both collectors and informants. Only Northamptonshire,[210] the Highlands,[211] and Eriskay in the Outer Hebrides[212] appear to have yielded information, the last two in the guise of *liath-lus*, a Gaelic name identified[213] with *Artemisia vulgaris*. Tansy's comparable role has already been referred to above.

In common with tansy once again (and wormwood, too) mugwort has also enjoyed a reputation for easing colds, heavy coughs and especially consumption (Cornwall,[214] South Wales,[215] 'Scotland',[216] Londonderry[217]) as well as sciatica (Cumbria[218]). With wormwood it seems to have served as a digestive interchangeably (Berwickshire,[219] the Highlands[220]) and as a diuretic like the other two it was once eaten as a vegetable in Devon in order to dissolve 'the stone'.[221] Finally, it is said to have shared in Ireland wormwood's apparently rare use there as a treatment for epilepsy.[222]

Artemisia absinthium Linnaeus
wormwood
temperate Eurasia; introduced into North and South America,
New Zealand

In contrast to mugwort (*Artemisia vulgaris*), another favourite of Classical medicine, *A. absinthium*, is everywhere an obvious cottage garden herb that has slipped out here and there into the wilds and in no part of the British

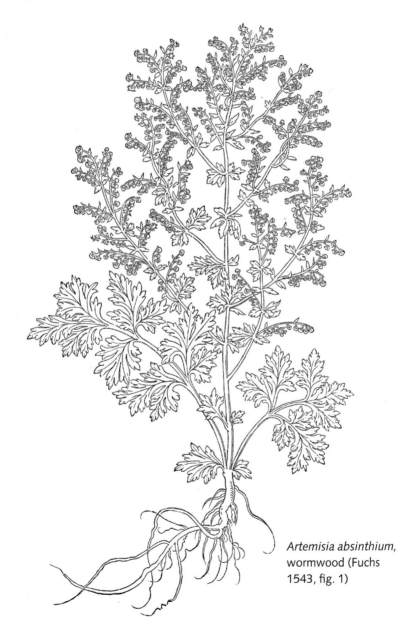

Artemisia absinthium,
wormwood (Fuchs
1543, fig. 1)

Isles is it anything like so common. It can only have been introduced for purposes for which that long-standing counterpart had shown itself inadequate.

Wormwood's main use has been as a digestive and for curing stomach upsets. This is outstandingly true of Wales, where it has been found fulfilling that function in every county—to an extent that it emerges as one of the most widely used of all contemporary herbal medicines in the rural parts of that country.[223] It has also found favour for the same purpose in Essex,[224] Derbyshire,[225] Berwickshire[226] and Orkney[227]—a curious scatter of counties which may merely be the fragments of a distribution formerly more general.

Only slightly less widespread has been wormwood's popularity as an insecticide (Wiltshire,[228] Sussex,[229] Suffolk,[230] parts of Wales[231]), which has considerably outstripped its deployment against intestinal worms (northern Wales,[232] Inverness-shire,[233] Orkney[234]). When taken internally, though, it has been well recognised as having risks: too large a dose (more than a tablespoonful in the case of adults) causes vomiting and pain.[235] In 'some parts of rural England' it has also served as a disinfectant: in one house with cases of scarlet fever the floor of the bedroom was washed with a strong decoction made from the achenes.[236]

The plant has also been valued almost as much as a tonic and purifier of the system (Essex,[237] Montgomeryshire,[238] Flintshire,[239] Cheshire,[240] Orkney[241]) and for rheumatic complaints (Essex,[242] Norfolk,[243] Pembrokeshire[244]). The exceptional strength of its following in Wales has found further reflection there in its use for colds in Pembrokeshire,[245] kidney trouble in Montgomeryshire[246] and—perhaps the same thing—colic (in combination with syrup of elderberries) in 'South Wales',[247] while as a narcotic it has served as a cure for insomnia in Cardiganshire.[248] Finally, a decoction of the plant has been taken for diabetes in the Isle of Man.[249]

The near-absence of Irish records for wormwood (and mugwort, too) is hard to explain. The sole ones traced are as a remedy for stomach pains in Mayo[250] and as an insecticide[251] and a cure for epilepsy (by pouring the juice into the sufferer's mouth) in unidentified parts of the country.[252]

Achillea ptarmica Linnaeus
sneezewort

Europe, south-western Asia, Siberia; introduced into North America, New Zealand

Despite its English name, no folk records of the use of *Achillea ptarmica* for colds have been discovered, though it allegedly promoted the flow of saliva and has been claimed effective therefore against toothache.[253] An infusion made from the flowers and leaves was once a popular drink in Orkney, but apparently purely as a refreshment.[254] The sole medicinal records consist of boiling the juice for stomach trouble in the Highlands[255] and employing the plant as a specific for 'wild fire' (allegedly urticaria in this case) in one district in Donegal.[256]

Achillea millefolium Linnaeus

yarrow

Europe, western Asia; introduced into North America,
 Australasia

Long and very widely known—in many parts of the world—for its haemostatic properties, *Achillea millefolium* has been primarily valued for altering blood flow in a variety of beneficial ways. Of the total of 125 records traced of the use of yarrow in British or Irish folk medicine, 47, or rather more than a third, come broadly into that category. The greatest number of these (16) are for staunching bleeding from wounds, cuts, scratches or sores, usually by means of an ointment but sometimes by merely applying the fresh leaves as a poultice. Familiar to the Romans and doubtless for millennia before them, this function of the plant is reflected in the names it bears in Welsh and Gaelic as well as such English ones as 'soldiers' woundwort' and 'carpenter's grass'. These names imply a once more general use than that limited number of records suggests. Other, more specialised applications of this property of the plant are for stopping nosebleeds (10 records, more particularly Welsh and Scottish and noticeably non-Irish), reducing high blood pressure (Gloucestershire,[257] Carmarthenshire[258]), for uterine haemorrhaging (Devon[259]) and cramp (Somerset—solved there by wearing

Achillea millefolium, yarrow
(Green 1902, fig. 320)

a leaf inside the shoes[260]). If put up the nostrils, as John Ray observed,[261] the leaves can also *provoke* a nosebleed and by thus reducing congestion in the blood vessels relieve migraine and headache, a practice recorded from Kent (?)[262] and Norfolk[263] as far as Britain is concerned. Similarly, by chewing the leaves or smoking them in a pipe, toothache can be made to disappear, but that essentially Irish remedy has apparently extended eastwards only to the Isle of Man.[264]

With a reputation as well for opening the pores and inducing sweating, yarrow has also been widely valued for coughs, heavy colds, bronchitis, asthma, fevers and catarrh (25 records). As with so many other cold-curing herbs, it has been hardly less in demand as a treatment for rheumatic complaints (21 records, mostly Irish) and probably for the same reason it has enjoyed popularity in some areas as a stimulating tonic, countering depression and cleansing the system (13 records, including, noticeably, from three areas of heavy Norse settlement (Isle of Man,[265] Orkney,[266] Shetland[267]).

Other, minor applications recorded from Britain include for kidney trouble in Pembrokeshire,[268] to improve an oily complexion and to help children to sleep in Gloucestershire,[269] to cystitis[270] and measles in Norfolk,[271] to rid children of intestinal worms in Yorkshire's North Riding[272] and, not altogether surprisingly in view of this versatility, to 'all diseases' in the Isle of Man.[273]

Ireland has made up for that apparently rare use of the plant for *stopping* nosebleeds by a disproportionately wide popularity for *inducing* them as a cure for migraine and headaches (Cavan,[274] Mayo,[275] Carlow,[276] Limerick[277]), while as a toothache remedy yarrow has been even more emphatically Irish (those same counties plus Offaly[278]). Though known in parts of the country as the 'herb of the seven cures', its repertory has clearly extended well beyond that limited, clearly magical number of lesser applications as well: for kidney trouble in 'Ulster'[279] and Tipperary,[280] jaundice and sore eyes in Cavan,[281] boils in Cork[282] and—echoing the optimism among the Manx—'all pains' in Co. Dublin.[283]

Chamaemelum nobile (Linnaeus) Allioni

Anthemis nobilis Linnaeus

chamomile

south-western Europe, north-western Africa, Azores; introduced
　　into North America, Australasia

Sometimes called 'Roman chamomile' or 'English chamomile' to distinguish it from 'German chamomile' (*Matricaria recutita* Linnaeus, which as a field weed or a crop has stood in for it medicinally in many parts of Europe but has apparently never featured in the British Isles as a folk cure), *Chamaemelum nobile* has a strongly south-western distribution in both Britain and Ireland in so far as it appears to be a native. It has a secondary area of frequency in Ulster but is absent from Scotland and most of northern England except where introduced. Though sufficiently abundant in part of that native range to have met medicinal demand locally—William Borlase reported it in eighteenth-century Cornwall as 'transplanted into gardens, for a strengthening emetic tea'[284]—extensive folk use in many other areas implies that its source was largely or wholly cottage gardens, at any rate in later centuries. In other words, this can have been a wild herb only to a relatively limited extent, and latterly it may even have become a semi-commercial one.

The greatest number of folk uses recorded for the plants are as a relaxant: for soothing the stomach (Devon,[285] Wiltshire,[286] Essex,[287] Gloucestershire,[288] Nottinghamshire,[289] the Highlands[290]); easing nervous pains in the head, teeth or ears (Wiltshire,[291] Essex,[292] Warwickshire,[293] Norfolk[294]) or period pains (Dorset[295]) or those accompanying pleurisy (Hertfordshire[296]); and inducing sleep or preventing nightmares (Norfolk[297]).

A secondary focus has been on colds, coughs of all kinds and sore throats. The treatment of these has usually taken the form of drinking a hot infusion of the flowers or

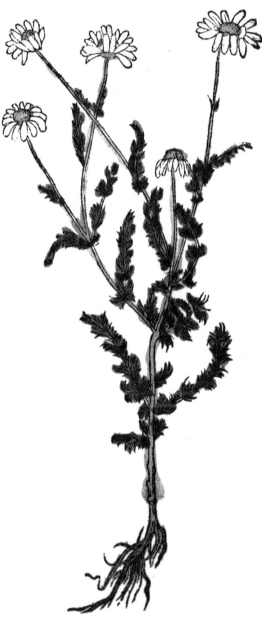

Chamaemelum nobile, chamomile (Bock 1556, p. 56)

inhaling just the steam from that (Norfolk,[298] Glamorgan, Montgomeryshire[299]), though for asthma in Norfolk[300] the plant was smoked and no more than the dew shaken from the flowers was once reckoned enough in South Wales to cure tuberculosis.[301]

The flowers have also been employed in the form of an infusion to poultice swellings and inflammation (Suffolk,[302] Orkney[303]) or infused and applied as a wash to sore or tired eyes (Norfolk[304]); mixed with cream they have served as an ointment for boils, too (Brecknockshire[305]), though whether that was the treatment for abscesses recorded for some part of Yorkshire[306] is unclear. In Kent an infusion was drunk at one time as a regular morning tonic,[307] while a recent discovery made in Suffolk is that the oil from the flower-heads appears to mitigate psoriasis.[308]

Ireland's spread of records for the two main uses of the plant equals Britain's: it is known as a relaxant from 'Ulster',[309] Cavan,[310] Westmeath,[311] Co. Dublin[312] and Limerick,[313] as a painkiller from Cavan,[314] Co. Dublin,[315] Limerick[316] and Cork[317] and as a soporific from Wicklow.[318] While it has been less favoured than in Britain for colds and the like, with records traced for use for those from Cavan[319] and Carlow[320] only, it has been applied markedly more widely in Ireland to swellings and inflammation (Londonderry,[321] Sligo,[322] Laois,[323] Co. Dublin,[324] Wicklow[325]) or boils (Cavan,[326] Cork[327]); boils, moreover, seem to have been poulticed with the plant's flower-heads whereas the ointment for those recorded from Wales has had a parallel only as an application to whitlows on fingers in Westmeath,[328] so far as has been traced. A jaundice cure reported from Cork,[329] however, involving boiling the plant in wine or porter and drinking the liquid over a period of ten days, would appear to be uniquely Irish.

Anthemis arvensis Linnaeus
corn chamomile
Europe, Asia Minor, North Africa; introduced elsewhere

(Name confusion) *Anthemis arvensis* is specifically named in one printed source as the chamomile on Colonsay in the Inner Hebrides used with other herbs in poultices for promoting suppuration and drunk as an infusion for strengthening the stomach. That the recorder describes it as a perennial and flowering in late summer, however, shows that it must have been *Chamaemelum nobile*, which happens to be anomalously widespread on that island, as the legacy of introduction for a lawn.[330]

Anthemis cotula Linnaeus
stinking chamomile
Europe, northern and western Asia; introduced elsewhere

(Folk credentials questionable) 'Some of our English housewives call it Iron Wort, and make an unguent for old sores', John Josselyn recorded in seventeenth-century New England.[331] *Anthemis cotula* was a sufficiently abundant cornfield weed in southern Britain in medieval times to have acquired an Anglo-Saxon name, but though long notorious for blistering the hands of harvesters and reputedly a powerful insect repellent, published assertions that it was used in folk medicine[332] are too unspecific to be accepted without fuller evidence.

Chrysanthemum segetum Linnaeus
corn marigold
Europe, western Asia; introduced into North Africa, North and
   South America

(Folk credentials questionable) Folk records of the use of marigolds probably relate to the common garden plant, *Calendula officinalis* Linnaeus, rather than to the once common cornfield weed *Chrysanthemum segetum*. Suspiciously, though a decoction drunk as a cure for measles in Wicklow has been attributed to the wild plant,[333] comparable drinks feature for that among the uses of 'marigolds' (which are more likely to have been the garden plant) in Norfolk[334] and Montgomeryshire.[335] The cornfield weed has passed simply as 'marigold' in parts of the north of England, but elsewhere it has tended to have at least 'wild' or 'field' preceding that.

Leucanthemum vulgare Lamarck
Chrysanthemum leucanthemum Linnaeus
ox-eye daisy
Europe, Siberia; introduced into North America, Australasia

Though found over much of the British Isles, *Leucanthemum vulgare* appears, curiously, to have been recorded as a folk herb only from the Highlands and limited areas of Ireland. Some of the recorded uses are shared with the ordinary daisy, *Bellis perennis*, for which this large-flowered relative may have served in part as an alternative; for others, however, it seems to have been targeted specifically.

In the Highlands a tea made from the plant has been drunk for asthma, while the juice has been not only mixed with honey as a cough cure but applied to wounds as well.[336] The Gaelic name has been interpreted as implying a one-time widespread use for scrofula,[337] though that is perhaps questionable.

In Ireland the boiled juice has similarly been applied for coughs, more especially tubercular ones, in the Aran Islands in the remoteness of Galway Bay, where this species was looked upon as the 'female' version of chamomile (*Chamaemelum nobile*).[338] Both there and in Limerick[339] sore eyes were also bathed with the cooled boiled juice. In Tyrone and Monaghan, on the other hand, a tea formerly much drunk there (to ward off a chill) was made from an infusion of the ray florets.[340]

Matricaria discoidea de Candolle

> *M. matricaroides* (Lessing) Porter, in part; *M. suaveolens* (Pursh)
> Buchenau
> pineapple weed
> north-eastern Asia; introduced into Europe, North and South
> America, Australasia

Under the Welsh name *pe-felen*, *Matricaria discoidea* is on record as used in Caernarvonshire some time before World War II for a leaf poultice in a case of severe boils on the neck (which it was seemingly successful in clearing up).[341] As this alien is not known to have reached the British Isles before 1869—though for long now a common weed of barish places—this is a rare instance of a folk use of demonstrably recent origin. The species was presumably standing in for *Chamaemelum nobile,* which is recorded from several counties, one of them Welsh, as the source of an ointment for boils.

Senecio aquaticus Hill

> water ragwort; *buachalán* (Ireland)
> western and central Europe; introduced into New Zealand

Senecio jacobaea Linnaeus

> ragwort, ragweed; *buachalán* (Ireland)
> Europe, western Asia, North Africa; introduced into North America,
> Australasia

Unexpectedly, ragwort emerges from the folk records as almost wholly an Irish herb. Both *Senecio aquaticus* and *S. jacobaea* occur there in abundance and hybridise with each other so extensively that it is surprising that in Tipperary what is manifestly *S. aquaticus* from the habitat description has acquired a name of its own in Irish Gaelic (translating as 'fisherman's ragwort') and been preferred to *S. jacobaea* at least for use on cuts.[342] That dif-

ferentiation may well have come about, though, merely through the fact that
S. aquaticus has the more succulent basal leaves, making it more suitable for
poultices (as observed on Clare Island, off the Galway coast).[343] More usually, rather than distinguishing between these two species, the folk tendency
has been to make a distinction between plants with flowers on the one hand
and plants displaying just a leaf rosette on the other. In the west of Ireland and
the Hebrides one of these was considered to be 'male' ragwort and the other
'female'—but accounts differ as to which was which. In Skye, the 'female' kind
was the one selected for healing women's breasts when swollen,[344] in keeping
with that folk belief, so often recorded elsewhere, that many herbs exist as gender pairs and cure effectively only if applied to the ills of the appropriate sex.

Those who subscribe to the belief that many of the practices of folk medicine were given direction by plant characters supposed to reveal the plant's
utility through their form (the Doctrine of Signatures) may consider that
ragwort with its yellow flowers has been used more for jaundice than for anything else lends support to that. If so, however, it is hard to see why the records
traced for that use should be from Ireland only: 'Ulster',[345] Cavan,[346] Sligo,[347]
Leitrim,[348] Westmeath,[349] Meath,[350] Mayo,[351] Wicklow,[352] Limerick[353] and
Tipperary.[354]

Less widespread but apparently more frequent locally is ragwort's popularity for colds, coughs and especially sore throats (Cavan,[355] Sligo,[356]
Meath,[357] Clare,[358] Limerick[359]). Use for cuts, sores and inflammation of various kinds matches that but with a more southerly distribution (Mayo,[360]
Wicklow,[361] Wexford,[362] Waterford,[363] Tipperary[364]); application to burns or
scalds (Sligo,[365] Westmeath[366]) could be regarded as a special subcategory of
that, however, as could the poulticing of boils or abscesses (Fermanagh,[367]
Cavan[368]).

Ragwort has also been valued, but less widely, for rheumatic complaints
(Ulster,[369] Clare,[370] Limerick[371]) and for sprains or swollen joints ('Ulster',[372]
Cavan,[373] Wicklow,[374] Kilkenny[375]). Dropsy (in Cavan[376]), measles (in
Sligo[377]), bowel hives in children (in Antrim[378]), warts and nettle stings (in
Limerick[379]) are further ailments for which it has had devotees, too.

The curiously rare records from Britain seem to be limited to Scotland
apart from a solitary one of rheumatism treatment from Hampshire.[380] In
the Inner Hebrides, as in Skye[381] and Colonsay,[382] the first year's growth or a
barren form of the plant was at one time cut into pieces, mixed with butter
and (sometimes with other herbs) applied as a warm plaster to bring a boil to
a head and 'draw' it quickly and without pain. In the Hebrides there has also

existed a firm belief that the smell of the plant, especially while green and flowerless, deters rats and mice[383] and in Uist, if not elsewhere, corn stacks were frequently layered with it.[384]

Senecio vulgaris Linnaeus
groundsel
Eurasia; introduced widely elsewhere

Very common as a weed of cultivation but with clearly native populations on coastal sand dunes, *Senecio vulgaris* once proclaimed its principal value

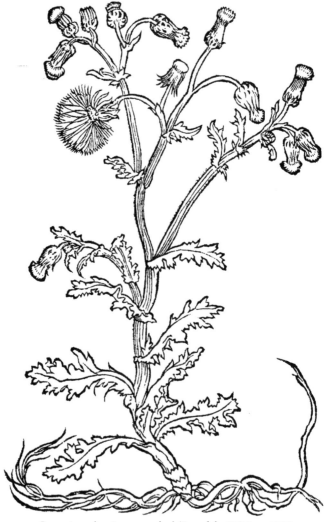

Senecio vulgaris, groundsel (Brunfels 1530, p. 120)

medicinally in the name it bore in Old English: 'groundsel' meant pus-absorber.[385] A minor virtue of its close relation, ragwort, the ability to draw matter out of wounds, blisters, boils and the like has been for this species its pre-eminent function, recorded from various parts of Ireland and most parts of Britain. In Carmarthenshire and Cardiganshire that reputation extends even to the extraction of thorns.[386]

No other uses of the plant come near that in popularity. In Britain, those have included healing inflammation, bruises and swellings when applied externally (Norfolk,[387] Berwickshire,[388] Aberdeenshire,[389] the Highlands,[390] Colonsay in the Hebrides,[391] Isle of Man[392]) as well as chapped hands when made into a lotion (Devon,[393] Norfolk,[394] the Highlands[395]); teething in infants, by including the juice in their milk (Suffolk,[396] Norfolk[397]); curing ague, by wearing a handful of the pulped plant in a bag against the bare breast or stomach and thereby inducing powerful vomiting some hours afterwards (Cornwall,[398] Isle of Man,[399] Edinburgh[400]); allaying rheumatism, especially by soaking the feet in a preparation (Fens of East Anglia,[401] the Highlands[402]); as a diuretic (Devon[403]) and as a wart cure (Essex[404]).

Ireland's subsidiary uses have been about as numerous—but almost all of them different: applied as a hot poultice to the face to ease toothache (Galway[405] and some other unspecified area[406]), taken as a tonic to cleanse the blood (Limerick[407]) and to staunch nosebleeds by drinking the juice mixed with water and a drop of turpentine (Offaly[408]). Before the advent of castor oil, a sprig or two added to babies' milk and that given to them once boiled and strained also seems to have been peculiarly Irish, though information is lacking on how widespread that was.[409] Only the use for chapped hands ('felons') in Co. Dublin[410] and as a diuretic for removing gravel in Donegal[411] have counterparts in the records traced from Britain.

Tussilago farfara Linnaeus
colt's-foot
Europe, northern and western Asia, North Africa; introduced into
North America, New Zealand

Tussilago farfara is the age-old folk cure for coughs *par excellence*. The properties which cause it to be valued for those have recommended it as well for colds, catarrh, sore throats and lung and chest complaints, and for some at least of those it has been recorded from most parts of the British Isles. Soaking the leaves (more rarely, the roots) in water specifically for asthma has also been a widespread practice, reported from areas in Britain as far apart as

Herefordshire,[412] Suffolk,[413] Fife[414] and the Highlands.[415] In Oxfordshire,[416] on the other hand, the plant's reputation has extended to that of a blood purifier, while an ointment made from the roots, with other ingredients added, was once in great repute for curing sprains and all swellings of the joints in Roxburghshire.[417]

Ireland has shared that use for asthma, with records from a similarly scattered set of counties (Antrim,[418] Wicklow,[419] Tipperary,[420] Cork[421]), but for

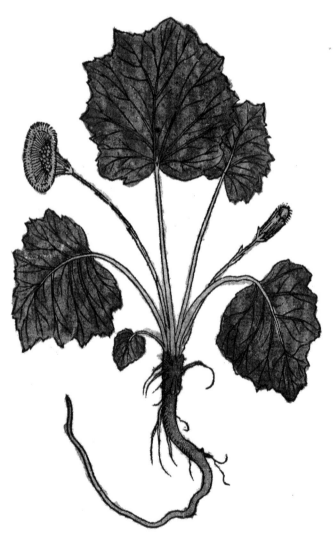

Tussilago farfara, colt's-foot (Bock 1556, p. 158)

children the leaves, instead of being smoked, were boiled in milk.[422] The oint-ment for swellings once popular on the Scottish border was also much employed in 'Ulster'[423] in the past. Britain has apparently had no counterpart, though, to the valuing of the plant for earache in Wicklow[424] and neuralgia in Limerick.[425]

Petasites hybridus (Linnaeus) P. Gaertner, Meyer & Scherbius
butterbur, thunder-dock, wild rhubarb
Europe, northern and western Asia; introduced into North America
An odd feature of *Petasites hybridus* is that the male and female plants are very different in appearance and, in Britain at least, have very different dis-tributions, the females restricted mainly to the northern half of England, the males found much more widely. Preferential planting of the male seems the only way to account for this, but evidence of that has yet to be discovered. Beekeepers may have valued the male for the profusion of its flowers, it has been suggested, or farmers may have found the greater vegetative vigour resulting from its not setting seed produced larger leaves in which to pack butter.[426] That it may have had some special role in folk medicine is clearly another possibility. The bitter, very resinous root of butterbur was at one time valued for its sweat-inducing action (like that of thrift) and caused it to be used extensively for plague and fevers, bringing it the name *Pestilenzwurz* in German. If the roots of the male plant gained a reputation as the more effec-tive, that might have been the one chosen for cultivating (or even importing from the Continent). In one Cornish village a tradition persisted that the but-terbur owed its presence in the churchyard to having sprung from the graves of the victims of an especially severe outbreak of plague in which this herb proved its worth.[427] As that is only one of two records traced in the folklore lit-erature (the other from the Highlands[428]) of the employment of the species for that purpose in Britain or Ireland, the far-fetched explanation to account for the plant's presence suggests that it was a use that was unfamiliar.

It is in quite other connections, rather, that butterbur features in the folk records. Suggestively, three of those are from the region to which the female plant is mainly restricted: Durham, as a treatment for spots and sores,[429] Berwickshire, for white swellings on the knees,[430] and Roxburghshire, for scurvy.[431] Elsewhere in Britain the species has been valued for shingles in Cornwall[432] (but combined with brambles), rheumatism in Somerset[433] and dropsy in the Highlands.[434]

The sole Irish records traced (Mayo,[435] Limerick[436]) are both, as in Somerset, as a rheumatism treatment.

Eupatorium cannabinum Linnaeus
hemp-agrimony
Europe, western and central Asia, North Africa; introduced into
   North America, New Zealand
(Folk credentials questionable) *Eupatorium cannabinum* was so widely recommended in the books that its apparent absence from the Irish folk records

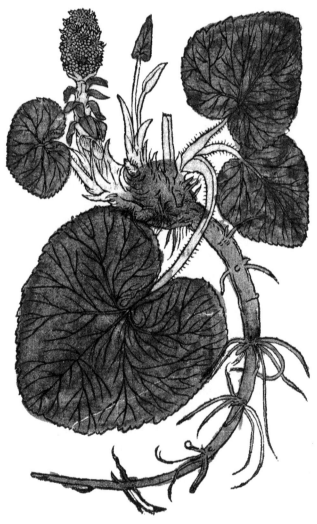

Petasites hybridus, butterbur (Bock 1556, p. 157)

and near-absence from the British ones leads one to suspect that, except in the case of a veterinary use mentioned by John Parkinson in 1640,[437] it may have been wholly borrowed from the learned tradition—and that despite the fact that Dutch peasants are known to have taken a preparation of the plant as an alterative and antiscorbutic,[438] and Belgian ones as a cure for jaundice.[439] John Lightfoot described it as a rough medicine sometimes favoured by 'the lower classes of people' (for jaundice and dropsy)[440] but left it unclear whether that statement was referring to Britain. More persuasively, a poultice of the leaves saved from amputation the severely poisoned arm of a Cornish fisherman in the 1930s, a remedy later copied with claimed success by a Middlesex acquaintance of his to extract pus from boils.[441] Because that was a function of the plant popularised by the influential Dutch physician Herman Boerhaave, however, even in that case an element of doubt must attach to the folk credentials of the remedy.

Notes

1. IFC S 485: 191
2. Deane & Shaw
3. Collyns
4. Johnston 1853, 129
5. McNeill
6. Moore 1898
7. Davies1938, 167
8. Jobson 1967, 57
9. Vickery MSS
10. Carmichael, ii, 349
11. Johnston 1853, 129
12. Quincy, 156
13. Moore 1898
14. Quelch, 50
15. Johnson 1862
16. IFC S 710: 43
17. McClafferty
18. IFC S 657: 248
19. McGlinchey, 86
20. IFC S 157: 463
21. Wilde, 34
22. Moloney
23. IFC S 657: 216
24. IFC S 710: 49
25. IFC S 1043: 265

26. Moore MS
27. IFC S 657: 248
28. IFC S 524: 119
29. IFC S 657: 248
30. IFC S 132: 97; 137: 135
31. Egan
32. IFC S 657: 248
33. IFC S 914: 555
34. Maloney
35. Ó hEithir MS
36. IFC S 672: 205, 206, 210, 258, 259; 673: 155
37. Farrelly MS
38. Maloney
39. Vickery MSS
40. IFC S 786: 116
41. IFC S 483: 300
42. IFC S 780: 243
43. Beith
44. A. Allen, 185
45. Hatfield, 28
46. Gerard, 166
47. Hatfield, 27
48. Egan
49. Maloney

50. IFC S 820: 277
51. IFC S 825: 60, 94, 117
52. McClafferty
53. IFC S 523: 271
54. McClafferty
55. Gregory
56. McGlinchey, 87
57. IFC S 412: 107
58. Colgan 1904
59. Hart 1898
60. Davies 1938
61. Newman & Wilson
62. Newman & Wilson
63. Moore 1898
64. MacFarlane
65. Moloney
66. Pratt 1850–7
67. Britten & Holland, 354
68. IFC S 888: 108
69. IFC S 571: 149, 170
70. Withering 1787–92, 859
71. Woodruffe-Peacock
72. Trevelyan, 91
73. Buchanan-Brown, 339
74. IFC S 747: 187
75. Vickery MSS
76. Newman & Wilson
77. Lafont
78. Tongue
79. Bethell
80. Hatfield, 25
81. Fairweather
82. Macdonald
83. Maloney
84. IFC S 921: 12
85. IFC S 481: 48; 483: 84
86. IFC S 413: 226
87. Maloney
88. IFC S 913: 64
89. IFC S 484: 220
90. IFC S 794: 35
91. IFC S 907: 368
92. IFC S 491: 57
93. IFC S 771: 173
94. IFC S 483: 271

95. IFC S 484: 41
96. IFC S 412: 194
97. IFC S 968: 225
98. IFC S 480: 374
99. IFC S 862: 152
100. IFC S 268: 63
101. IFC S 904: 454
102. Ó Súilleabháin, 311
103. IFC S 550: 274
104. IFC S 1090: 274
105. IFC S 907: 209
106. IFC S 797: 13
107. Sargent
108. IFC S 519: 230
109. Vickery 1995
110. Vickery 1995
111. Evans 1969, 88
112. Hackwood, 150
113. Morrison; Paton MS
114. Moore 1898
115. Garrad MS
116. Couch, 177
117. IFC S 710: 48
118. IFC S 510: 95
119. IFC S 250: 62, 223, 237
120. IFC S 747: 590
121. McClafferty
122. McClafferty
123. IFC S 689: 261
124. Maloney
125. Sargent
126. Turner 1568, part 1, 119
127. e.g. Britten & Holland, 96
128. e.g. Ray 1690, 279
129. Gerard, 515
130. Britten & Holland, 136
131. de l'Obel 1576, 255
132. Paton
133. Jobson 1967, 59
134. IFC S 897: 238
135. IFC S 601: 51
136. Bardswell; Taylor MS (Hatfield, 29)
137. Neill, 12; Spence; Leask, 72
138. Garrad 1976
139. A. Allen, 185

140. Wright, 248
141. Maloney
142. IFC S 888: 109
143. IFC S 22: 238; 617: 78
144. IFC S 497: 132
145. Hewett, 66
145a. A. Allen, 185
146. A. Allen, 185
147. CECTL MSS (Vickery 1995)
148. Martin, 94, 230
149. Martin, 94, 230
150. Maloney
151. IFC S 385: 55
152. IFC S 672: 257
153. Moore MS
154. Purdon
155. Turner 1568, part 1, 78
156. Vickery MSS
157. McNeill: Beith
158. Whitlock 1992, 106
159. Pennant 1776, ii, 42
160. Lafont, 32
161. Rawlence
162. Newman & Wilson
163. Maloney
164. IFC S 132: 97
165. IFC S 269: 105
166. IFC S 897: 93
167. Maloney
168. IFC S 191: 90
169. IFC S 710: 43
170. IFC S 690: 41
171. IFC S 907: 156
172. McGlinchey, 83
173. Taylor MS (Hatfield, appendix)
174. Martin, 226
175. Spence
176. informant in a television interview, Sept. 1993
177. Woodward, 25–6, 103
178. Johnston 1853
179. Carmichael, iv, 120
180. Leask, 77
181. Boase, 126
182. Latham, 39; Quelch, 153
183. Whitlock 1992, 114
184. Palmer 1994, 122
185. Porter 1969, 10
186. Palmer 1994, 122
187. Newman & Wilson
188. Hatfield, appendix
189. Quelch, 152
190. Pratt 1850–7
191. Moore MS
192. Synnott
193. Purdon
194. Egan
195. IFC S 1: 195
196. Moloney
197. Maloney
198. Johnston 1853, 129
199. Parkinson, 101, 104
200. A. Allen, 183
201. *Hardwicke's Science-gossip* (1875), 34
202. Mason, 558
203. Newman & Wilson
204. Armstrong
205. Druce
206. Pennant 1771, 311
207. Lafont
208. A. Allen
209. Johnston 1853
210. Hatfield MS
211. Carmichael, vi, 83
212. McDonald, 151
213. Cameron
214. Deane & Shaw
215. Trevelyan, 91
216. Wright, 241
217. Moore MS
218. Short 1746
219. Johnston 1829–31, i, 181
220. Beith
221. Lafont
222. Moloney
223. Williams MS
224. Newman & Wilson

225. CECTL MSS
226. Johnston 1829–31, i, 181
227. Spence
228. Whitlock 1992, 115
229. A. Allen, 72, 74
230. Hatfield, appendix
231. Williams MS
232. Williams MS
233. McCutcheon
234. Spence; Firth, 96; Leask, 78
235. McCutcheon
236. Quelch, 164
237. Hatfield, appendix
238. Evans 1940
239. Williams MS
240. Wright, 239
241. Spence
242. Newman & Wilson
243. Harland, 83
244. Williams MS
245. Williams MS
246. Williams MS
247. Trevelyan, 315
248. Williams MS
249. Fargher
250. IFC S 93: 528
251. Moloney
252. Wood-Martin, 188
253. Pratt 1850–7
254. Spence
255. Beith
256. Hart 1898
257. Ibbott, 64
258. Williams MS
259. Collyns
260. Tongue
261. Ray 1690, 290
262. Pratt 1850–7
263. Bardswell
264. Fargher
265. Paton
266. Neill, 28
267. Tait
268. Williams MS

269. Ibbott, 64
270. Hatfield MS
271. Hatfield, 43
272. Blakeborough, 134
273. Fargher
274. Maloney
275. IFC S 137: 210
276. IFC S 908: 133
277. IFC S 498: 314
278. IFC S 820: 212, 225
279. Egan
280. IFC S 550: 274
281. Maloney
282. IFC S 286: 25
283. IFC S 787: 52
284. Borlase 1758, 229
285. Collyns
286. Whitlock 1992, 105
287. Newman & Wilson
288. Gibbs, 57; Palmer 1994, 123
289. Vickery MSS
290. MacFarlane
291. Whitlock 1992, 105
292. Newman & Wilson
293. Vickery MSS
294. Bardswell
295. Dacombe
296. Ellis, 317
297. Bardswell
298. Taylor MS (Hatfield, 28)
299. Williams MS
300. Bardswell
301. Trevelyan, 315
302. Jobson 1959, 144
303. Spence
304. Hatfield, 37
305. Williams MS
306. Vickery MSS
307. Pratt 1850–7
308. Hatfield, 87
309. Egan
310. IFC S 933: 154
311. IFC S 736: 137
312. IFC S 795: 191

313. IFC S 523: 169
314. Maloney
315. IFC S 795: 191
316. IFC S 485: 56
317. IFC S 287: 67; 1128: 26
318. IFC S 914: 322
319. IFC S 933: 154
320. IFC S 907: 267
321. Moore MS
322. IFC S 170: 259
323. IFC S 825: 74
324. IFC S 795: 191
325. IFC S 920: 69
326. Maloney
327. IFC S 337: 77
328. IFC S 736: 22, 23
329. IFC S 287: 180
330. McNeill; R. L. Gulliver, oral information
331. Josselyn
332. e.g. Pratt 1850–7; Cameron
333. McClafferty
334. Taylor MS (Hatfield, 42)
335. Evans 1940
336. Beith
337. Cameron
338. Ó hEithir
339. IFC S 484: 220
340. Hart 1898, 373
341. *PLNN*, no. 6 (1999), 289
342. IFC S 572: 297
343. Colgan 1911
344. Martin, 231
345. Purdon
346. Maloney
347. IFC S 171: 337
348. IFC S 226: 506
349. IFC S 746: 238, 456; 747: 30
350. IFC S 689: 2
351. IFC S 132: 37
352. IFC S 888: 202; 920: 70
353. IFC S 485: 52
354. IFC S 550: 275
355. Maloney

356. IFC S 158: 120
357. IFC S 690: 39; 710: 48
358. IFC S 589: 62
359. IFC S 497: 371; 504: 27, 135; 521: 149
360. IFC S 132: 98
361. IFC S 914: 283, 553
362. IFC S 897: 238
363. IFC S 636: 191, 355
364. IFC S 550: 284
365. IFC S 170: 256
366. IFC S 746: 456
367. Barbour
368. Maloney
369. Egan
370. IFC S 616: 48
371. IFC S 522: 197
372. Egan
373. Maloney
374. McClafferty
375. IFC S 849: 315
376. Maloney
377. IFC S 170: 196
378. Vickery MSS
379. IFC S 504: 27
380. Kingsley
381. Martin, 231
382. McNeill
383. Carmichael, iv, 120
384. Carmichael, vi, 25
385. Palmer 1904, 34
386. Williams MS
387. Pigott
388. Johnston 1853, 129 footnote
389. Henderson & Dickson, 155
390. Beith
391. McNeill
392. Fargher
393. Vickery MSS
394. Bardswell
395. Beith
396. Jobson 1967, 58
397. Wigby, 65; Hatfield, appendix
398. Deane & Shaw

399. Moore 1898
400. Stedman
401. Randell, 86
402. Cameron, 56 footnote
403. Lafont
404. Newman & Wilson
405. IFC S 60: 302
406. Sargent
407. IFC S 481: 143; 483: 369
408. IFC S 820: 173
409. Moloney
410. IFC S 787: 367
411. McGlinchey, 84
412. Jones-Baker, 101
413. Jobson 1959, 144
414. Simpkins, 133
415. Beith
416. 'E.C.'
417. Johnston 1853, 129
418. Vickery MSS
419. McClafferty
420. IFC S 550: 274

421. IFC S 287: 180
422. Logan, 26
423. Purdon
424. McClafferty
425. IFC S 506: 743
426. Walters
427. Polwhele 1816, 69
428. Beith
429. Vickery 1995
430. Johnston 1853, 129
431. Johnston 1853, 129
432. *Folk-lore,* 19 (1887), 200
433. Palmer 1976, 115
434. Beith
435. IFC S 138: 100
436. IFC S 499: 201
437. Parkinson, 597
438. Withering 1787–92, 502
439. Ray 1670, 332
440. Lightfoot, 464
441. *PLNN,* no. 66 (2001), 313

CHAPTER 16

Pondweeds, Grasses, Lilies and Orchids

Monocotyledonous flowering plants in the orders (and families) Alismatales (Alismataceae, water-plantains), Najadales (Potamogetonaceae, pondweeds), Arales (Araceae, arums; Lemnaceae, duckweeds), Juncales (Juncaceae, rushes), Cyperales (Cyperaceae, sedges; Poaceae, grasses), Typhales (Typhaceae, reedmaces), Liliales (Liliaceae, lilies; Iridaceae, irises; Dioscoreaceae, yams) and Orchidales (Orchidaceae, orchids) are included in this chapter.

ALISMATACEAE

Sagittaria sagittifolia Linnaeus
arrowhead
temperate Eurasia
In Devon a cupful of tea made of nine leaves of *Sagittaria sagittifolia* to a pint of boiled water was reckoned a good strengthening medicine, if taken every day in spring and autumn.[1]

Alisma plantago-aquatica Linnaeus, in the broad sense
water-plantain
Eurasia, North Africa; introduced into west North America,
    Australasia
Though a highly valued folk herb in other parts of the world, *Alisma plantago-aquatica* appears to have had only a marginal presence in that capacity in the British Isles—and that only in Ireland. Apart from an unlocalised record of its use in the latter for a sore mouth,[2] its juice has had a reputation in Londonderry as able to stop the spitting of blood.[3]

POTAMOGETONACEAE

Potamogeton natans Linnaeus
broad-leaved pondweed
northern temperate zone

Potamogeton polygonifolius Pourret
bog pondweed
Europe, north-western Africa, eastern North America

Both common, *Potamogeton natans* and *P. polygonifolius* have been used, doubtless interchangeably, for healing burns and scalds—either by simply placing a relay of leaves on them or by boiling the leaves in cream and apply-ing the product as an ointment. In two counties in south-eastern Wales (Monmouthshire,[4] Brecknockshire[5]) the plant in question, known as *dail llosg[y]tân*, fire-burn leaves, has been botanically identified as *P. natans*. In the island of Colonsay in the Inner Hebrides, where the waters by contrast are all acid and peaty, *duilleaga-bhàite*, drowned-leaf, proved to be *P. polygonifolius*, that member of the genus abundant there.[6]

The 'broad leaf from the pond' formerly placed on burns in the Lleyn Peninsula of Caernarvonshire[7] seems likely to have been *Potamogeton natans*, too, while *P. polygonifolius* is suggested by the 'penny leaves that are got in the bog' rated very highly in Limerick for the same purpose[8]—though marsh pennywort (*Hydrocotyle vulgaris*) is a more dubious candidate for the latter.

ARACEAE

Acorus calamus Linnaeus   PLATE 28
sweet flag
southern Asia, Africa; introduced into Europe, North America

In Britain, as elsewhere in Europe, the populations of *Acorus calamus* are ster-ile triploids and accepted as wholly introduced. The rhizome contains a gly-coside, acorin, and has been valued medicinally since Classical times. Well established in the wild by 1668 in Norfolk, the only part of the British Isles where the plant has been abundant, it was long prized there by the country folk as a remedy for 'ague' (credibly, in this marshy county, benign tertiary malaria rather than other kinds of fever in this instance).[9] The rhizome was cut into pieces, dried and then ground into a powder.

Arum maculatum Linnaeus
lords-and-ladies, cuckoo-pint
Europe, North Africa

Though *Arum maculatum,* a common plant of hedge bottoms, is dangerously poisonous, rich in compounds capable of causing death, the acrid juice of the berries has been valued as a wart cure in Worcestershire.[10] The acridity, however, is lost when the fresh root is reduced to powder and in that form it has constituted a highly rated remedy for rheumatism in Devon.[11] Success has also been claimed in Somerset for poulticing abscess swellings with (the leaves of?) the plant.[12]

The sole Irish record traced comes from Wexford, where the powder from the root placed under the tongue and swallowed with the saliva has been held to relieve 'palsy'.[13]

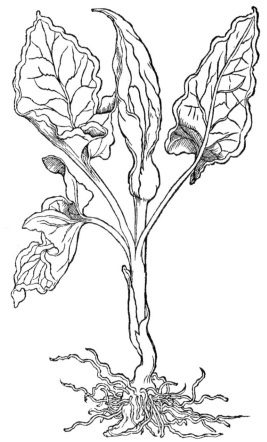

Arum maculatum, lords-and-ladies (Brunfels 1530, p. 56)

LEMNACEAE

Lemna minor Linnaeus; and other species
duckweed
cosmopolitan except for polar regions and tropics
Allegedly once a cure in the Highlands for headaches and inflammation,[14] a
record of *Lemna minor* in Leitrim to bathe a swelling[15] may be confirmatory
evidence of that. In Cavan,[16] however, and in some other unidentified part of
Ireland[17] the plant's value has been as a tonic to cleanse the system. 'Duck's
weed' was also formerly a popular healing herb in Lewis in the Outer Hebrides for some unspecified purpose.[18]

JUNCACEAE

Juncus inflexus Linnaeus
hard rush
Europe, western and central Asia, Macaronesia, northern and
    southern Africa, Java; introduced into eastern North America,
    Australasia
It may or may not have been mere chance that it was *Juncus inflexus* that
proved to be in use in parts of Ulster at one time for jaundice.[19] Usually, folk
records refer only to 'rushes' unspecifically. In various parts of Ireland, those
have been burnt and the ashes put to service: as a cure for ringworm in
Offaly[20] and Waterford[21] or, mixed with lard and made into an ointment
applied to 'wildfire'—presumably shingles—in Westmeath,[22] or to the pustules of chickenpox, to prevent scarring, in some other, unidentified area.[23]

The sole British record traced of a medical use of 'rushes' is as a wart cure
in Cheshire.[24]

CYPERACEAE

Eriophorum angustifolium Honckeney
cottongrass
northern and central Europe, Siberia, North America
(Name confusion) The misattribution to *Eriophorum angustifolium* of the
Irish Gaelic name for self-heal (*Prunella vulgaris*) has led to erroneous records
of its use in Wicklow[25] and, probably from the same cause, in the Aran
Islands, too.[26]

POACEAE

'Grass' in a vague, generic sense features here and there in the folk medicine records, especially the Irish ones: stuffed in shoes to remedy corns in Roscommon,[27] used to bandage severe cuts in Waterford[28] or staunch a haemorrhage in Tipperary[29] or, torn up for the roots, a source of a rheumatism cure in Kerry.[30] Though other records are more specific, they are scarcely more helpful. All that we are told of a wart cure in Hampshire's New Forest is that it was a preparation of 'a certain kind of grass'.[31] Even a name is not necessarily any advance: What, for example, is 'cough grass', employed for colds in Limerick?[32] 'Cough' seems unlikely to have been a slip for 'couch', for colds are not one of the ailments for which *Elytrigia repens* is known to have been used. In some cases, however, the kind of grass in question can be pinned down to a particular species with more or less certainty.

Briza media Linnaeus
   quaking-grass
   Europe, temperate Asia; introduced into eastern North America
   (Misidentification suspected) *Briza media* has been recorded as used in Kirkcudbrightshire for some unspecified medicinal purpose under the unlikely-sounding name 'mountain flax'[33]—which ordinarily belongs to *Linum catharticum* and raises the suspicion that some mix-up in identification may have occurred. There can hardly be any doubt, though, that it *was* this that enjoyed the reputation in the East Riding of Yorkshire of keeping away mice, to which end bunches of it were dried and hung up on the mantelpieces.[34]
   The claims of this to be Ireland's mysterious 'hungry grass' are discussed under *Agrostis stolonifera*, following.

Agrostis stolonifera Linnaeus
   A. alba Linnaeus
   creeping bent, fiorin grass
   Europe, central and eastern Asia, North Africa; introduced into
      North America and elsewhere
Irish folklore collectors have been much exercised over the identity of the *feargorta(ch)* or *fairgurtha*, variously described as 'a long blade of grass' which 'grows up through whins'[35] and 'a peculiar grass that grows on the mountains'[36] (both of Connemara and Kerry) and said to be the cause, once stepped on, of violent hunger, abnormal craving and—by the more scientifically inclined—diabetes. In Monaghan it has been used in combination with

the roots of other herbs for a particular kind of sore like a boil occurring on fingers and toes.[37] At least one authority[38] has plumped for quaking-grass (*Briza media*) as the solution of the mystery, but that could hardly be considered a species of mountains. It has been widely overlooked, however, that one of Ireland's finest field botanists had *fear gorta* pointed out to him, in Tyrone, and found that it was the common *Agrostis stolonifera*.[39] It does not necessarily follow, though, that the name has been applied consistently, and it also remains to be demonstrated that creeping bent is capable of producing the bodily effects described.

Phleum pratense Linnaeus
timothy
Europe, northern Asia, Algeria; introduced into North America and
   elsewhere.
A use of *Phleum pratense* recorded from Waterford[40] involved placing a leaf round a cut on a finger to keep the cloth from adhering to the wound.

Elytrigia repens (Linnaeus) Desvaux ex Nevski
Agropyron repens (Linnaeus) P. Beauverd, *Elymus repens*
   (Linnaeus) Gould
common couch, twitch, squitch-grass, scutch-grass, dog-grass,
   foul-grass
Europe, Siberia, North Africa; introduced into North America
Renowned since Classical times for its claimed efficacy against disorders of the kidney and genitourinary infections, an infusion derived from the bruised rhizomes of *Elytrigia repens* enjoyed such sustained popularity for those purposes in learned medicine that it was no doubt from that source that it acquired its scattered following for them in the folk tradition in the British Isles, too. There are British records from Essex and Norfolk.[41]

Irish records are more widespread: from 'Ulster',[42] Cavan,[43] Kilkenny[44] and Waterford.[45]

Phragmites australis (Cavanilles) Trinius ex Steudel
P. communis Trinius
common reed
cosmopolitan
Martin Martin, in the course of his Hebridean travels in 1695, learned of a cough cure in Lewis in the Outer Hebrides made from boiling together the roots of reeds and of nettles and leaving the liquid to ferment by adding yeast to it.[46]

TYPHACEAE

Typha latifolia Linnaeus
   great reedmace
   most of northern hemisphere, South America
Supplying a toothache remedy in an unidentified part of Ireland,[47] *Typha latifolia* was once also in high repute as a cure for epilepsy in the south-western Highlands, under a Gaelic name translating as 'fairy wives' spindle'. Evidently more of a charm, though, than a medicine, it was held to be most potent if gathered at Midsummer midnight (with a prescribed ritual) before being wrapped in a shroud—for keeping a dead stem and root of the plant in 'dead-clothes' ensured freedom from every ailment for the rest of one's life.[48]

LILIACEAE

Narthecium ossifragum (Linnaeus) Hudson
   bog asphodel
   Atlantic Europe, allied species in North America
Under the name *limerik, Narthecium ossifragum* was formerly used in Shetland as a substitute for 'saffron' (see the following), standing in for that medicinally as well as a dye.[49]

Colchicum autumnale Linnaeus
   meadow saffron
   central and south-eastern Europe; introduced into North America,
      New Zealand

Crocus sativus Linnaeus
   saffron crocus
   horticultural

Crocus vernus (Linnaeus) Hill
   spring crocus
   south-eastern Europe; introduced into North America
The word saffron is a potential source of much confusion. Most Irish folk cures apparently mean by it sheep droppings, records of it as an abortifacient are based on mishearings of 'savin', i.e. juniper,[50] and even when correctly applied herbally it can mean any of three species: the saffron crocus (*Crocus sativus*, of the family Iridaceae), once extensively grown as a crop in East Anglia, the spring crocus (*C. vernus*), anciently a stand-in for that in the

bleaker north of England and surviving there today in one or two meadows, and meadow saffron (*Colchicum autumnale*), alone accepted as native. The main English populations of this last species, east of the Severn estuary, have been raided down the years to supply the druggists, but that it was often used instead of *Crocus sativus* for the saffron cakes eaten in Essex for rheumatism (imparting a different colour and taste)[51] suggests that it may have enjoyed a more purely folk following as well. Possibly it was also the source of the saffron tea formerly much given in Norfolk to children to bring out sweating in fevers or the spots in cases of measles.[52]

It was for measles, too, that 'saffron' was used in one of only two instances traced in the Irish folk records (Tipperary[53]) that are explicitly herbal. In the other (Carlow[54]) the plant was boiled in milk and drunk for jaundice. These two counties fall within the area in which meadow saffron is accepted as native in Ireland. But that *Colchicum autumnale* is poisonous even after being boiled would imply that, if indeed it did have a place in the folk repertory, it must have been used only with great discretion.

Convallaria majalis Linnaeus
lily-of-the-valley
Europe, north-eastern Asia; introduced into North America
(Folk credentials questionable) No less poisonous than *Colchicum autumnale,* containing glycosides which in small amounts both purge and slow the heartbeat and in larger ones cause convulsions and even death, *Convallaria majalis* has probably always been too scarce in the wild in Britain to be utilised from that source herbally even if it was not avoided as too dangerous. Two Irish records (Antrim,[55] Cavan[56]) of its use for heart trouble must surely be borrowings from the learned tradition, but binding a leaf on to a cut or abrasion to 'draw' or otherwise heal it (Gloucestershire,[57] Cambridgeshire[58]) sounds like genuine folk applications even though garden-based.

Polygonatum multiflorum (Linnaeus) Allioni
Solomon's-seal
Europe, temperate Asia to Japan; introduced into North America

Polygonatum ×hybridum Bruegger
horticultural
In Hampshire, where *Polygonatum multiflorum* is commoner than anywhere else in Britain and an indicator of ancient woodland, 'the vulgar sort of people', according to John Gerard, were in his day in the habit of drinking a decoction of the powdered root, or applying it as a poultice, to heal broken

bones.[59] No later record of that use has been traced; instead, the crushed roots have been valued mostly for drawing the blackness out of a bruise (Kent,[60] Gloucestershire,[61] East Anglia,[62] Cumbria[63]) or for removing suntan, freckles or spots on the face (Hampshire,[64] Norfolk[65]). The plant has also been credited with an astringent property which has won it favour in Sussex as an application to wounds[66] and in Cumbria, under the name 'vagabond's friend', to sores.[67]

Away from south-eastern and south-central England and southern Wales, *Polygonatum multiflorum* is regarded as probably only a naturalised introduction, a status which is shared more generally by the Solomon's-seal more often grown in gardens, *P. ×hybridum.* Those uses in Cumbria are thus likely to have been based on plants imported from farther south or derived from books.

That same explanation must hold, too, for the only record traced from Ireland: a one-time popularity in 'Ulster' of a decoction of this herb for staunching haemorrhages and diarrhoea.[68] No species of this genus are accepted as other than introduced in that region of the country.

Paris quadrifolia Linnaeus
herb Paris
Europe, Siberia
(Folk credentials questionable) An important herb in traditional medicine in Asia and recommended in later European herbals, *Paris quadrifolia* would surely have been too scarce in English woods to have sustained any use here based on native populations. A claim that it has been applied in Sussex[69] to wounds is credible only if knowledge of its healing potential was taken from books.

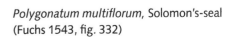

Polygonatum multiflorum, Solomon's-seal
(Fuchs 1543, fig. 332)

Hyacinthoides nonscripta (Linnaeus) Chouard ex Rothmaler
Endymion nonscriptus (Linnaeus) Garcke
bluebell
Atlantic Europe; introduced into North America, New Zealand
It would be remarkable if so abundant and conspicuous a member of the flora of the British Isles as *Hyacinthoides nonscripta* had not had its sticky juice put to some medicinal purposes at least. That only two folk records that have been traced of the use of that, however, both Irish—boiled for throat ailments in Cavan[70] and applied to whitlows in Monaghan[71]—suggests that it has largely been found ineffective.

In Inverness-shire, though, the roots when chopped, fried and applied as a plaster at one time had a reputation for promoting suppuration speedily.[72]

Allium ursinum Linnaeus   PLATE 29
ramsons, wild garlic
Europe, Asia Minor
Allium ursinum occurs in such profusion in much of the west of the British Isles that, as the folk records suggest, many there have probably always been content to gather it from the wild: transplanting it to the garden would bring only a marginal gain in convenience. Outside that region, though, gardens are likely to have been the usual source.

Predominantly Irish as a folk medicine and invested there with a sprinkling of semi-magical beliefs indicative of ancient usage, ramsons has a reputation as a preventative of infection as well as a source of cures. A west-of-England saying ran, 'Eat leeks in Lide [March] and ramsins in May, and all the year after physitians may play'.[73] More specifically, 'nine diseases shiver before the garlic', it was held in Sligo, where faith in the plant's ability to ward off illness was still so widespread at the time of the 1918 influenza pandemic that many carried a piece around with them in a pocket.[74] That practice was not as far-fetched as it may sound, for one of the traditional, if less usual, ways of bringing garlic to bear on a cough or a cold has been to wear strips of the leaves under the soles of the feet, and in Lincolnshire,[75] Galway[76] and Clare,[77] if not elsewhere, that has extended to walking around with them inside one's shoes or socks. Mostly, though, the plant is either eaten raw or boiled (usually in milk) and the liquid then rubbed into the skin.

The prolonged burning sensation left by the juice has naturally made this plant an age-old favourite for treating ailments most obviously responsive to that. Straightforward applications externally, however, seem to have been very much an Irish speciality: for easing toothache (all 11 records out of the total of 112 logged for uses of every kind in Britain and/or Ireland), rheumatism ('Ulster',[78] Tipperary[79]), the inflamed sores on the fingers popularly known as felons (Wicklow[80]) and the poulticing of mumps and swellings round the neck (Galway[81]). The herb is more effective, though, if crushed or chewed and digested, for that releases a substance called allicin which has been found to act against micro-organisms. That would seem to justify the beliefs in parts of Ireland (Cavan,[82] Louth,[83] Laois,[84] Tipperary[85]) that garlic purifies the blood, cures boils (Kilkenny[86]) and heals sore eyes (Kilkenny also[87]). It must also justify in part the plant's popularity for chest and lung infections, which together with sore throats, colds and coughs of every kind account form by far the largest number (75) of uses—if the 9 relating to asthma are included in that broad category as well. On the other hand, that explanation will hardly do for the mainly Irish conviction that garlic is good for indigestion and stomach-ache (Clare,[88] Tipperary,[89] Cork[90]), nor for its use to counter intestinal worms in Roscommon[91] or warts and corns in Offaly,[92] or to alleviate measles in Mayo.[93] But because allicin has been discovered also to lower cholesterol, and more particularly the low-density lipoprotein, a persistent belief in the Aran Islands[94] that the plant is effective against blood clots has now received impressive confirmation.

There can be no surprise that the recommendation of garlic by Dioscorides for the bites of snakes finds no reflection in Ireland, though it has found some in Cheshire (as 'churl's treacle').[95] This use may well have come through the herbals, but that seems less likely as regards knowledge of the plant's action as a diuretic. Early travellers in the Hebrides found an infusion of the leaves of wild garlic being drunk there extensively for gravel or the stone: Martin Martin encountered this in Skye and Harris,[96] and John Lightfoot in Arran,[97] Thomas Pennant adding that the potion was taken in the latter in brandy.[98] There is a more recent record of employment for kidney trouble in Shetland,[99] too. Yet nothing under that head has turned up in the Irish records, contrary to what one might have supposed—even though the Highlands have shared with Ireland that faith in the plant's power to purify the blood and in its ability to clear infected matter from wounds.[100] The British also seem to have applied it externally much less widely than the Irish, aching joints and bruised limbs in Cumbria[101] alone falling into that category.

Allium ampeloprasum Linnaeus var. *babingtonii* (Borrer) Syme
wild leek
south-western England, western Ireland

In the west of Ireland *Allium ampeloprasum* var. *babingtonii* shares the name 'wild garlic' with *A. ursinum* and has doubtless shared some of the uses of that there, too. It has been identified botanically as the plant applied under that name to a cattle disease in Donegal.[102]

Allium oleraceum Linnaeus
field garlic
Europe to Caucasus; introduced into North America, Australia

In Devon the young shoots of both *Allium oleraceum* and *A. vineale* at one time enjoyed a reputation among agricultural labourers of acting on the kidneys to cure gravel[103] (a use found recorded only from Scotland in the case of *A. ursinum*).

Allium vineale Linnaeus
wild onion, crow garlic
Europe, south-western Asia, North Africa; introduced into North
   America, Australasia

In the New Forest in Hampshire, where *Allium vineale* largely replaces *A. ursinum*, a woman claimed to have cured herself of tuberculosis by living on a diet of this plant, bread, spring water and little else.[104] The dried bulbs crushed to a powder and then worn on a flannel inside a shoe have also featured as a cold cure in Warwickshire.[105]

Narcissus Linnaeus
daffodil

As no records of folk uses of the wild daffodil, *Narcissus pseudonarcissus* Linnaeus, have been traced from those parts of England and Wales where, alone in the British Isles, that is accepted as native, it can only have been garden or naturalised examples of one or other of the numerous cultivated species or hybrids that have been employed in Donegal as an emetic[106] and in some unidentified part of Ireland made into hot fomentations to cure colds,[107] uses which can hardly have had any lengthy history. The same applies to a veterinary use of the Spanish daffodil, *N. pseudonarcissus* subsp. *major*, recorded from Colonsay in the Inner Hebrides.

Ruscus aculeatus Linnaeus
butcher's-broom
central and southern Europe, Azores

The reputation of the diuretic action of *Ruscus aculeatus,* and its consequent recommendation for kidney and urinary complaints, can be traced back through the herbals to Dioscorides. That would be reason enough to suspect the few instances in which this species has been traced in the folk medicine records represent no more than borrowings from the learned tradition. Heightening that suspicion is the fact that, with only one exception, none of those records comes from areas where the plant is accepted as native. The exception is Devon, where an infusion was made from the leaves and stems, which were chopped and dried. This potion was drunk for jaundice as well.[108] It contrasts with the Classical recommendation of a decoction of the rhizomes and may therefore be of genuinely folk origin. That the plant's use in the county may go back a long way is perhaps given added credence by the fact that the its prickly leaves have also stood in there for those of holly as a painful means of healing chilblains.[109] On the other hand, the seeming lack of records from anywhere farther east in England, especially from Hampshire, where the plant is locally common in woods and hedgerows, does not help that case.

It is damning, moreover, that all the other folk records are from Ireland. That those should be relatively widespread in a country in which the species is not considered native has a parallel in the case of barberry (*Berberis vulgaris*). The standard use as a diuretic is known from Cavan[110] and Galway,[111] and there is a third, unlocalised record for that as well.[112] In Down, on the other hand, the preparation has been applied as a poultice in cases of dropsy.[113]

IRIDACEAE

In addition to *Iris* the family Iridaceae includes *Crocus,* but records for that genus are given under the discussion of *Colchicum autumnale,* included above under Liliaceae.

Iris pseudacorus Linnaeus

yellow iris, yellow flag, flagger; *feileastram* (Ireland)
Europe, western Asia, North Africa; introduced into North America,
   Australasia

The highly acrid rhizomes of *Iris pseudacorus* are strongly purgative and were in use c. 1700 in Skye for enemas.[114] A more prevalent use for the plant in northern Scotland, however, has been for colds,[115] throat inflammations[116] and, in particular, toothache. As originally reported by the Rev. John Stuart from Mull and certain parts of the Highlands, a teaspoonful of the juice was poured into both nostrils, producing a copious flow of mucus and saliva which often effected a cure.[117] Alternatively, as in Orkney,[118] the liquid itself was snorted up the nose. For toothache in Argyllshire, on the other hand, the rhizome itself was chopped up and chewed[119]—a practice frowned on in Orkney, where it was held to cause stammering[120]—but elsewhere (as also in Ireland) a piece was kept against the particular tooth affected.

None of these applications appears to be on record from southern Britain. Instead, it has been for kidney trouble that the plant has been valued in Cardiganshire,[121] while in Sussex it has featured in a list of wound plants,[122] and in Kent (?) an ointment made from the flowers served as a popular village cosmetic in the early nineteenth century.[123]

The Irish, however, have shared to some extent (Wicklow,[124] Galway,[125] Kerry[126]) that Scots faith in the plant's effectiveness against toothache and have also used it for mumps (Meath,[127] Offaly[128]). Apparently unique, though, is a record from the area just south of western Ulster of the inclusion of these yellow flowers in a mixture taken there for jaundice.[129]

Iris foetidissima Linnaeus
stinking iris, gladdon, gladwin
western and central Europe, North Africa; introduced into
North America, New Zealand

Popular as a purge since Anglo-Saxon times, *Iris foetidissima* was still in use for that purpose in England as late as the early nineteenth century. William Turner found that in the Isle of Purbeck in Dorset it was locally known as 'spurgewort' for that reason[130]; John Gerard knew it only as a Somerset remedy,[131] but by the time of John Parkinson it was described as a herb of 'many of our country people in many places'.[132] Those who found the traditional decoction of the sliced rhizome acted too violently drank instead an infusion of the bitter leaves in ale. This latter method was in favour in the south of England at the time when the last reports were published.[133] By the twentieth century, however, the country folk of Somerset had apparently shifted to using the rhizome only for cramp,[134] while in the Isle of Man the plant was valued as a diuretic.[135]

That purging tradition has seemingly been absent (or died out) from Ireland, where this plant is much scarcer and not considered native. Instead, in 'several parts' of that country in the nineteenth century, 'gladum' or 'glading root' was esteemed for dropsy (as in Tyrone[136]) and for applying to fresh wounds.[137] By the 1930s, however, the Irish country people talked of it mainly if not solely as a treatment for mumps or a throat swollen from other causes.

The remedy involved heating the leaves or their stalks and then tying them round the neck. Records of this have been traced from four counties in the vicinity of Dublin as well as from Roscommon,[138] Galway[139] and Kilkenny.[140] Such widespread knowledge of one particular application seems indicative either of a relatively recent origin and spread or of considerable antiquity. The latter explanation seems more likely in view of the fact that one informant knew of a special ritual with which the plant had to be gathered for use for this purpose.[141]

DIOSCOREACEAE

Tamus communis Linnaeus
  black bryony
  southern and western Europe, south-western Asia, North Africa

In common with its 'gender pair', white bryony (*Bryonia dioica*), *Tamus communis* has had a history of being misidentified as, or mischievously substituted for, the true mandrake plant (*Mandragora* spp.) on account of its large taproot and has owed to that mistake a reputation as a powerful aphrodisiac. Lincolnshire is one county where that belief has been found surviving.[142] More generally, though, black bryony has had a role in folk medicine in its own right, under the name oxberry. The fresh rhizome, scraped and sliced, has enjoyed at least a regional popularity (Wiltshire,[143] Worcestershire,[144] Herefordshire,[145] Shropshire[146]) as an acrid, counter-irritant plaster for rheumatism and gout, while the juice of the berries, preferably after a soaking in gin or brandy, has been valued in parallel for rubbing on chilblains (Devon,[147] the Isle of Wight,[148] Wiltshire,[149] Worcestershire[150]). Both berries and rhizome have also been used in the Isle of Wight to remove skin discolouring caused by bruises, suntan and the like.[151]

In Ireland the plant is restricted to just one small area in the west and is unlikely to have been utilised there—unless indeed it owes its very presence to ancient introduction medicinally.

ORCHIDACEAE

Listera ovata (Linnaeus) R. Brown
  common twayblade
  Europe, Siberia

Listera ovata has featured in a Sussex list of wound cures.[152] It has also been identified with the *dà-dhuilleach,* a principal ingredient in salep, a well-known Highlands remedy for soothing stomach and bowel irritation.[153] The plant's very wide, if rather sparse, distribution throughout the British Isles would make that feasible.

Platanthera chlorantha (Custer) Reichenbach
greater butterfly-orchid
Europe, Siberia
An ointment of a delicate green colour was at one time made in Dorset from *Platanthera chlorantha* and applied to ulcers.[154]

Dactylorhiza purpurella (Stephenson & T. A. Stephenson) Soó
northern marsh-orchid
north-western Europe

Dactylorhiza maculata (Linnaeus) Soó subsp. **ericetorum**
(E. F. Linton) P. F. Hunt & Summerhayes   PLATE 30
heath spotted-orchid
north-western Europe

Orchis mascula (Linnaeus) Linnaeus   PLATE 31
early-purple orchid
Europe, northern and western Asia, North Africa ·
A decoction of the testicle-like roots of purple-spiked species belonging to *Dactylorhiza* or *Orchis* has enjoyed an age-old reputation as a love-philtre, with an allegedly aphrodisiac effect on women. If there is a case for believing that there was a Doctrine of Signatures, this would seem the most persuasive example. The plant in Galloway credited with this power, known there as *dodjell reepan* and as 'rocket-juice',[155] has been identified botanically as one or more of the marsh-orchids[156] (of which *D. purpurella* is the most likely there). Its counterpart in Wicklow, however, *mogra-myra*—apparently a corruption of an old Irish name—has been referred by a folklorist with botanical expertise to *O. mascula*.[157] Probably because this latter is the species usually cited in books in this connection, at least one other Irish author[158] has settled for the same identity; it has also been taken to be the orchid species which was once highly valued in the Highlands for soothing, or providing a protective lining to, the alimentary canal.[159] It is certainly sufficiently widespread and locally plentiful in Scotland and Ireland for that assumption to be made. On the other hand, an orchid used in the Highlands as a poultice for 'drawing' thorns or splinters has been identified as one of the spotted-orchids, which in that geographical context is most likely to be *D. maculata*

subsp. *ericetorum*, the common one there of wet, heathy ground and bogs. The majority of those recording the use as a love-charm, however, have attributed it just to 'orchids' generically.

Notes

1. Friend 1882
2. Ó Súilleabháin, 314
3. Moore MS
4. *Phytologist*, 1 (1843), 583
5. Williams MS (Welsh Folk Museum tape no. 6571B)
6. McNeill
7. Anne E. Williams, in litt.
8. IFC S 483: 329, 369
9. Pratt 1850–7; Johnson 1862
10. Chamberlain 1882
11. Collyns
12. Tongue
13. IFC S 897: 235
14. Cameron
15. IFC S 226: 22
16. Maloney
17. Wilde, 28
18. Parman
19. Barbour
20. IFC S 812: 440
21. IFC S 655: 150, 267
22. IFC S 737: 107
23. Logan, 76
24. Baker, 57
25. McClafferty
26. Ó hEithir
27. IFC S 251: 173
28. IFC S 654: 89
29. IFC S 512: 523; 572: 70
30. IFC S 476: 91
31. de Crespigny & Hutchinson, 106
32. IFC S 484: 42
33. *Scottish Naturalist*, 1 (1871), 54
34. Robinson 1876, 202
35. IFC S 932: 32
36. *Folk-lore Record*, 4 (1881), 96–125
37. IFC S 931: 26
38. Cameron
39. Hart 1898
40. IFC S 636: 133
41. Hatfield, 41
42. Purdon
43. Maloney
44. IFC S 850: 113
45. IFC S 654: 242; 655: 175
46. Martin, 93
47. Ó Súilleabháin, 314
48. Stewart, 110
49. Tait
50. *PLNN*, no. 36 (1994), 172
51. Newman & Wilson
52. Taylor MS (Hatfield, 42)
53. IFC S 550: 283
54. IFC S 907: 267
55. Harris
56. Maloney
57. Palmer 1994, 122
58. *PLNN*, no. 9 (1989), 40
59. Gerard, 758
60. Pratt 1850–7
61. Gibbs, 57
62. Porter 1974, 46
63. *PLNN*, no. 46 (1996), 223
64. Read, 305
65. Harland
66. A. Allen, 185
67. Wright, 247
68. Purdon
69. A. Allen, 185
70. Maloney
71. IFC S 931: 304
72. Henderson & Dickson, 33
73. Wright, 238
74. IFC S 170: 47, 205, 257
75. Taylor MS (Hatfield, 30)

76. IFC S 5: 163
77. IFC S 617: 222
78. Egan
79. IFC S 550: 275
80. IFC S 914: 284
81. IFC S 21: 248; 59: 217
82. Maloney
83. IFC S 672: 211
84. IFC S 826: 22
85. IFC S 550: 288
86. IFC S 862: 151
87. IFC S 849: 82
88. IFC S 601: 51
89. IFC S 550: 100
90. IFC S 287: 67
91. IFC S 250: 273
92. IFC S 820: 176; 821: 4
93. IFC S 132: 37
94. Ó hEithir
95. Wright, 240
96. Martin, 117, 225
97. Lightfoot, 180
98. Pennant 1774, 175
99. Jamieson
100. Beith
101. Freethy, 82
102. Hart 1898, 367
103. Collyns
104. de Baïracli-Levy, 66
105. Bloom, 29
106. Hart 1898, 372
107. Wilson
108. Lafont
109. Lafont
110. Maloney
111. Logan, 38
112. Purdon
113. Vickery 1995
114. Martin, 231
115. MacFarlane
116. Lightfoot, 1078
117. Lightfoot, 1078

118. Spence; Leask, 79
119. Black, 203
120. Leask, 79
121. Williams MS
122. A. Allen, 185
123. Pratt 1850–7
124. McClafferty
125. IFC S 60: 44
126. IFC S 412: 286
127. IFC S 690: 42
128. IFC S 811: 63
129. Logan, 46
130. Turner 1568, part 2, 171 verso
131. Gerard, 54
132. Parkinson, 259
133. Banks; Pratt 1850–7
134. Tongue
135. Cregeen
136. *Hardwicke's Science-gossip* (1877), 46
137. Moore MS
138. IFC S 268: 230
139. IFC S 21: 216, 248; 60: 46, 50, 51
140. IFC S 849: 84
141. IFC S 849: 84
142. Woodruffe-Peacock; Rudkin
143. Whitlock 1992, 104
144. *Phytologist*, n.s. 5 (1861), 159
145. *Phytologist*, n.s. 5 (1861), 159
146. *Phytologist*, n.s. 5 (1861), 159
147. Friend 1882
148. *Phytologist*, 3 (1849), 893
149. Whitlock 1992, 104
150. *English Dialect Dictionary*
151. Bromfield
152. A. Allen, 185
153. Beith, 232
154. Udal 1889, 31
155. Mactaggart, 174–5
156. Britten & Holland
157. Kinahan, 117
158. Moloney
159. Beith

CHAPTER 17

Distribution Patterns of Folk Medicinal Uses

Because the records of folk uses are for the most part so fragmentary, chrono-logically as well as spatially, and in particular largely lacking for sizeable areas of England and Scotland (in contrast to Ireland), distribution patterns of the degree of completeness to which botanists or epidemiologists are accustomed are too much to hope for. That very incompleteness means that some of the patterns that have emerged in the foregoing pages may well be illusory, des-tined to dissolve if and when additional records accumulate. This important caveat needs to be borne in mind throughout what follows.

It also needs to be stressed that a herbal tradition based on plants available in the wild will to a large extent have been shaped by the natural ranges of the plant species concerned. The distribution patterns exhibited by many folk remedies are thus products at one remove of those factors of climate or ter-rain that set more or less strict limits to where the species can occur in the quantity necessary to enable them to be exploited herbally. Outside those limits the species are likely to have been too scarce, at least in more recent times, to be reliably on hand whenever needed and to justify the effort required to search for them. Though that restriction imposed by nature can be overridden in many cases by taking the plants from the wild and growing them domestically, cottage gardens tend to be relatively tiny and congested, with food plants necessarily accorded priority; moreover, the same adverse factors that render a herb scarce in the wild can make it resistant to attempts to bring it into cultivation successfully.

The majority of the distribution patterns that emerge from the data, how-ever, do not coincide, even very roughly, with the natural ranges of the spe-cies concerned. Many herbal plants are to be found in some degree of plenty over much or all of both Britain and Ireland, yet if the records of their use for therapeutic purposes are broadly representative of the whole, in many areas—and some of those very extensive ones—their potential has been ignored. Some herbs will have failed to penetrate some areas fully suited to them because an alternative with a similar action was well established there already; others may have gained favour through being sponsored by a particular forceful individual or dominant social group; still others may be the legacy of some past wave of incomers, their utilisation preserved by mere habit down through the centuries since.

Some of these patterns are relatively limited in their extent; others, however, can be traced across some major portion of either Ireland or Britain. It is tempting to assume that a wide distribution is indicative of considerable age, but such an assumption may be misplaced: we have no means of knowing how rapidly in the past herbal novelties were able to spread. Rural societies tend to be extremely retentive of the practices they are used to, but a demonstrably more effective cure for an ailment possessed by a neighbouring, more sophisticated culture has probably always had the power to break down resistance, especially at times of crisis, when an epidemic occurs that exposes the ineffectiveness of a tried-and-tested nostrum and the helplessness of those whose healing knowledge had hitherto been regarded as infallible.

In some cases it is just one particular application of a herb, out of the full range of its recorded functions, that has thrown up a pattern worthy of note. One or two of these patterns are fully as clear-cut, in a stark all-or-nothing type of occurrence, as any displayed at the level of the herb as a whole. Thus as a remedy for skin troubles, *Geranium robertianum* (herb-Robert) has emerged as exclusively British, whereas as a treatment for coughs or as a cure for kidney complaints it has come to light as equally exclusively Irish. *Veronica chamaedrys* (germander speedwell), similarly, features mainly as a cure for jaundice in the Irish records, yet its British records are wholly as an eye lotion and wholly from the south of England at that. *Iris foetidissima* (stinking iris) has been widely recorded in Ireland as in use for mumps or a swollen throat, whereas in the older English records it receives mention only as a purge. *Sambucus nigra* (common elder) provides a fourth, less extreme example. Though one of the most widely used of all British and Irish folk herbs and applied to a great variety of ailments, its flowers or berries have been looked to for ameliorating colds and the like in numerous counties and other areas in Scotland, Wales and especially England but in relatively very few in Ireland. Contrariwise, this tree's employment in a salve for burns or scalds has been recorded very widely in Ireland but scarcely at all in Britain.

An alternative form in which countrywide contrasts are found is diagonally: between Ireland plus Scotland on the one hand and England (plus in some cases Wales) on the other. Three herbs exhibit this pattern, each in rather different ways. In *Potentilla anserina* (silverweed) the dichotomy is a wholesale one, embracing all the recorded uses; in *Iris pseudacorus* (yellow iris) it is between just a single use (for toothache) in the north and west and several uses in the south and east; while in *Glechoma hederacea* (ground-ivy) just two uses out of a diversity of known ones constitute the polar opposites: it is a cold cure in the 'Celtic' countries (that useful term popularly employed in a non-linguistic sense to cover Ireland, Scotland, Wales, the Isle of Man and Cornwall) and a tonic in central and southern England.

That use of *Iris pseudacorus* to ease toothache is one of quite a number of instances of therapeutic properties that would otherwise be wholly Irish extending across to the Western Isles and/or Highlands of Scotland. Others are the valuing of *Rorippa nasturtium-aquaticum* (water-cress) and *Asplenium trichomanes* (maidenhair spleenwort) for feverish complaints, and *Senecio jacobaea* (common ragwort) for drawing boils and the like. In addition, Ireland and that stretch of Scotland appear to have had more or less exclusive monopolies of several plants as herbs: *Leucanthemum vulgare* (oxeye daisy), *Lathyrus linifolius* (bitter-vetch), *Lemna* species (duckweed), *Sphagnum* species (bog-moss), *Parmelia* species (the lichens generically known as crotal)—and *Palmaria palmata* (dulse), and *Chondrus crispus* and *Mastocarpus stellatus* (Irish moss) among the seaweeds. Most if not all these range far more widely in the British Isles as a whole and can be found elsewhere in them in at least comparable quantities, so a general similarity in the natural environment can hardly stand up as an explanation for that shared legacy of use. That the pattern is the result of cultural links, going back perhaps many centuries, does seem more likely; and that likelihood is strengthened by the fact that it is in just its northernmost counties of Donegal and Londonderry—in so far as the records traced go—that Ireland has shared with either northern or western Scotland faith in the healing powers of *Asplenium trichomanes* and *Lathyrus linifolius*.

Cultural links, too, rather than floristic or environmental affinities must surely be the explanation for certain uses being common to Ireland and the 'Celtic fringe' of Britain as a whole. For how else are we to account for the restriction of records for applying *Rumex* species (docks) to burns or scalds to seven widely separated Irish counties and in Britain only to three of its westernmost extremities (Cornwall, Pembrokeshire, Scotland's Outer Hebrides)? Though no other use exhibits this pattern with such precision, there are several more that broadly approximate to it: the pondweeds *Potamogeton natans* and/or *P. polygonifolius* for burns, *Linum catharticum* (fairy flax) for menstrual irregularity and species of *Arctium* (burdock) as a purifying tonic. Other plants such as *Sorbus aucuparia* (rowan), *Myrica gale* (bog-myrtle), *Rumex acetosa* (common sorrel) and the Lycopodiaceae (clubmosses) are broadly 'Celtic fringe' across the full range of their herbal functions, but except in the case of *R. acetosa* those are ones restricted to Ireland and north and west Britain already by habitat and climate requirements.

Neither environmental determinants nor cultural links, however, seem capable of explaining why both Wales and the south-west of England stand well apart in certain respects not only from the rest of the 'Celtic fringe' but from other parts of the British Isles as a whole. Apparently peculiar to Cornwall and Devon, for example, has been the very extensive drinking of 'organ tea' made from *Mentha pulegium* (pennyroyal), partly just as a refreshment but mostly to clear the nasal and bronchial passages whenever colds or related complaints occur. Though a plant rather specialised in its habitat demands, this species of mint formerly grew naturally in much of lowland England, so it is hard to understand how it came to be preferred over other members of the mint family that have a similar therapeutic property so widely and so persistently in just that one corner of the country. No less hard to explain is the seeming near-restriction of the herbal use of *Anagallis arvensis* (scarlet pimpernel), a plant far more common and generally distributed than *M. pulegium*, to that same corner of England (and to some extent the neighbouring parts of Wales as well). Even more inexplicable is the uniquely wide range of uses to which the multitudinous microspecies of *Rubus fruticosus* (blackberry) have been put in that region—one of them, the application of the leaves to skin complaints, seemingly unrecorded anywhere else. Yet those plants are no more nor less ubiquitous in the West Country than in most other lowland areas of England, Wales and Ireland, nor is there any evidence that any of the microspecies special to that region are particularly endowed with properties that make them more rewarding for herbal purposes than elsewhere. Why, too, is it virtually only on the stony beaches of England's south-west that another widespread plant, *Glaucium flavum* (yellow horned-poppy), has been sought out for the putative healing power of its latex? Are what we confronted with in cases such as these the relics of uses that originated in the particular area in question but subsequently failed to spread much more widely, perhaps as a result of poor communications? Or are they the relics of once much more general uses that, through the accidents of time, have chanced to survive only peripherally?

Wales seems to owe its distinctiveness in part to a tradition of herb *cultivation* in which there has been a strong preference for certain introduced species at the expense of native ones. Only that could explain why the alien *Artemisia absinthium* (wormwood) has been found in use there so exceptionally widely and for a markedly greater variety of ailments than elsewhere—and why another foreign import, more strictly confined to gardens, *Tanacetum parthenium* (Linnaeus) Schultz 'Bipontinus' (feverfew), has attracted folk applications there, too, that are sharply different from those recorded for it elsewhere in Britain and in Ireland. The Welsh, though, are hardly likely to have taken into cultivation the unquestionably indigenous *Menyanthes trifoliata* (bogbean), that favourite bitter of the entire 'Celtic fringe', and some other explanation is needed to account for their esteeming that for rheumatism to a particularly wide extent while showing a singular lack of interest in it as a tonic and digestive in marked contrast to their fellow 'Celts' elsewhere in the British Isles.

A particularly suggestive distribution pattern is to be found among the many records and uses of *Umbilicus rupestris* (navelwort), a common and very widespread plant of western Britain and Ireland. Only in the south-eastern corner of the latter and in the south-western corner of Wales, directly opposite, does that appear to have been recorded as supplying a treatment for chilblains. In those same two areas, but some way beyond them as well, the plant has served as a corn cure, too. It is tempting to look to the Irish settlement of Dyfed in the fourth and fifth centuries A.D. as the explanation in this case.

In the same way it is tempting to ascribe to past Norse influence a number of herbal practices for which records have been traced only—and otherwise inexplicably—from areas where that influence is known to have been particularly long-lasting and pronounced. Apparently in the Hebrides and Shetland alone has *Allium ursinum* (ramsons) been brought to bear on urinary-cum-kidney troubles; only from the Hebrides and the Isle of Man have records emerged for the application of one or more species of *Equisetum* (horsetails) to bleeding; only in Orkney and the Outer Hebridean island of South Uist does that near-ubiquitous decorator of maritime turf, *Armeria maritima* (thrift), appear to have had a herbal role at all. Similarly, it seems to have been only in the Isle of Man, Orkney, Shetland and (even more tellingly) the Faeroe

Islands as well that the fleshy leaves of *Rumex acetosa* (common sorrel) have been eaten to counter scurvy, and only in that same quarter plus the Highlands, Sligo and Pembrokeshire that the even fleshier *Cochlearia officinalis* (scurvy-grass), the more usual weapon in Europe against this sickness, has apparently been reported in use, too. Again, it is from the Isle of Man, Orkney and Shetland that a noticeably disproportionate number of the records come for the taking of a tonic made from *Achillea millefolium* (yarrow) to lift the spirits from depression.

Much more resistant to any explanation, cultural or environmental, is the seeming restriction just to England of a number of remedies obtained from plants that occur commonly over much of both Britain and Ireland in the wild. Thus it is only from a wide scatter of English counties, almost all in the southern half of the country, that the prickly leaves of *Ilex aquifolium* (holly) appear to have featured as a painful cure for chilblains. It is also as a treatment for chilblains and the like that *Solanum dulcamara* (bittersweet) has yielded records from England alone. Could it be that the English have traditionally found it especially hard to bear that particular torment of the flesh—or is it one to which their climate (or diet?) has made them more than ordinarily prone? A further geographical oddity is the pattern of the records that have survived for the wearing of pieces of *Potentilla anserina* (silverweed) in footwear to prevent or ease sore feet: all are from the eastern stretch of England between London and Yorkshire. Was this a practice that arose somewhere within that area and then gradually spread through it over the years (for the records go back nearly three centuries)? Or was it a once much more general use that has merely chanced to linger on in just this portion of its range?

There are other plants that are common in Britain and Ireland alike that in certain of their medicinal roles appear to have featured in the southern half of England mainly or even wholly. Among these are *Glechoma hederacea* (ground-ivy) as a tonic, species of *Ranunculus* (buttercups), *Prunus spinosa* (blackthorn) and *Silene dioica* (red campion) as cures for warts, *Veronica chamaedrys* (germander speedwell) as an eye lotion, species of *Plantago* (plantains) as soothers of stings and species of *Salix* (willows) in their aspirin-like functions. Restriction to southern England is easier to understand in the case of *Viscum album* (mistletoe), for it is only in parts of there that this long-valued herb occurs naturally in the British Isles in any quantity; yet why have the virtues of *Calystegia soldanella* (sea bindweed) apparently remained unappreciated elsewhere, and why should the tradition of using quite a range of plants as a teething necklace for babies have been exclusively English, too?

Unsurprisingly, it is between Britain and Ireland that the greatest number of differences are to be found. For millennia the two have been isolated from each other by geography in a far more thoroughgoing way than Wales has been from England or the northern half of Scotland from the parts of Britain to its south. For much of that time, too, Ireland has enjoyed a substantial degree of cultural autonomy. The Irish flora lacks a third of Britain's species, principally on account of its greater distance from the European mainland and its much more limited upland terrain. Basically, though, the Irish flora is similar to Britain's. This has not prevented the two countries diverging very considerably in the ways in which they have exploited the natural botanical heritage for therapeutic purposes. Ireland's lengthier history of poverty and, especially in the west, greater remoteness from the Classical herbal tradition introduced to England by the Romans and subsequently perpetuated and widely diffused there have compelled in this respect a self-sufficiency that has been both more extensive and longer-lasting.

At the same time that comparative freedom from Continental influence must not be exaggerated. More records have proved forthcoming from Ireland than from Britain of the herbal use of two plants, *Berberis vulgaris* (barberry) and *Ruscus aculeatus* (butcher's-broom), that are not accepted by botanists as other than human introductions in the former. The impressively wide scatter of those Irish records can only therefore be the product of monkish or later usage.

Even if a plant features on the list of unquestioned Irish natives, it does not follow that any or of all the medicinal purposes to which it may have been put are themselves Irish in origin. Remedies on record largely or wholly from the area around Dublin—such as those described for *Pilosella officinarum* (mouse-ear hawkweed)—particularly invite suspicion in this connection. At the same time some distribution patterns that appear suspicious may have quite innocent explanations. Thus all the records traced of the use of *Rumex acetosa* (common sorrel) to poultice boils and other septic sores are from the south-eastern counties, seemingly pointing to an infiltration of that use from Wales or England, yet no evidence has been found that that has ever been one of the functions of this plant in either of those countries. Alien influences, though, do not all have to come from those quarters of the compass. There are records from six Irish counties, all of them in Leinster, of a cure for earache or a headache involving dropping into the ear sap from a twig of *Fraxinus excelsior* heated in a fire. This tree, the ash, was prominent in Norse mythology and, if that remedy had other than an Irish origin, it seems more likely to have come from northern Europe, directly or indirectly, than been devised in one or other of the neighbours immediately to the east.

Only two native flowering plants that are common on both sides of the Irish Sea appear to have had major roles as herbs in Ireland yet no herbal role whatever in Britain. These are *Caltha palustris* (marsh-marigold) and *Ulex gallii* (western gorse); Ireland's other gorse, the much taller *U. europaeus*, is apparently a late introduction but has doubtless come to share the folk attentions of its fellow species. It may be more than coincidence that these bear golden yellow flowers very conspicuously, which would make them prime choices for magico-religious rituals in which that colour had some special significance (and from which its use could have carried over into the medicinal sphere). Perhaps lending support to that notion is that the shrubby counterpart of the *Ulex* species, *Cytisus scoparius* (broom), while not similarly exclusive to Ireland as a herbal remedy, appears to have been applied to a markedly wider range of ailments there than in Britain. It may be more than coincidence, too, that in contrast to the wide medicinal use made of *Prunus spinosa* (blackthorn) in England and Wales, particularly in the form of juice from its sloes, that tree features in the Irish records anomalously slightly. Was that because of the malignant power with which that and its counterpart, *Crataegus monogyna* (whitethorn), were at one time in Ireland so widely and emphatically credited?

But if there are hardly any widely used Irish herbs that appear to have had no history in Britain of any medicinal function at all, there are quite a number that the two countries have shared that have had at least one application seemingly exclusive to Ireland. Apart from the three extreme cases of *Geranium robertianum*, *Veronica chamaedrys* and *Iris foetidissima*, mentioned earlier, in which Britain has reciprocated with an application equally exclusive to itself, these include

Betula (birch) bark for eczema
Fraxinus excelsior (ash) leaves for rheumatism
Lonicera periclymenum (honeysuckle) for 'thrush'
Prunella vulgaris (self-heal) for heart trouble
Quercus (oak) bark for sore feet
Rumex (dock) roots for jaundice and liver trouble
Sedum acre (biting stonecrop) for intestinal worms

Senecio jacobaea (common ragwort) for jaundice
Stellaria media (common chickweed) for cuts or sores and for coughs
  or sore throats
Symphytum officinale (common comfrey) for burns and scalds
Taraxacum officinale (dandelion) for consumption and heart trouble
Teucrium scorodonia (wood sage) for colds and coughs

One or two further applications that come into this Ireland-only category have distribution patterns that are sufficiently intriguing to call for some special comment. The most remarkable is that of the drinking of a tea made from *Urtica dioica* (common nettle) to bring out the rash in measles. For this there is a striking density of records in the far north-western corner of the country and in a band extending eastwards along both sides of the present-day border, yet none has been traced from anywhere else. Could it be that there was a measles epidemic in that region at some time in the past, possibly even in the fairly distant past, in the course of which this tea was found to have such an effect and thereafter gained an enduring reputation for it locally? The one thing that is certain is that a special abundance of the herbal plant in question cannot be responsible for the intense localisation of the use, for the common nettle occurs almost everywhere on suitable terrain throughout Britain and Ireland below a certain altitude.

The relative remoteness of that north-western corner of Ireland has tended to leave it culturally rather self-contained and one where old practices have persisted on a perhaps more than ordinarily extensive scale. That is doubtless why the records of three other folk medical applications rise to a marked peak in the same region: a cold cure made from the boiled seeds of *Rumex* species (docks), a tonic from *Menyanthes trifoliata* (bogbean) for cleansing the system of impurities, and a poultice for sprains and other swellings from that specially Irish herb, *Scrophularia nodosa* (common figwort).

That region is by no means the only part of Ireland to have had a herbal use seemingly largely or wholly exclusive to it. *Prunella vulgaris* (self-heal), for example, though common and more or less countrywide in its distribution botanically, appears to have been used for easing tubercular coughs uniquely in the British Isles in a group of counties in Ireland's centre, in three or four of which the records rise to a more than proportional frequency. That, again, has the look of a remedy that originated in that area at some past point in time, proceeded to acquire an extensive and faithful following, but failed to spread further—perhaps, similarly, as the result of a measure of socioeconomic isolation.

Another speciality of that same central belt is the valuing of *Primula vulgaris* (primrose) as a treatment for jaundice. Yet that is the part of Ireland where that plant is at its most scarce, on account of the high lime content of the soils, and yet, paradoxically, where its sister species, *P. veris* (cowslip), which is preferred to the other as a jaundice cure elsewhere, attains its greatest Irish plenty. No less difficult to account for is the marked concentration along that country's western coast of the records for the employment of *Taraxacum officinale* (dandelion) for heart trouble as well as for tuberculosis. Equally hard to explain is the restriction to the three adjacent border counties of Cavan, Monaghan and Louth of the records for boiling 'thistles' (apparently *Silybum marianum*) in milk as a remedy for whooping cough.

More unexpected than any of those, however, is the chequer-board pattern revealed by studying in tandem the distributions of their recorded use in folk medicine of two herbs not previously thought of as being in any way associated. Though these are alike in having foliage of a kind that botanists term 'fleshy', one of them, *Umbilicus rupestris* (navelwort), is unquestionably a native whereas the other, *Sempervivum tectorum* (house-leek), is equally unquestionably an ancient introduction, for it is apparently always sterile and is believed to have originated in central Europe, perhaps as a hybrid; it has also been widely known by an alternative name, sengreen, that appears to be Anglo-Saxon in origin. When the overall herbal distributions of these two are compared in detail, they turn out to be mirror images of one another: where one county has seemingly specialised in the *Umbilicus* species, a neighbour of that has seemingly chosen the *Sempervivum*—and presumably instead. Because the *Umbilicus* can flourish only in the wetter climate of the western half of the British Isles, there was a vacant niche in the east for a herb of vaguely similar character (though not appearance) and credited with similar healing properties. But the *Sempervivum* had the edge in also being credited with magico-religious power, and after its introduction from the European mainland (presumably by post-Roman Germanic immigrants) it was evidently taken far and wide into the territory of the *Umbilicus*. The age-old attachment to the *Umbilicus* species in the west, though, must have been sufficiently deep to prevent a total replacement occurring. Closer analysis may one day demonstrate that it has been in those parts of Ireland where English penetration has been longest and most pronounced that the *Sempervivum* attained its principal distribution.

The greater completeness of the Irish records geographically and the greater scale on which reliance on folk medicinal herbs has persisted in that country till very recently have the results that regional peculiarities are easier to detect there and less likely to be the product of accidental bias in coverage. For the same reasons it is more probable than not that the extent of Irish distinctiveness identified in the foregoing paragraphs is a reasonable approximation to reality. That distinctiveness might have been considerably greater, indeed, had it not been for the massive movements of population from Ireland into Britain in the course of the past two centuries. These have made it impossible to tell how far the numerous mainly Irish uses that have been recorded in Britain are merely late transfers from one country to the other or whether they constitute the fragments of distributions that were genuinely common to the two previously. The more rural a record, however, the more likely it is to belong in the second of these categories, for that immigration has been very heavily concentrated in the larger towns and cities.

The superior quality of the Irish folk records may partly, but only partly, account for the rather large number of plants that are widely plentiful members of the native flora of both Ireland and Britain yet as medicinal herbs emerge as Irish in the main. These include *Rorippa nasturtium-aquaticum* (water-cress), *Alchemilla vulgaris* in the broad sense (lady's-mantle), *Hedera helix* (ivy), *Verbascum thapsus* (great mullein), *Veronica beccabunga* (brooklime), *Centaurea nigra* (common knapweed), *Allium ursinum* (ramsons) and the genera *Polypodium* (polypodies) and *Juncus* (rushes). The bark of trees as a source of remedies turns out to be a predominantly Irish trait, too. In the case of *H. helix* not only are the majority of the records for the principal uses of that particularly popular medicinal plant Irish ones, but in Ireland it has been noted in use for a considerably wider range of afflictions. There is a strongly Irish tilt, similarly, to the distribution of just certain applications of herbs that overall, across the British Isles as a whole, are more evenly spread: of that of *Primula vulgaris* (primrose) and *Phyllitis scolopendrium* (hart's-tongue) in so far as they have been applied to burns or scalds, of *Primula veris* (cowslip) when brought to bear on insomnia, of *Stellaria media* (chickweed) as a cure for swellings, *Taraxacum officinale* (dandelion) for jaundice or liver trouble, and *Geranium robertianum* (herb-Robert) for bleeding. In all of these cases the patterns that have emerged in this study may be no more than accidental, the product of the comparative insufficiency, or at any rate much greater patchiness, of the British data. Equally, though, they may reflect reality. Only when much fuller information for Britain becomes available will the uncertainties on this score have a chance of being resolved.

Veterinary Remedies

Considerably more than a hundred different herbs are on record as having been used in Britain or Ireland to treat ailments of animals. Almost all are ones that have been applied in one or both countries to human ailments as well—though not necessarily the same ones. Many of the afflictions that animals suffer from are common to humanity, too, and it is only to be expected that remedies tried and tested on them will have been shared. Even if the veterinary ailments are not ones ordinarily met with in human beings, it is equally predictable that herbs credited with effectiveness against a particularly wide range of human ills will have come into play in the veterinary area as well. By no means all the main multi-purpose stand-bys, however, feature in the list that follows: noteworthy absentees include *Arctium* (burdock), *Centaurium erythraea* (centaury), *Chamaemelum nobile* (chamomile), *Primula vulgaris* (primrose), *Prunella vulgaris* (self-heal) and *Valeriana officinalis* (valerian); even the outstandingly versatile *Sempervivum tectorum* (houseleek) can claim a place only marginally. The failure of such herbs to appear in the records could merely be a result of the very much more limited number of veterinary remedies that have been recorded, given that the primary interest of folklore collectors is in what people do to or believe about themselves. Yet it is quite likely that these non-appearances are not accidental and that the herbs in question have been tried over the centuries but found wanting. In some cases they may simply have been rejected as just too mild, for animals have traditionally been regarded as having stronger constitutions than human beings and therefore able to endure, and perhaps indeed requiring, potions of a more drastic character.

Unlike human ailments, many veterinary ones are not generally familiar. Those that feature most prominently in the list that follows are

blackhead. A disease of the liver and caecum in turkeys, caused by a protozoan parasite carried by earthworms.

black-leg. Clostridial myositis, a quickly fatal, soil-borne bacterial infection of ruminants (mainly cattle) characterised by swellings and often severe lameness. Traditional 'black-leg land' tends to be periodically flooded or poor-quality moors.

botts. Inflammation of the digestive tract in horses resulting from infection by larvae of the botfly.

farcy. A contagious bacterial disease of horses and donkeys characterised by nasal mucus ('horse' cold) and swellings under the jaw which develop discharging abscesses.

fluke (otherwise 'rot'). A sometimes fatal infestation of ruminants with parasitic flatworms, following ingestion of the snails that act as intermediate host.

foul (otherwise 'scald'). Interdigital necrobacillosis, severe lameness in cattle caused by swelling of bacterial origin in the cleft of the hoof.

gapes. Infestation of young birds by nematode worms in the bronchial tubes and trachea, causing frequent gasping.

laminitis. Acutely painful inflammation of the vascular tissues of horses' hooves.

mastitis (formerly 'garget'). Acute inflammation of the mammary gland, usually the result of bacterial infection; widely known as 'felon' in eastern Ulster, as 'start' in Leinster and Munster, and as 'blast' in east Leinster (Doherty, 45).

pip. A fatal disease of young birds, reputedly the result of a worm in the windpipe, characterised by thick mucus in the mouth and throat.

red-water fever (otherwise 'red disease', 'blood murrain' or 'red murrain'). A disease of cattle and sheep caused by a tick-borne protozoan parasite which attacks the red blood corpuscles, turning the urine red or blackish. Particularly occurs in moorland areas and especially prevalent in Ireland, where records of 'the murrain', marked with a dagger (†) in the list that follows, normally refer to this.

sheep scab (properly, psoroptic mange). A serious contagious disease caused by a species of mite, the bites of which raise itching scabs that drop off with the wool.

strangles. A commonly fatal, highly contagious bacterial infection of the lymph glands round the neck and jaw of horses, typically characterised by monstrous swelling followed by a necklace of discharging abscesses.

white scour. Severe whitish diarrhoea and progressive emaciation in cattle, especially young calves, sometimes the result of a contagious bacterial disease, sometimes a dietary disorder.

As the records are too few and scattered to yield distribution patterns other than very exceptionally, a simple listing—by scientific names in alphabetical sequence (under vascular plants, algae and fungi) for ease of reference—has to do duty in this instance for substantive entries species by species. An asterisk (*) indicates a species not among records of human ailments.

VASCULAR PLANTS

Achillea millefolium, yarrow (figure on page 301). Red-water fever (Caernarvonshire,[1] in mixtures in Merionethshire[2] and Cavan[3]); diarrhoea in rabbits (Norfolk[4]).

Agrimonia eupatoria (figure on page 147), *A. procera,* agrimony. Cuts in horses and cattle (Norfolk[5]).

Alchemilla spp., lady's-mantle. 'Moorl', unidentified cattle ailment (Donegal[6]), probably a version of the name used in Ulster for red-water fever (cf. Doherty, 43).

Allium ursinum, ramsons (Plate 29). 'Hoose', worm-induced lung disease in calves (Cavan[7]); coughs in horses and cattle (four Irish counties); worms (six Irish counties); ringworm in calves (Mayo[8]); farcy (Wicklow[9]); black-leg (twelve Irish counties, normally by binding a piece into a slit in the tail); fits in dogs (Galway,[10] Carlow,[11] Limerick[12]); canine distemper (Norfolk, in a mixture[13]); pip (four Irish counties).

Anemone nemorosa, wood anemone. Sheep scab (Wicklow[14]).

Angelica sylvestris, wild angelica. Black-leg (Sutherland[15]).

Anthriscus sylvestris, cow parsley. Laminitis in a pony (Norfolk, combined with Sambucus nigra[16]).

*Arrhenatherum elatius (Linnaeus) P. Beauverd ex J. S. & C. Presl, false oat-grass (Poaceae). Europe, western Asia, North Africa; introduced into North America and Australia. Variety *bulbosum* (Wildenow) St Amans (onion couch). White 'scale' on eyes of dogs and horses (Londonderry[17]).

Artemisia absinthium, wormwood (figure on page 299). Cuts on cows' udders (Carmarthenshire, in a mixture[18]).

Artemisia vulgaris, mugwort. Gangrene in horses (Donegal[19]).

Berberis vulgaris, barberry. Jaundice in cattle (Ireland, unlocalised[20]).

Bryonia dioica, white bryony (figure on page 113). Tonic for pigs (Fens of East Anglia[21]); to add gloss to horses' coats (Oxfordshire,[22] Norfolk,[23] Lincolnshire[24]).

Capsella bursa-pastoris (Linnaeus) Medikus, shepherd's-purse. Cosmopolitan weed. Diarrhoea in calves (Isle of Man[25]).

Chelidonium majus, greater celandine (figure on page 79). Warts in cattle (Ireland, unlocalised[26]).

Cirsium spp., thistles. To staunch bleeding in cattle or horses after lancing (Limerick[27]).

Cirsium vulgare, spear thistle. 'Sick cattle' (Wexford[28]).

Conium maculatum, hemlock (Plate 18). Fluke (Louth[29]); sheep scab (Kildare, in a mixture[30]); cuts (Tipperary[31]), sore breasts (Kilkenny, combined with *Malva*[32]; Carlow[33]), swollen feet (Mayo[34]), farcy (Londonderry[35])—all in horses; swellings in 'animals' ('Ulster'[36]). Some of these may be *Anthriscus sylvestris* or even *Heracleum sphondylium.*

Conopodium majus, pignut. To lower urine flow in horses (Isle of Man[37]).

Corylus avellana, hazel. Adder bites (Glamorgan, in a mixture[38]).

Crataegus monogyna, hawthorn (Plate 13). Diarrhoea in bullocks (Longford[39]).

Cytisus scoparius, broom. Dropsy in sheep (Suffolk[40]); worms or botts (five Irish counties); gravel (Sligo[41]) and broken wind (Co. Dublin[42]) in horses; fits in dogs (Louth[43]).

Daphne laureola, spurge-laurel. Purge for horses (Isle of Man[44]); to add gloss to horses' coats (Hampshire[45]).

Daucus carota, wild carrot. 'Diseases in horses' (Carlow[46]).

Digitalis purpurea, foxglove (figure on page 255). Sheep scab (Berwickshire, in a mixture[47]; Isle of Man[48]); eczema in 'livestock' (Somerset[49]); mange or fleas in dogs (Gloucestershire[50]); strangles (Cumbria[51]); red-water fever (Merionethshire, in a mixture[52]).

Dryopteris filix-mas, male-fern (figure on page 63). Red-water fever (Cavan,[53] Laois,[54] Tipperary[55]); fluke (four Irish counties). 'Fern' for white scour (Cavan[56]) and kidney disease in horses (Limerick[57]) may be this or *Pteridium aquilinum.*

Euonymus europaeus, spindle. Fleas and lice in dogs (unlocalised[58]).

Eupatorium cannabinum, hemp-agrimony. Cough in cattle 'and other beasts' (England, unlocalised[59]).

Euphorbia spp., spurges. Black-leg (Cavan[60]).

Euphorbia hyberna, Irish spurge. Purge for horses and cattle (Galway[61]).

Euphrasia officinalis, eyebright (figure on page 261). Red-water fever (Donegal[62]).

Filago vulgaris, common cudweed. Red-water fever (unlocalised[63]).

Filipendula ulmaria, meadowsweet. Diarrhoea in calves (Armagh[64]).

Fragaria vesca, wild strawberry (Plate 11). Red-water fever (Cavan[65]); constipation in rabbits and guinea pigs (Cambridgeshire[66]).

Fraxinus excelsior, ash. Adder bites (Dorset,[67] Galloway[68]).

Fumaria spp., fumitory. Worms in foals (Orkney[69]).

Galium aparine, cleavers (figure on page 269). Ringworm in dogs (Norfolk[70]); to increase sperm in a stallion (Norfolk[71]).

Galium verum, lady's bedstraw. Fits in dogs (Westmeath[72]).

Gentianella campestris, field gentian. Rickets-like disease in cattle enforcing crouching, known as the *chrùbain,* nowadays attributed to phosphorus deficiency (Highlands[73]); to bring on oestrus in cows (Shetland[74]).

Geranium robertianum, herb-Robert (figure on page 175). Red-water fever (throughout Ireland); worms in horses and cattle (Limerick[75]); 'drymurrain', i.e. constipation (Waterford[76]); diarrhoea in calves (Limerick[77]); tuberculosis in dogs (Ireland, unlocalised—root tied to leg[78]).

Glechoma hederacea, ground-ivy (figure on page 220). Kidney trouble in cattle (Kilkenny[79]); white specks on eyes of horses (Kent[80]); 'pink eye' in sheep (East Riding of Yorkshire[81]).

Hedera helix, ivy. Eye trouble in cows and sheep (four Irish counties); warts in cattle (Kildare[82]); fluke (Longford[83]); expelling afterbirth (Hampshire,[84] Norfolk,[85] Limerick[86]); digestive troubles in goats (Norfolk[87]); loss of appetite in ruminants (Somerset,[88] Norfolk[89]); 'start', i.e. mastitis, in cattle (Cavan[90]); pain in sheep (Offaly[91]); 'sick' animals (Aran Islands,[92] Wicklow[93]).

Helleborus foetidus, stinking hellebore. Foot-and-mouth disease (Leicestershire[94]); mastitis in calves (Norfolk[95]); draining 'bad humours' from ruminants by 'settering' or 'felling', involving insertion of this in open wound made in ear, dewlap or above forelegs (England, unlocalised[96]; Cumbria[97]).

Helleborus viridis, green hellebore. Swollen udder in cows (Cumberland[98]); to add gloss to a horse's coat (Suffolk[99]).

Heracleum sphondylium, hogweed. Winter rheumatism in cows (Ireland, unlocalised[100]).

Huperzia selago, fir clubmoss. Lice in cows and pigs (England, unlocalised[101]); perhaps also the unspecified clubmoss applied to 'some cattle diseases' in Orkney.[102].

Hypericum elodes, marsh St John's-wort. Diarrhoea in cows (Donegal[103]).

Hypericum pulchrum, slender St John's-wort. Red-water fever (Donegal[104]).

Inula helenium, elecampane (figure on page 292). Horse tonic (Isle of Man[105]); lameness in horses (Shropshire[106]); hydrophobia (Glamorgan[107]).

Iris pseudacorus, yellow iris. To increase flow of urine in a horse (Cardiganshire[108]).

Juniperus communis, juniper (Plate 1). Botts and worms ('Wales' and Cumbria,[109] Galloway[110]); tonic for horses (Lincolnshire,[111] East Anglia[112]).

Lamium purpureum, red dead-nettle. Blackhead (Suffolk[113]); gapes (Norfolk, in a combination[114]).

Lemna spp., duckweed. Diarrhoea in 'animals' (Wicklow[115]).

Ligusticum scoticum, lovage. Cough in sheep (Skye[116]); purge for cattle (Skye, sometimes with *Sedum rosea*[117]; Eriskay in the Outer Hebrides[118]).

Linaria vulgaris, common toadflax. 'Drooping' in birds (Sussex[119]).

Linum catharticum, fairy flax. Purge for cows (Isle of Man[120]).

Lonicera periclymenum, honeysuckle. Farcy (Tipperary,[121] Limerick[122]).

Lotus corniculatus, common bird's-foot-trefoil. Cut legs of horses (Somerset[123]).

Malva sylvestris, common mallow (figure on page 107). Sore, swollen or 'flagged' udders of cows (Cavan,[124] Wicklow,[125] Limerick[126]); cattle scabs and sores in general (Wicklow[127]); sprains in animals (Dorset,[128] Radnorshire[129]); swelling under jaw in cattle at start of winter (Cork[130]); to prevent cattle disease (Devon[131]); sore breast on a horse (Kilkenny, combined with *Conium maculatum*[132]). Records for 'marsh-mallow' assumed to refer to this and not *Althaea officinalis.*

Mentha spp., 'peppermint'. Fits in dogs and pigs (Leitrim[133]).

Menyanthes trifoliata, bogbean (figure on page 202). Bovine tuberculosis (Kent,[134] Orkney[135]); purge for calves (South Uist in the Outer Hebrides[136]); settling stomach in calves (Fife[137]); removing afterbirth from cows (Leitrim[138]); 'pine', i.e. trace-element deficiency (Doherty, 46) in cattle and sheep (Mayo[139]); cattle disease called 'darn' (Highlands[140]).

Myrica gale, bog-myrtle. Red-water fever and collar sores on horses (Mayo[141]); fluke in calves (Leitrim[142]); fits in dogs, and worms (Westmeath[143]); gravel in horses (Mayo[144]); appetiser for horses (Limerick[145]).

Myrrhis odorata, sweet cicely (Plate 16). Inducing flow of milk in cows (Teesdale[146]).

* *Narcissus pseudonarcissus* Linnaeus subsp. *major* (Curtis) Baker, Spanish daffodil. South-western Europe; introduced elsewhere. Worms (Colonsay in the Inner Hebrides[147]).

Oenanthe crocata, hemlock water-dropwort (figure on page 185). Saddle galls (Cumberland[148]); 'foul' (Westmoreland[149]).

Ophioglossum vulgatum, adder's-tongue. Inflamed ulcers of cows (Surrey and Sussex[150]).

Origanum vulgare, marjoram. Stitches and pains in horses (Highlands[151]).

Oxalis acetosella, wood-sorrel. Ticks and lice in sheep (Wicklow[152]).

Peucedanum ostruthium, masterwort. Tonic for sick cattle and to induce milk in cows (Teesdale[153]); sore udders of cows (Cumberland[154]). 'Fellon-grass', a name recorded for this in Cumbria and Roxburghshire and assumed to be applied to the cold-induced skin sores on cows known as felons,[155] seems more probably a corruption of 'felling-girse', a name in that region of *Helleborus* species once used there for 'felling'.

Pinguicula vulgaris, common butterwort. Chapped udders of cows (West Riding of Yorkshire[156]); cattle bitten 'by any venomous worm' (Yorkshire[157]).

Plantago spp., plantain. Cuts on legs of horses (Somerset[158]).

Plantago coronopus, buck's-horn plantain (figure on page 246). Bites by rabid dogs (Cornwall, in a mixture[159]; Norfolk,[160] Suffolk[161]).

Plantago lanceolata, ribwort plantain. Coughs in wild birds (Devon[162]).

Polygonum aviculare, knotgrass. Swine fever (Kilkenny, as 'pigroot'[163]— most likely this—widely known in England by similar names).

Potentilla erecta, tormentil (figure on page 145). Diarrhoea in cattle and horses (Colonsay in the Inner Hebrides,[164] Orkney,[165] Donegal,[166] Wicklow[167]) and in cats (Isle of Man[168]); red-water fever (Londonderry[169]); white scour (Cavan[170]); braxy, a fatal bacterial infection of sheep, and 'louping ill', acute encephalitis in sheep resulting from a tick-borne virus, characterised by leaps and jerks (Berwickshire[171]).

Potentilla reptans, creeping cinquefoil. Diarrhoea in kittens (Isle of Man[172]).

Primula veris, cowslip. Coughs in cattle (Cumbria, in combination with *Symphytum*[173]).

Primula vulgaris, primrose (Plate 9). Bites by rabid dogs (Cornwall, in a mixture[174]).

Prunus padus, bird cherry. 'Certain diseases in cattle' (parts of the Highlands[175]).

Prunus spinosa, blackthorn (figure on page 152). Diarrhoea in 'animals' (Wicklow[176]).

* *Puccinellia maritima* (Hudson) Parlatore, common saltmarsh-grass (Poaceae). Coasts of western Europe, north-eastern Asia, North America. Mild purge for cattle (Donegal[177]).

Quercus petraea, Q. robur, oak. Harness sores on horses (Donegal,[178] Cavan[179]); cuts on horses (Colonsay in the Inner Hebrides[180]); diarrhoea in cattle (Norfolk,[181] Cavan[182]).

Ranunculus spp., buttercup, including records for 'crowfoot'. Black-leg (Cavan[183]); red-water fever (†Limerick,[184] †Wicklow[185]).

Ranunculus flammula, lesser spearwort. To raise blisters on ponies (Somerset[186]).

Rhamnus cathartica, buckthorn. 'Dry murrain' in cattle (Mayo[187]).

Rubus fruticosus, bramble (Plate 10). Diarrhoea in cattle (four Irish counties) and goats (Norfolk[188]); 'hide-bound' cattle (Berwickshire[189]); thrush in horses (Norfolk[190]); purge for rabbits and guinea pigs (Cambridgeshire[191]); 'pod belly' in rabbits (Norfolk[192]); pip (Meath[193]).

Rumex spp., dock. Coughs in horses and cattle (Monaghan,[194] Louth,[195] Longford[196]); farcy (Louth,[197] Kilkenny[198]); to wrap greasy fetlocks in horses (Norfolk[199]); sheep scab (Isle of Man[200]); nettle stings in dogs (Hampshire[201]).

Salix alba, white willow. Pip (Ireland, unlocalised[202]).

Sambucus ebulus, dwarf elder. Ulcerated udders and teats of cows (Louth[203]); to improve horses' coats (Isle of Wight[204]).

Sambucus nigra, elder (figure on page 271). Sore teats in cows (Dorset[205]); cuts on cows' udders (Carmarthenshire, in a mixture[206]); foot-rot in sheep (Norfolk[207]); 'to dose pigs' (Longford[208]); coughs in wild birds (Devon[209]); laminitis in ponies (Norfolk, combined with *Anthriscus sylvestris*[210]).

Samolus valerandi, brookweed. 'Any malady affecting swine' (England, unlocalised[211]).

Sanicula europaea, sanicle (frontispiece). Gapes in young pheasants (Donegal[212]).

Scrophularia nodosa, common figwort (Plate 24). Scab in pigs (England, unlocalised[213]); farcy (Ireland, unlocalised[214]); expulsion of afterbirth in cows (Londonderry[215]); red-water fever (Wicklow, combined with *Stellaria media*[216]).

Scutellaria galericulata, skullcap. Distemper in dogs (Norfolk, in a mixture[217]).

Sedum acre, biting stonecrop (figure on page 138). Worms in 'animals' (Cavan,[218] Longford[219]).

Sedum anglicum, English stonecrop. Swellings on horses (Colonsay in the Inner Hebrides, combined with *Senecio vulgaris*[220]).

* *Sedum rosea* (Linnaeus) Scopoli, roseroot. Arctic and mountains of northern temperate zone. Purge for calves (Skye, combined with *Ligusticum*[221]).

Sempervivum tectorum, house-leek (figure on page 136). Diarrhoea in cattle (Wicklow[222]); expulsion of afterbirth in cows (Mayo[223]); cuts or sores in 'any animal' (Montgomeryshire[224]); 'windgall', distension of tendon sheaths round fetlock in horses (Cumbria[225]).

Senecio aquaticus, S. jacobaea, ragwort. 'Staggers', neuromuscular affliction of horses characterised by stumbling (England, unlocalised[226]); wounded or broken horse's leg (Cork[227]); cuts on 'animals' (Tipperary[228]); gripes in horses (Norfolk[229]); windgall (see preceding entry) (Cavan[230]); 'blasts', inflammation caused by wind (Wicklow, in a mixture[231]); red-water fever (Wicklow[232]); gapes (Limerick[233]).

Senecio vulgaris, groundsel (figure on page 308). Purge for cows (Isle of Man[234]); cuts on cows' udders (Carmarthenshire, in a mixture[235]); red-water fever (†Wicklow, in a mixture[236]); black-leg (Wicklow[237]); botts (England, unlocalised[238]); tonsillitis in horses (Norfolk[239]); 'festilow', sore eruption between ears and shoulders in horses (Devon[240]); swellings on horses (Colonsay in the Inner Hebrides, combined with *Sedum anglicum*[241]); aperient in birds (Isle of Man[242]); pip (Limerick[243]).

* *Silene vulgaris* Garcke, bladder campion. Europe, temperate Asia and North Africa; introduced into Australasia. To make a cow desire a bull (England, unlocalised, as 'Spatling Poppy'[244]).

Smyrnium olusatrum, Alexanders. Mouth sores in cattle (Isle of Man[245]).

Solanum dulcamara, bittersweet. For pigs 'whenever badly' (Lincolnshire[246]).

Sorbus aucuparia, rowan. Strangles (Limerick[247]—smoke of burnt wood inhaled).

Stellaria media, chickweed. Red-water fever (†Wicklow, combined with *Scrophularia nodosa*[248]); black-leg (Cavan[249]); moulting in cagebirds (Ireland, unlocalised[250]); convulsions in pigs (Leitrim[251]); pip (Sligo[252]); gapes (Norfolk,[253] Cavan[254]).

Symphytum officinale, common comfrey (figure on page 208). Sprains and broken legs (Limerick[255]); swellings in horses (Limerick[256]); swollen udders of cows (Monaghan,[257] Meath[258]); sore feet in 'animals' (Long-ford[259]); swine fever (Leitrim[260]); diarrhoea in cattle (Cavan region[261]); 'blood scour' (Limerick[262]); coughs in cows (Cumbria, combined with *Primula veris*[263]); digestive problems in horses and poultry (Norfolk[264]); tonic for horses and geese (Norfolk[265]); tonic for pigs (Fens of East Anglia[266]).

* *Symphytum ×uplandicum* Nyman, Russian comfrey. Caucasus?; widely introduced elsewhere. Foot-and-mouth disease (England, unlocal-ised[267]).

Tamus communis, black bryony. Barrenness in cows (Cheshire[268]); stimu-lant for mares (Lincolnshire[269]); tonic for pigs (Fens of East Anglia[270]); stiff joints of animals, especially of pigs lame from an unidentified dis-ease called 'broyant' (Montgomeryshire[271]).

Tanacetum vulgare, tansy (figure on page 295). Red-water fever (South Uist in the Outer Hebrides,[272] †Kerry[273]); worms in horses (Galway[274]); pip (Cork[275]); adder bites (Glamorgan, in a mixture[276]).

Taraxacum officinale, dandelion (figure on page 288). Fluke in calves (Limerick[277]); black-leg (Cavan[278]); diarrhoea in calves (Limerick[279]); cowpox (Roscommon[280]); pain in horses (Offaly[281]); pip (Co. Dublin[282]); 'pine' (see entry for *Menyanthes trifoliata*) in turkeys (Limerick[283]).

Taxus baccata, yew. To make horses' coats shine (Montgomeryshire[284]—the 'dust' given in tiny quantities).

Teucrium scorodonia, wood sage. Worms in horses (Skye[285]); mastitis (Hampshire[286]); sore udders of cows (three counties of north-western Wales[287]); blindness in cows and sheep (Skye and Harris in Heb-rides[288]—juice put into ears).

Thymus spp., thyme. Unspecified ailment(s) of ponies (Hampshire[289]).

Trifolium pratense, red clover. Sore tongue in cattle (Tipperary[290]); fever in heifers (Monmouthshire[291]).

Ulex spp., gorse. Worms (Isle of Man,[292] six Irish counties); botts (Monaghan[293]); coughs in cattle (Cavan[294]); pains in horses (Galway[295]); swellings (Meath[296]).

Ulmus glabra, wych elm. Expulsion of afterbirth in cows (Berwickshire[297]).

Umbilicus rupestris, navelwort (figure on page 135). Expulsion of afterbirth in cows (Mayo,[298] Wicklow[299]); sore udders of cows (Merionethshire[300]); 'sick cattle' (Kerry[301]); saddle galls on horses (Isle of Man[302]); scruff on legs of a horse (Wicklow[303]).

Urtica dioica, common nettle (figure on page 85). Red-water fever (Kerry[304]); 'teart', deficiency disease in cattle (Colonsay in the Inner Hebrides[305]); tonic for pigs, goats and rabbits (Norfolk[306]); to ensure pregnancy in a mare that has been served (Norfolk[307]); blackhead (Norfolk[308]); pip (Tipperary[309]).

Valeriana officinalis, common valerian. Distemper in dogs (Norfolk, in a mixture[310]).

Verbascum thapsus, great mullein (figure on page 251). Bovine tuberculosis (Kent[311]); diarrhoea in cattle (England, unlocalised[312]); sores on 'animals' (Co. Dublin[313]).

Veronica spp., speedwell. Worms (Isle of Man[314]).

Viscum album, mistletoe (figure on page 166). Barrenness in cows (Isle of Man[315]); expulsion of afterbirth in cows (Essex,[316] Herefordshire[317]); purge for sheep, and a gentle tonic for ewes after lambing (Herefordshire[318]).

ALGAE

*Characeae, stoneworts. 'Gaa', obscure disease of cattle supposedly of bilious origin (Shetland[319]).

Pelvetia canaliculata, channelled wrack. 'Dry disease' in cows (South Uist in the Outer Hebrides[320]).

Porphyra spp., slake. Spring purge for cows (Skye[321]).

FUNGI

Lycoperdaceae, puffballs. Collar and saddle sores on horses, and to staunch bleeding in cattle when polled (Wicklow[322]).

Tremella spp., jelly fungus. Purge for cattle (Skye[323]).

Notes

1. Williams MS
2. Williams MS
3. IFC S 969: 28
4. Hatfield, appendix
5. Hatfield, appendix
6. Hart 1898, 380
7. IFC S 993: 70
8. IFC S 93: 132, 156
9. IFC S 913: 96
10. IFC S 60: 32
11. IFC S 907: 30
12. IFC S 524: 14
13. Hatfield MS
14. IFC S 920: 71
15. Henderson & Dickson, 55
16. Hatfield, appendix
17. Moore MS
18. Williams MS
19. IFC S 1090: 437
20. Moloney
21. Randell, 86
22. Vickery MSS
23. Hatfield MS; *PLNN*, no. 8 (1989), 36
24. Rudkin; Baker
25. Vickery 1995
26. 'Jude', 11
27. IFC S 483: 300
28. IFC S 903: 464
29. IFC S 672: 257
30. IFC S 771: 51
31. IFC S 550: 274
32. IFC S 850: 114
33. IFC S 903: 464
34. IFC S 138: 314
35. Moore MS
36. Foster, 61
37. Fargher
38. *Folk-lore*, 7 (1896), 89
39. *PLNN*, no. 22 (1991), 101
40. Cullum MS
41. IFC S 170: 196
42. IFC S 794: 442
43. IFC S 658: 129
44. Garrad 1985, 41
45. *Hampshire Review*, no. 1 (1949), 42
46. IFC S 907: 414
47. Johnston 1853
48. Quayle, 93
49. Tongue
50. Hopkins, 52; Palmer 1994, 122
51. Rollinson, 77
52. Williams MS
53. Maloney
54. IFC S 826: 31
55. Vickery MSS
56. Maloney
57. IFC S 519: 115
58. Maloney
59. Parkinson, 597
60. Maloney
61. Hart 1873
62. Hart 1898, 381
63. Withering 1787–92
64. *PLNN*, no. 57 (1998), 274
65. IFC S 993: 125
66. Vickery MSS
67. Vickery 1995
68. MacKerlie, 305
69. Spence
70. Hatfield, appendix
71. Hatfield, 87
72. IFC S 736: 191
73. Cameron; MacFarlane
74. Vickery 1995
75. IFC S 510: 291
76. IFC S 637: 7
77. IFC S 509: 410
78. Wood-Martin
79. IFC S 850: 114
80. Pratt 1850–7
81. Woodward, 83
82. IFC S 771: 9
83. IFC S 762: 158
84. de Baïracli-Levy, 125

85. Taylor MS; Hatfield, appendix
86. IFC S 512: 98
87. Hatfield MS
88. Palmer 1994, 111
89. Hatfield, 79, appendix
90. Maloney
91. IFC S 812: 441
92. IFC S 1: 196
93. McClafferty
94. Tuckwell, 57
95. Britten & Holland
96. Turner 1568, part 1, 161; Parkinson, 216; Coles, 110
97. Duncan & Robson, 62; Rollinson, 76
98. Hodgson
99. Evans 1969
100. *PLNN*, no. 55 (1998), 265
101. Withering 1787–92
102. Pratt 1859, 125
103. Hart 1898, 381
104. Hart 1898, 365
105. Garrad 1985, 17
106. Mabey, 364
107. Trevelyan, 314
108. Williams MS
109. Ray 1670, 183
110. Mactaggart, 418
111. Woodruffe-Peacock
112. Kightly, 61
113. Hatfield, appendix
114. Hatfield, appendix
115. McClafferty
116. Martin, 226
117. Henderson & Dickson, 94; Pennant 1774, 310
118. Goodrich-Freer, 206
119. Pratt 1850–7
120. Fargher
121. IFC S 572: 70
122. IFC S 512: 523
123. Tongue
124. Maloney
125. IFC S 914: 322
126. IFC S 484: 412

127. IFC S 920: 71
128. Dacombe
129. Vickery 1995
130. IFC S 385: 57
131. Lafont
132. IFC S 850: 114
133. IFC S 226: 22
134. Gerard, 630
135. Spence
136. Shaw, 50
137. Simpkins, 132
138. IFC S 226: 25
139. IFC S 133: 339
140. Hooker
141. IFC S 92: 132
142. IFC S 226: 482
143. IFC S 747: 51
144. IFC S 1337: 134
145. IFC S 523: 272
146. *Botanical Locality Record Club Report* for 1875, 141
147. McNeill
148. Threlkeld
149. Withering 1796, 302
150. Britten, 182
151. MacFarlane
152. McClafferty
153. *Botanical Locality Record Club Report* for 1875, 141
154. Hodgson
155. Britten & Holland
156. Gerard, 646; de l'Écluse, 311
157. Gerard, 646
158. Tongue
159. *Gentleman's Magazine*, 5 (1735), 619
160. de Grey, 160
161. Steward 1739
162. Vickery MSS
163. IFC S 849: 322
164. McNeill
165. Elaine R. Bullard, in litt., 1989
166. Hart 1898
167. McClafferty

168. Fargher
169. Moore MS
170. Maloney
171. Johnston 1853
172. Vickery 1995
173. Freethy, 73
174. *Gentleman's Magazine*, 5 (1735), 619
175. Carmichael, ii, 290
176. McClafferty
177. Hart 1898, 382
178. IFC S 825: 217, 1075: 135
179. Maloney
180. McNeill
181. Hatfield, 79
182. IFC S 993: 137
183. Maloney
184. IFC S 483: 369
185. McClafferty
186. Tongue
187. Vickery MSS
188. Hatfield MS
189. Johnston 1853
190. Hatfield, appendix
191. Vickery MSS
192. Hatfield, appendix
193. IFC S 710: 41
194. IFC S 932: 311
195. IFC S 657: 217
196. IFC S 163: 265
197. IFC S 658: 138
198. IFC S 861: 212
199. Hatfield MS
200. Moore 1898
201. Mabey, 111
202. Moloney
203. Synnott
204. Broomfield
205. Dacombe
206. Williams MS
207. Hatfield, appendix
208. *PLNN*, no. 20 (1991), 91
209. Vickery MSS
210. Hatfield, appendix
211. Pratt 1850–7

212. Hart 1898, 387
213. Withering 1787–92
214. Moloney
215. Moore MS
216. McClafferty
217. Hatfield MS
218. Maloney
219. IFC S 752: 23
220. McNeill
221. Henderson & Dickson, 94
222. McClafferty
223. Vickery 1985
224. Kightly, 224
225. Duncan & Robson, 65
226. Gerard, 219; Parkinson, 671
227. IFC S 386: 117
228. IFC S 572: 297
229. Hatfield MS
230. Ó Súilleabháin, 315
231. McClafferty
232. McClafferty
233. IFC S 484: 92
234. Moore 1898
235. Williams MS
236. McClafferty
237. IFC S 914: 322
238. Ray 1670, 281
239. Hatfield, 77
240. Lafont
241. McNeill
242. Moore 1898
243. IFC S 514: 27
244. Lisle, ii, 106
245. Moore 1898, wrongly ascribed to *Aegopodium podagraria;* Kermode MS
246. Woodruffe-Peacock
247. IFC S 524: 34
248. McClafferty
249. Maloney
250. Moloney
251. IFC S 226: 391
252. IFC S 158: 120
253. Hatfield, appendix

254. Maloney

255. IFC S 482: 60; 515: 148; 524: 82

256. IFC S 483: 368

257. IFC S 932: 217

258. Farrelly MS

259. IFC S 762: 158

260. Logan, 173

261. Maloney; Logan, 170

262. IFC S 520: 15; 521: 149

263. Freethy, 73

264. Hatfield, 54

265. Hatfield MS

266. Randell, 90

267. Quelch, 74

268. Britten & Holland, 364

269. Rudkin

270. Randell, 86

271. Britten & Holland, 516

272. Shaw, 50

273. IFC S 413: 228

274. IFC S 22: 224

275. IFC S 350: 75

276. *Folk-lore*, 7 (1896), 89

277. IFC S 482: 358

278. Maloney

279. IFC S 499: 298

280. IFC S 250: 273

281. IFC S 812: 441

282. IFC S 795: 110

283. IFC S 483: 209

284. Kightly, 61

285. Martin, 227

286. de Baïracli-Levy, 130

287. Williams MS

288. Martin, 227

289. de Baïracli-Levy, 130

290. IFC S 572: 71

291. Hughes, 144

292. Moore 1898

293. IFC S 932: 220

294. Maloney

295. IFC S 59: 88

296. Lucas, 185

297. Johnston 1853

298. Vickery MSS

299. McClafferty

300. Williams MS

301. IFC S 476: 89, 90

302. Vickery 1995

303. McClafferty

304. IFC S 412: 197

305. McNeill

306. Hatfield, appendix

307. Hatfield, 61

308. Hatfield MS

309. IFC S 530: 192

310. Hatfield MS

311. Gerard, 630

312. Parkinson, 63

313. IFC S 787: 278

314. Fargher

315. Fargher

316. Vickery 1995

317. Bull

318. Bull

319. Tait

320. Shaw, 50

321. Martin, 229

322. McClafferty

323. Henderson & Dickson, 94

Reference Sources

Printed Works

Allen, Andrew (1995). *A Dictionary of Sussex Folk Medicine*. Newbury: Countryside Books.

Allen, D. E. (1980). A possible scent difference between *Crataegus* species, *Watsonia*, 13: 119–20.

Allen, D. E. (1986 ['1984']). *Flora of the Isle of Man*. Douglas: Manx Museum.

Anon. (c. 1830). *New Cyclopaedia and Complete Book of Herbs*. 2 vols. London: W. M. Clark

Anon. (1906). The physicians of the Western Isles, *Blackwood's Magazine*, 1906: 264–72.

Archer, Fred (1990). *Country Sayings*. Stroud: Alan Sutton.

Armstrong, E. A. (1944). Mugwort lore, *Folk-lore*, 55: 22–42.

Arthur, Dave, ed. (1989). *A Sussex Life: the Memories of Gilbert Sargent, Countryman*. London: Barrie and Jenkins.

Baker, Margaret (1980). *Discovering the Folklore of Plants*. Ed. 2. Aylesbury: Shire Publications.

Banks, George (1830–2). *The Plymouth and Devonport Flora*. Devonport: privately published.

Barbour, John H. (1897). Some country remedies and their uses, *Folk-lore*, 8: 386–90.

Bardswell, Frances Anne (1911). *The Herb-garden*. London: A. and C. Black.

Barnes, William (1886). *A Glossary of the Dorset Dialect*. London, Trübner.

Barrington, John (1984). *Red Sky at Night*. London: Michael Joseph.

Beddington, Winifred G., and Eliza B. Christy (1937). *It Happened in Hampshire*. Winchester: Hampshire Women's Institutes.

Beith, Mary (1995). *Healing Threads: Traditional Medicines of the Highlands and Islands*. Edinburgh: Polygon.

Belcher, Hilary, and Erica Swale (1984). Catch a falling star, *Folklore*, 95: 210–20.

Bethell, W. (1866). Rural natural history, *Hardwicke's Science-gossip*, 1866: 163.

Black, William George (1883). *Folk-medicine: a Chapter in the History of Culture*. London: Folk-lore Society.

Blakeborough, Richard (1911). *Wit, Character, Folklore and Customs of the North Riding of Yorkshire*. Ed. 2, Saltburn: W. Rapp and Sons.

Bloom, J. Harvey (1830). *Folk Lore, Old Customs and Superstitions in Shakespeare Land*. London: Mitchell Hughes and Clark.

Boase, Wendy (1976). *The Folklore of Hampshire and the Isle of Wight*. London: Batsford.

Bock, Hieronymus (1556). *Kreüter Buch*. Strassburg: J. Rihel.

Borlase, William (1756). *Observations on the Ancient and Present State of the Islands of Scilly*. Oxford: W. Jackson.

Borlase, William (1758). *The Natural History of Cornwall*. Oxford: privately published.

Boulger, G. S. (1889). *The Uses of Plants*. London: Roper and Drowley.

Bradshaw, M. E. (1962). The distribution and status of five species of the *Alchemilla vulgaris* L. aggregate in Upper Teesdale, *Journal of Ecology*, 50: 681–706.

Bray, [A. E.] (1838). *Traditions . . . of Devonshire on the Borders of the Tamar and the Tavy*. 3 vols. London: Murray.

Briggs, T. R. Archer (1872). Notes respecting some Plymouth plants, *Journal of Botany*, 10: 259–61.

Briggs, T. R. Archer (1880). *Flora of Plymouth*. London: Van Voorst.

Britten, James (1879–81). *European Ferns*. London: Cassell.

Britten, James, and Robert Holland (1878–86). *A Dictionary of English Plant Names*. London: Trübner for English Dialect Society.

Bromfield, William Arthur (1856). *Flora Vectensis*, ed. Sir William Jackson Hooker and Thomas Bell Salter. London: Pamplin.

Brunfels, Otto (1530). *Herbarium Vivae et Eicones ad Naturae Imitationem*. Strassburg: J. Schott.

Bryant, Charles (1783). *Flora Dietetica*. London: Benjamin White.

Buchanan-Brown, J., ed. (1972). *John Aubrey: Three Prose Works*. Fontwell: Centaur Press.

Buckley, Anthony D. (1980). Unofficial healing in Ulster, *Ulster Folklife*, 26: 15–34.

Bull, H. G. (1907). The mistletoe in Herefordshire, *Transactions of the Woolhope Naturalists' Field Club* for 1852–65: 312–47.

Burne, Charlotte Sophia, ed. (1883). *Shropshire Folk-lore*. London: Trübner and Co.

Cameron, John (1900). *The Gaelic Names of Plants*. Ed. 2. Glasgow: John Mackay.

Campbell, J. L. (1976). Unpublished letters of Edward Lluyd in the National Library of Scotland, *Celtica*, 11: 34–42.

Carmichael, Alexander (1900–71). *Carmina Gadelica: Hymns and Incantations.* 6 vols. (3–4 ed. J. Carmichael Watson, 5–6 ed. Angus Matheson). Edinburgh: Constable (1900); Oliver and Boyd (1940–54); Scottish Academic Press (1971).

Chamberlain [Edith L.] (1882). *A Glossary of West Worcestershire Words.* London: English Dialect Society.

Chamberlain, Mary (1981). *Old Wives' Tales: Their History, Remedies and Spells.* London: Virago Press.

Cockayne, T. Oswald (1864–6). *Leechdoms, Wortcunning and Starcraft of Early England.* 3 vols. London: Longman. [reprinted 1961 by Holland Press]

Coles, William (1656). *The Art of Simpling.* London: Nathaniel Brook.

Colgan, Nathaniel (1892). The shamrock: an attempt to fix its species, *Irish Naturalist,* 1: 95–7.

Colgan, Nathaniel (1904). *Flora of the County Dublin.* Dublin: Hodges, Figgis.

Colgan, Nathaniel (1911). A biological survey of Clare Island in the County of Mayo, Ireland. Part 4. Gaelic plant and animal names, *Proceedings of the Royal Irish Academy,* 31: 1–30.

Collyns, W. (1827). On ... the economical and medical uses to which various common wild plants are applied by the cottagers in Devonshire, *Gardener's Magazine,* 2: 160–2.

Comrie, John D. (1927). *History of Scottish Medicine to 1860.* London: Baillière, Tindall and Cox

Couch, Jonathan (1871). *The History of Polperro.* Truro: W. Lake.

Courtney, M. A. (1890). *Cornish Feasts and Folk-lore.* Penzance: Beare and Son.

Cregeen, Archibald (1835). *A Dictionary of the Manx Language.* Douglas: J. Quiggin.

Dacombe, Marianne R., ed. [1935]. *Dorset Up Along and Down Along.* Dorchester: Dorset Federation of Women's Institutes.

Dalyell, J. G. (1834). *The Darker Superstitions of Scotland.* Edinburgh: Waugh and Innes.

Dartnell, George Edward, and Edward Hungerford Goddard (1894 ['1893']). *A Glossary of Words Used in the County of Wiltshire.* London: Oxford University Press for English Dialect Society.

Darwin, Tess (1996). *The Scots Herbal: the Plant Lore of Scotland.* Edinburgh: Mercat Press.

Davey, F. Hamilton (1909). *Flora of Cornwall.* Penryn: F. Clegwidden.

Davies, Hugh (1813). *Welsh Botanology.* London: privately published.

Davies, W. Ll. (1938). The conjuror in Montgomeryshire, *Collections ... Montgomeryshire,* 45: 158–70.

Deane, Tony, and Tony Shaw (1975). *The Folklore of Cornwall.* London: Batsford.

de Baïracli-Levy, Juliette (1958). *Wanderers in the New Forest.* London: Faber.

de Crespigny, Rose C., and Horace Hutchinson (1895). *The New Forest.* London: John Murray.

Deering, G. C. (1738). *Catalogus Stirpium; or a Catalogue of Plants . . . More Especially About Nottingham.* Nottingham: privately published.

de Grey, Thomas (1652). *The Compleat Horse-man, and Expert Farrier.* Ed. 2. London: H. Moseley.

de l'Écluse, Charles (1601). *Rariorum Plantarum Historia.* Antwerp: J. Moret.

de l'Obel, Matthias (1576). *Plantarum seu Stirpium Historia.* Antwerp: Plantin.

Dickson, Camilla (1991). Memories of a midden mavis—the study of ancient diets and environments from plant remains, *Glasgow Naturalist,* 22: 65–76.

Dickson, Camilla, and James Dickson (2000). *Plants and People in Ancient Scotland.* Stroud: Tempus Publishing.

Dillenius, J. J., ed. (1724). *Synopsis Methodica Stirpium Britannicarum.* Ed. 3. London: Smith.

Doherty, Michael L. (2002). The folklore of cattle diseases: a veterinary perspective, *Béaloideas,* 70: 41–75.

Dony, J. G., S. L. Jury and F. H. Perring (1986). *English Names of Wild Flowers.* Ed. 2. London: Botanical Society of the British Isles.

Dorson, Richard M. (1968). *The British Folklorists: a History.* London: Routledge and Kegan Paul.

Druce, G. Claridge (1897). *Flora of Berkshire.* Oxford: Clarendon Press.

Duddridge, Margaret (1989). West Dorset's mystery saint, *Dorset County Magazine,* no. 131: 50–3.

Duncan, Joan E., and R. W. Robson (1977). *Pennine Flowers.* Clapham, Yorks.: Dalesman Publishing.

Dyer, T. F. Thistleton (1880). *English Folk-lore.* Ed. 2. London: Bogue.

Dyer, T. F. Thistleton (1889). *The Folk-lore of Plants.* London: Chatto.

'E.C.' (1951). Fragments of Oxfordshire plant-lore, *Oxford & District Folklore Society Annual Record,* no. 3: 12.

Edmondson, J. R. (1994). Snuffed out for snuff: *Meum athamanticum* in the Roberts Leyland herbarium, *Naturalist,* 119: 45–6.

Egan, F. W. (1887). Irish folk-lore. Medical plants, *Folk-lore Journal,* 5: 11–13.

Ellis, W. (1750). *The Country Housewife's Family Companion.* London: J. Hodges.

Emerson, P. H. (1887). *Pictures of East Anglian Life.* London: Sampson Low.

Evans, George Ewart (1966). *The Pattern Under the Plough.* London: Faber.

Evans, George Ewart (1969). *The Farm and the Village.* London: Faber.

Evans, John (1940). Folk-medicines, *Collections . . . Montgomeryshire,* 46: 98–9.

Eyre, William L. W. (1890). *A Brief History of the Parishes of Swarraton and Northington.* London: Simpkin; Winchester: Warren.

Fairweather, Barbara (1984). *Highland Heritage.* Glencoe: North Lorn Folk Museum.

Falconer, William (1792). *An Account of the Efficacy of the Aqua Nephritica Alkalina.* London: T. Cadell.

Fargher, D. C. (1969). *The Manx Have a Word for It. 5. Manx Gaelic Names of Flora.* Port Erin: privately published (mimeo).

Fernie, W. T. (1914). *Herbal Simples Approved for Modern Uses of Cure*. Ed. 3. Bristol: J. Wright.

Firth, John (1920). *Reminiscences of an Orkney Parish*. Stromness: J. Rae.

Folkard, Richard (1884). *Plant Lore, Legends and Lyrics*. London: Sampson Low.

Foster, Jeanne Cooper (1951). *Ulster Folklore*. Belfast: H. R. Carter.

Freethy, Ron (1985). *From Agar to Zenry*. Marlborough: Crowood Press.

Friend, Hilderic (1882). A glossary of Devonshire plant names, *Transactions of the Devonshire Association for the Advancement of Science, Literature, and Art*, 14: 529–91.

Friend, Hilderic [1883–4]. *Flowers and Flower Lore*. 2 vols. London: Swan Sonnenschein.

Fuchs, Leonhard (1543). *New Kreüterbuch*. Basel: M. Isingrin.

Gardiner, William (1848). *The Flora of Forfarshire*. London: Longman.

Garner, Robert (1844). *Natural History of the County of Stafford*. London: Van Voorst.

Garrad, Larch S. (1976). Walls, waysides and weeds, *Proceedings of the Isle of Man Natural History and Antiquarian Society*, 8: 27–35.

Garrad, Larch S. (1984). Some Manx plant lore, in Roy Vickery, ed., *Plant-lore Studies* (London: Folklore Society), 75–83.

Garrad, Larch S. (1985). *A History of Manx Gardens*. Douglas: Collector's Choice.

Gepp, Edward (1923). *An Essex Dialect Dictionary*. Ed. 2. London: Routledge.

Gerard, John (1597). *The Herball, or, Generall Historie of Plantes*. London: John Norton.

Gibbs, J. Arthur (1898). *A Cotswold Village*. London: John Murray.

Gifford, Isabella (1853). *The Marine Botanist*. Ed. 3. Brighton: R. Folthorp.

Gill, W. Walter (1932). *A Second Manx Scrapbook*. London and Bristol: Arrowsmith.

Glassie, Henry (1982). *Passing the Time: Folklore and History of an Irish Community*. Dublin: O'Brien Press.

Glyde, John (1866). *The New Suffolk Garland*. Ipswich: Simpkin, Marshall.

Godwin, H. (1975). *The History of the British Flora*. Ed. 2. Cambridge: Cambridge University Press.

Goodrich-Freer, A. (1902). *Outer Isles*. London: Constable.

Gordon, Ruth E. St Leger (1965). *The Witchcraft and Folklore of Dartmoor*. London: Robert Hale.

Grant, I. F. (1961). *Highland Folk Ways*. London: Routledge.

Grattan, J. H. G., and Charles Singer (1952). *Anglo-Saxon Magic and Medicine, Illustrated Specially from the Semi-pagan Text Lacnunga*. London: Oxford University Press.

Green, C. Theodore (1902). *The Flora of the Liverpool District*. Liverpool: D. Marples and Co.

Gregor, Walter (1881). *Notes on the Folk-lore of the North-east of Scotland*. London: Folk-lore Society.

Gregory, [Isabella Augusta], Lady (1920). *Visions and Beliefs in the West of Ireland*. First Series. New York and London: Putnam.

Grigson, Geoffrey (1955). *The Englishman's Flora*. London: Phoenix Press.

Groves, M. J., and N. G. Bisset (1991). A note on the topical use of *Digitalis* prior to William Withering, *Journal of Ethnopharmacology*, 35: 99–103.

Gunther, R. T. (1922). *Early British Botanists and Their Gardens*. Oxford: privately published.

Gutch [Eliza], and Mabel Peacock (1908). *County Folk-lore. Vol. V. Lincolnshire*. London: Folk-lore Society.

Hackwood, Frederick William (1924). *Staffordshire Customs, Superstitions and Folk-lore*. Lichfield: 'The Mercury' Press.

Haggard, Lilias Rider, ed. (1974). *I Walked by Night*. Woodbridge: Boydell Press.

Harland, Elizabeth M. (1951). *No Halt at Sunset: the Diary of a Country Housewife*. London: Benn.

Harris, K. M. (1960). Cures and Charms, *Ulster Folklife*, 6: 65–7.

Harrison, J. W. Heslop (1948). Introduced vascular plants in the Scottish Western Isles, *North Western Naturalist*, 23: 132–5.

Hart, Henry Chichester (1873). *Euphorbia hyberna, Equisetum trachyodon*, etc., in Co. Galway, *Journal of Botany*, 11: 338–9.

Hart, Henry Chichester (1898). *Flora of the County Donegal*. Dublin: Sealy, Bryers and Walker.

Hatfield, Gabrielle (1994). *Country Remedies: Traditional East Anglian Plant Remedies in the Twentieth Century*. Woodbridge: Boydell Press.

Hayward, L. H. (1938). Shropshire folklore of yesterday and to-day, *Folk-lore*, 49: 223–43).

Henderson, D. M., and J. H. Dickson (1994). *A Naturalist in the Highlands: James Robertson, His Life and Travels in Scotland 1767–1771*. Edinburgh: Scottish Academic Press.

Henslow, G. (1905). *The Uses of British Plants*. London: Lovell Reeve.

Herbert, George (1652). *A Priest to the Temple; or the Country Parson, His Character, and Rule of Holy Life*. London: Benjamin Tooke.

Hewett, Sarah (1973). *Nummits and Crummits*. Norwood, Penn.: Norwood Editions.

Hibbert, Samuel (1822). *A Description of the Shetland Islands*. Edinburgh: Constable.

Hodgson, William (1898). *Flora of Cumberland*. Carlisle: W. Meals.

Hole, Christina, ed. (1961). *Encyclopaedia of Superstitions*. London: Hutchinson.

Hooker, W. J. (1830). *The British Flora*. London: Longman.

Hopkins, Mary (1989). *Gloucestershire's Green Heritage*. Winchcombe: Barn Owl Books.

Howse, W. H. (1949). *Radnorshire*. Hereford: E. J. Thurston.

Hughes, Anne (1981). *The Diary of a Farmer's Wife 1796–7*. Ed. 3. Harmondsworth: Penguin Books. [considered by some to be fiction]

Humphries, Steve, and Beverley Hopwood (2001). *Green and Pleasant Land*. London: Channel 4 Books.

Hunt, Robert, ed. (1871). *Popular Romances of the West of England*. London: J. C. Hotten.

Hutchinson, Peggy (c. 1945). *More Home-made Wine Secrets*. London: W. Foulsham and Co.

Ibbott, Selena (1994). *Folklore, Legends and Spells* [of Gloucestershire]. Bath: Ashgrove Press.

Jamieson, Christina (1964). Old cures, *Shetland Folk Book,* 1: 59–60.

Jobson, Allan (1959). *An Hour-glass on the Run*. London: Michael Joseph.

Jobson, Allan (1967). *In Suffolk Borders*. London: Robert Hale.

Jóhansen, Jóhannes (1994). Medicinal and other useful plants in the Faroe Islands before A.D. 1800, *Botanical Journal of Scotland,* 46: 611–16.

Johnson, C. Pierpoint (1862). *The Useful Plants of Great Britain: a Treatise*. London: William Kent.

Johnson, Thomas, ed. (1633). *The Herball or Generall Historie of Plantes*. Ed. 2. London: Islip, Norton and Whitakers.

Johnson, Thomas, ed. (1636). *The Herball or Generall Historie of Plantes*. [Ed. 3]. London: Islip, Norton and Whitakers.

Johnston, George (1829–31). *A Flora of Berwick-on-Tweed*. 2 vols. Edinburgh: Carfrae.

Johnston, George (1849). On the medicinal properties of our geraniums, *History of the Berwickshire Naturalists' Club,* 2: 175–7.

Johnston, George (1853). *The Natural History of the Eastern Borders. Vol. 1. The Botany*. London: Van Voorst.

Jones, Dewi (1996). *The Botanists and Guides of Snowdonia*. Llanwrst: Gwasg Carreg Gwalch.

Jones, T. Gwynn (1930). *Welsh Folklore and Folk-custom*. London: Methuen.

Jones-Baker, Doris (1977). *The Folklore of Hertfordshire*. London: Batsford.

Josselyn, John (1672). *New-Englands Rarities Discovered*. London: G. Widdowes.

'Jude' (1933). *Medicinal and Perfumery Plants and Herbs of Ireland*. Dublin: Gill and Son.

Kent, D. H. (1992). *List of Vascular Plants of the British Isles*. London: Botanical Society of the British Isles.

Kightly, Charles (1984). *Country Voices: Life and Lore in Farm and Village*. London: Thames and Hudson.

Killip, Margaret (1975). *The Folklore of the Isle of Man*. London: Batsford.

Kinahan, G. H. (1881). Notes on Irish folk-lore, *Folk-lore Record,* 4: 96–125.

Kingsley, Rose G. (1917). The flora of Eversley and Bramshill fifty years ago, *Papers and Proceedings of the Hampshire Field Club,* 8: 129–38.

Kirby, Mary (1887). *Leaflets from My Life: a Narrative Autobiography*. London: Simpkin, Marshall.

Knight, Sid (1960). *Cotswold Lad*. London: Phoenix House.

Knights, B. A., et al. (1983). Evidence concerning the Roman military diet at Bearsden, Scotland, in the 2nd century A.D., *Journal of Archaeological Science*, 10: 139–52.

Lafont, Ann-Marie (1984). *Devon's Heritage: a Herbal Folklore*. Bideford: Badger Books.

Lankester, Edwin, ed. (1848). *The Correspondence of John Ray*. London: Ray Society.

Latham, C. (1878). Some West Sussex superstitions lingering in 1868, *Folk-lore Record*, 1: 1–67.

Leask, J. T. Smith (1931). *A Peculiar People and Other Orkney Tales*. Kirkwall: W. R. Mackintosh.

Leather, Ella Mary (1912). *The folk-lore of Herefordshire*. Hereford: Jakeman and Carver; London: Sidgwick and Jackson.

Lightfoot, John (1777). *Flora Scotica*. 2 vols. London: Benjamin White.

Lindsay, W. L. (1853). Medical properties of British ferns, *Phytologist*, 4: 1062–7.

Lisle, Edward (1777). *Observations in Husbandry*. Ed. 2. London: Hitch and Hawes.

Logan, Patrick (1972). *Making the Cure: a Look at Irish Folk Medicine*. Dublin: Talbot Press.

Long, D. J., et al. (2000). The use of henbane (*Hyoscyamus niger* L.) as a hallucinogen at Neolithic 'ritual' sites: a re-evaluation, *Antiquity*, 74: 49–53.

Lousley, J. E. (1964). The Berkshire records of Job Lousley (1790–1855), *Proceedings of the Botanical Society of the British Isles*, 5: 203–9.

Lucas, A. T. (1960). *Furze: a Survey and History of Its Uses in Ireland*. Dublin: Stationery Office.

Mabey, Richard (1996). *Flora Britannica*. London: Sinclair Stevenson.

McClafferty, George (1979). *The Folk Medicine of Co. Wicklow*. Master's thesis, National University of Ireland.

MacCulloch, Mary Julia (1923). Folk-lore of the Isle of Skye, IV, *Folk-lore*, 34: 86–93.

McCutcheon, Alexander (1919). Some Highland household remedies, *Pharmaceutical Journal*, 19 April 1919: 235.

McDonald, Allan (1958). *Gaelic Words and Expressions from South Uist and Eriskay*, ed. J. L. Campbell. Dublin: Dublin Institute for Advanced Studies.

Macdonald, Norman (1961). Notes on Gaelic folklore II, *Journal of Scandinavian Folklore*, 17: 193.

MacFarlane, A. M. (1929). Gaelic names of plants: study of their uses and lore, *Transactions of the Gaelic Society of Inverness*, 32: 1–48.

McGlinchey, Charles (1986). *The Last of the Name*, ed. Brian Friel. Belfast: Blackstaff Press.

McKay, Margaret M., ed. (1980). *The Rev Dr John Walker's Report on the Hebrides of 1764 and 1771*. Edinburgh: John Donald.

MacKerlie, P. H. (1891). *Galloway in Ancient and Modern Times.* Edinburgh and London: Blackwood.

MacNeill, Máire (1982). *The Festival of Lughnasa.* Dublin: University College.

McNeill, Murdoch (1910). *Colonsay: One of the Hebrides.* Edinburgh: David Douglas.

Mactaggart, John (1876). *The Scottish Gallovidian Encyclopaedia; or Curiosities of the South of Scotland.* Ed. 2. London: privately published.

Majno, Guido (1977). *The Healing Hand.* Cambridge, Mass.: Harvard University Press.

Maloney, Beatrice (1972). Traditional herbal cures in County Cavan: part 1, *Ulster Folklife*, 18: 66–79 (part 2 never followed).

Martin, Martin (1703). *A Description of the Western Isles of Scotland.* London: A. Bell. [page references cited are from the widely available 4th edition of 1934 (Stirling: Eneas Mackay), ed. Donald J. Macleod]

Mason, James (1873). The folk-lore of British plants, *Dublin University Magazine*, 82: 313–28, 424–40, 555–70, 668–86.

Meehan, Joseph (1906). The cure of elf-shooting in the north-west of Ireland, *Folk-lore*, 17: 200–10.

Merrett, Christopher (1666). *Pinax Rerum Naturalium Britannicarum.* London: C. Pulleyn.

Moffet, Thomas (1655). *Healths Improvement . . .* , ed. Christopher Bennet. London: S. Thomson.

Moloney, Michael F. (1919). *Irish Ethno-botany and the Evolution of Medicine in Ireland.* Dublin: M. H. Gill and Son.

Monteith, Robert (1711). *The Description of the Isles of Orknay and Zetland.* Edinburgh: privately published.

Moore, A. W. (1898). Folk-medicine in the Isle of Man, *Yn Lioar Manninagh*, 3: 303–14.

Moore, Thomas (1855). *A Popular History of British Ferns.* London: Lovell Reeve.

Morrison, Sophia (1911). A list of Manx plant names, in P. G. Ralfe, *Manx Wild Flowers.* Peel: Peel City Guardian.

Murray, Alexander (1836). *The Northern Flora.* Edinburgh: A. and C. Black.

Neill, Patrick (1805). Remarks made in a tour through some of the Shetland Islands in 1804, *Scots Magazine*, 67: 347–52, 431–5.

Nelson, E. Charles (1991). *Shamrock: Botany and History of an Irish Myth.* Aberystwyth and Kilkenny: Boethius Press.

Newall, Carol A., Linda A. Anderson and J. David Phillipson (1996). *Herbal Medicines: a Guide for Health-care Professionals.* London: Pharmaceutical Press.

Newman, Barbara, and Leslie Newman (1939). Some birth customs in East Anglia, *Folk-lore*, 50: 176–87.

Newman, Edward (1844). *A History of British Ferns.* Ed. 2. London: Van Voorst.

Newman, Leslie F. (1945). Some notes on folk medicine in the Eastern Counties, *Folk-lore*, 56: 349–60.

Newman, Leslie F. (1948). Some notes on the pharmacology and therapeutic value of folk-medicines, *Folk-lore*, 59: 118–35, 145–56.

Newman, L. F., and E. M. Wilson (1951). Folk-lore survivals in the southern 'Lake Counties' and in Essex: a comparison and contrast. Part I, *Folk-lore*, 62: 252–66.

'Ó Clara, Padraig' (1978). The big Mrs. Pearson, *Cork Holly Bough*, Christmas 1978: 35.

Ó Cléirigh, Tomás (1928). Gleanings in Wicklow, *Béaloideas*, 1: 245–52.

Ó Cuív, Brian (1962). Fragments of two mediaeval treatises on horses, *Celtica*, 2: 30–63.

Ó hEithir, Ruarí (1983). *Folk Medical Beliefs and Practices in the Aran Islands, Co. Galway*. Master's thesis, National University of Ireland.

Ó Síocháin, P. A. [1962]. *Aran, Islands of Legend*. Dublin: Foilsiúcháin Éireann.

Ó Súilleabháin, Seán (1942). *A Handbook of Irish Folklore*. Wexford: Educational Co. of Ireland.

O'Toole, Edward (1928). A miscellany of North Carlow folklore, *Béaloideas*, 1: 316–28.

Page, Christopher N. (1988). *Ferns: Their Habitats in the British and Irish Landscape*. London: Collins.

Palmer, A. Smythe (1904). *The Folk and their Word-lore*. London: Routledge.

Palmer, Kingsley (1976). *The Folklore of Somerset*. London: Batsford.

Palmer, Roy (1985). *The Folklore of Leicestershire and Rutland*. Wymondham: Sycamore Press.

Palmer, Roy (1994). *The Folklore of Gloucestershire*. Tiverton: Westcountry Books.

Parkinson, John (1640). *Theatrum Botanicum*. London: Thomas Cotes.

Parman, Susan (1977). Curing beliefs and practices in the Outer Hebrides, *Folklore*, 88: 107–9.

Paton, C. I. (1933). A list of the flowering plants, ferns, and horse-tails of the Isle of Man, *North Western Naturalist*, 8: supplement (1–67).

Payne, Joseph Frank (1904). *English Medicine in Anglo-Saxon Times*. Oxford: Clarendon Press.

Pena, Pierre, and Mathias de l'Obel (1571). *Stirpium Adversaria Nova*. London: Thomas Purefoy.

Pennant, Thomas (1771). *A Tour in Scotland 1769*. London: John Monk.

Pennant, Thomas (1774). *A Tour in Scotland and Voyage to the Hebrides*. Chester: John Monk.

Pennant, Thomas (1776). *A Tour in Scotland and Voyage to the Hebrides, 1772*. Ed. 2. 2 vols. London: Benjamin White.

Pennant, Thomas (1784). *A Tour in Wales*. Ed. 2. 2 vols. London: Benjamin White.

Perring, F. H. (1975). *Symphytum* survey, *Watsonia*, 10: 296–97.

Pickells, W. (1844). On the deleterious effects of *Oenanthe crocata*, *Report of 13th Meeting, British Association for the Advancement of Science*. London: John Murray.

Pigott, B. A. F. (1882). *Flowers and Ferns of Cromer and Its Neighbourhood.* Norwich: Jarrold.

Polson, Alexander (1926). *Our Highland Folklore Heritage.* Dingwall: George Souter; Inverness: Northern Chronicle.

Polwhele, Richard (1816). *The History of Cornwall.* Ed. 3. 5 vols. London: Law and Whittaker.

Polwhele, Richard (1826). *Traditions and Recollections; Domestic, Clerical, and Literary.* 2 vols. London: J. Nichols and Son.

Porter, Enid (1964). Some old Fenland remedies, *Education Today,* July 1964: 9–11.

Porter, Enid (1969). *Cambridgeshire Customs and Folklore.* London: Routledge.

Porter, Enid (1974). *The Folklore of East Anglia.* London: Batsford.

Praeger, R. Lloyd (1909). *A Tourist's Flora of the West of Ireland.* Dublin: Hodges, Figgis.

Pratt, Anne [1850–7]. *The Flowering Plants and Ferns of Great Britain.* 5 vols. London: Society for Promoting Christian Knowledge.

Pratt, Anne [1852]. *Wild Flowers.* 2 vols. London: Society for Promoting Christian Knowledge.

Pratt, Anne [1857]. *The Poisonous, Noxious and Suspected Plants of Our Fields and Woods.* London: Society for Promoting Christian Knowledge.

Pratt, Anne [1859]. *The Grasses, Sedges, and Ferns of Great Britain.* London: Society for Promoting Christian Knowledge.

Purdon, Henry S. (1895). Notes on old native remedies, *Dublin Journal of Medical Science,* ser. 3, 100: 214–18.

Quayle, George E. (1973). *Legends of a Lifetime: Manx Folklore.* Douglas: Courier Herald.

Quelch, Mary Thorne (1941). *Herbs for Daily Use.* London: Faber.

Quincy, John (1718). *Pharmacopeia Officinalis et Extemporanea.* London: A. Bell et al.

Quinlan, F. J. B. (1883a). A note upon the use of the mullein plant in the treatment of pulmonary consumption, *British Medical Journal,* 1883 (I): 149–50.

Quinlan, F. J. B. (1883b). *Galium aparine* as a remedy for chronic ulcers, *British Medical Journal,* 1883 (I): 1173–4.

Randell, Arthur R. (1966). *Sixty Years a Fenman,* ed. Enid Porter. London: Routledge.

Rawlence, E. A. (1914). Folk-lore and superstitions still obtaining in Dorset, *Proceedings of the Dorset Natural History and Antiquarian Field Club,* 35: 81–7.

Ray, John (1670). *Catalogus Plantarum Angliae, et Insularum Adjacentium.* London: John Martyn.

Ray, John (1690). *Synopsis Methodica Stirpium Britannicarum.* London: Samuel Smith.

Read, D. H. Moutray (1911). Hampshire folklore, *Folk-lore,* 22: 292–329.

Reynolds, Sylvia (1993). A botanist's understanding of the names used for native Irish plants in the Schools' Collection, Department of Irish Folklore, *Sinsear,* no. 7: 22–9.

Riddelsdell, H. J., G. W. Hedley and W. R. Price (1948). *Flora of Gloucestershire.* Arbroath: Buncle.

[Roberts, Mary] (1831). *The Annals of My Village.* London: Hatchard.

Robinson, D. (1994). Plants and Vikings; everyday life in Viking Age Denmark, *Botanical Journal of Scotland,* 46: 542–51.

Robinson, F. K. (1876). *A Glossary of Words Used in the Neighbourhood of Whitby.* London: Trübner for English Dialect Society.

Roe, Helen M. (1939). Tales, customs and beliefs from Laoghis, *Béaloideas,* 9: 21–35.

Roeder, C. (1897). Contribution to the folk lore of the south of the Isle of Man, *Yn Lioar Manninagh,* 3: 129–91.

Rollinson, William (1974). *Life and Tradition in the Lake District.* London: Dent.

Rootsey, Samuel (1834). Observations upon some of the medical plants mentioned by Shakspeare, *Transactions of the Royal Medico-botanical Society,* 1832–3: 83–96.

Rudkin, Ethel H. (1933). Lincolnshire folklore, *Folk-lore,* 44: 189–214.

Rymer, L. (1976). The history and ethnobotany of bracken, *Journal of the Linnean Society, Botany,* 73: 151–76.

St Clair, Sheila (1971). *Folklore of the Ulster People.* Cork: Mercier Press.

Salter, Thomas (1849–50). On the cure of epilepsy by the expressed juice of the Cotyledon Umbilicus, *London Medical Gazette,* n.s. 8: 367–70; 10: 1025–7.

Sargent, Maud E. (1908). Irish cures and charms, *New Ireland Review,* 29: 287–93.

Shaw, Margaret Fay (1955). *Folkways and Folklore of South Uist.* London: Routledge.

Sherratt, A. S. (1991). Sacred and profane substances: the ritual use of narcotics in later Neolithic Europe, pages 50–64 in P. Garwood et al., eds., *Sacred and Profane: Proceedings of a Conference on Archaeology, Ritual and Religion.* London: Oxford University Press.

Short, Edward (1983). *I Knew My Place.* London and Sydney: Macdonald.

Short, Thomas (1746). *Medicina Britannica; or, a Treatise on Such Physical Plants as Are Generally to Be Found in the Fields or Gardens of Great-Britain.* London: R. Manby.

Simpkins, John Ewart (1914). *Examples of Printed Folk-lore Concerning Fife, with Some Notes on Clackmannan and Kinross-shire.* London: Sidgwick and Jackson.

Simpson, Eva Blantyre (1908). *Folk Lore in Lowland Scotland.* London: Dent.

Singer, Charles, ed. (1961). Introduction: T. Oswald Cockayne's *Leechdoms, Wortcunning and Starcraft of Early England.* Ed. 2. 3 vols. London: Holland Press.

Smith, Henry (1817). *Flora Sarisburiensis.* London: Wilkie.

Spence, Magnus (1914). *Flora Orcadensis.* Kirkwall: D. Spence.

Spooner, B. C. (1930). Fragments that are left in north-east Cornwall, pages 187–98 in *Papers and Transactions—Jubilee Congress of the Folk-lore Society, 1928.* London: William Glaisher.

Stace, Clive (1997). *New Flora of the British Isles.* Ed. 2. Cambridge: Cambridge University Press.

Stedman, John (1737). Remarks on the external use of tobacco and groundsel . . . , *Medical Essays & Observations* (Ed. 2), 2: 45–8.

Steward, Alexander (1885). *'Twixt Ben Nevis and Glencoe: the Natural History, Legends, and Folk-lore of the West Highlands.* Edinburgh: William Paterson.

Steward, Thomas (1739). The virtues of the star of the earth, *Coronopus,* or buck-shorn plantain, in the cure of the bite of the mad-dog. *Philosophical Transactions of the Royal Society,* 40: 449–62.

Stone, Edward (1763). An account of the success of the bark of the willow in the cure of agues, *Philosophical Transactions of the Royal Society,* 53: 195–200.

Sullivan, D. J., and A. W. Stelfox (1943). Survey of Inishtrahull, II. A list of flowering plants and ferns, *Irish Naturalists' Journal,* 8: 116–23.

Sullivan, W. K. (1873). Introduction, in Eugene O'Curry, *On the Manners and Customs of the Ancient Irish.* 3 vols. London: Williams and Norgate.

Svabo, Jens Christian (1959). *Indberetninger fra en Reise I Færøe 1781 og 1782,* ed. N. Djurhuus. Copenhagen: Selskabet til Udgivelse af Færøske Kildeskrifter og Studier.

Swanton, E. W. (1915). Economic and folklore notes, *Transactions of the British Mycological Society,* 5: 408–9.

Swire, Otta F. (1964). *The Inner Hebrides and Their Legends.* London: Collins.

Synnott, D. M. (1979). Folk-lore, legend and Irish plants, pages 37–43 in E. Charles Nelson and Aidan Brady, eds., *Irish Gardening and Horticulture.* Dublin: Royal Horticultural Society of Ireland.

Tait, Robert W. (1947). Some Shetland plant names, *Shetland Folk Book,* 1: 73–88.

Taylor, Alfred S. (1848). *On Poisons, in Relation to Medical Jurisprudence and Medicine.* London: John Churchill.

Taylor, Francis Edward (1901). *The Folk-speech of South Lancashire.* Manchester: John Heywood.

Taylor, Mark R. (1929). Norfolk folklore, *Folk-lore,* 40: 113–33.

Threlkeld, Caleb (1726). *Synopsis Stirpium Hibernicarum.* Dublin: F. Davys et al.

Tongue, R. L. (1965). *Somerset Folklore,* ed. K. M. Briggs. London: Folk-lore Society.

Townsend, Frederick (1884). *Flora of Hampshire, Including the Isle of Wight.* London: Lovell Reeve.

Trevelyan, Marie (1909). *Folk-lore and Folk-stories of Wales.* London: Elliot Stock.

Tuckwell, W. (1891). *Tongues in Trees and Sermons in Stones.* London: George Allen.

Turner, L., and T. D. Turner (1983). The pharmacy of the physicians of Myddfai, *Pharmaceutical Historian*, 13(2): 2–5.

Turner, William (1548). *The Names of Herbes*. London: John Day and William Seres.

Turner, William (1568). *A New Herball*. Completed edition. Cologne: Arnold Birckman.

Tynan, Katharine, and Frances Maitland (1909). *The Book of Flowers*. London: Smith, Elder.

Udal, John Symonds (1889). Dorsetshire folk-speech and superstitions relating to natural history, *Proceedings of the Dorset Field Club*, 10: 19–46.

Udal, John Symonds (1922). *Dorsetshire Folk-lore*. Hertford: privately published.

Vickery, Roy (1981). Traditional uses and folklore of *Hypericum* in the British Isles, *Economic Botany*, 35: 289–95.

Vickery, Roy (1985). *Sempervivum tectorum* as an abortifacient, *Folklore*, 96: 253.

Vickery, Roy (1995). *A Dictionary of Plant-lore*. Oxford: Oxford University Press.

Wallace, James (1693). *A Description of the Isles of Orkney*. Edinburgh: John Reid.

Walters, S. M. (1991). Ray's butterbur still in Paradise! *Nature in Cambridgeshire*, no. 33: 25–6.

Warner, Joseph (1754). Two letters concerning the use of agaric, as a styptic, *Philosophical Transactions of the Royal Society*, 48(2): 813–18.

Watling, Roy (1974). Prehistoric puff-balls, *B.S.E. News*, no. 14: 12–13; and *Bulletin of the British Mycological Society*, 9: 112–14.

Watling, R., and M. R. D. Seaward (1976). Some observations on puff-balls from British archaeological sites, *Journal of Archaeological Science*, 3: 165–72.

Watson, J. (1775). *The History and Antiquities of the Parish of Halifax*. London: T. Lowndes.

Watson, W. (1746). Critical observations concerning the *Oenanthe aquatica, succo viroso crocante* of Lobel. . . . , *Philosophical Transactions of the Royal Society*, 44: 227–42.

Webb, D. A., and Mary J. P. Scannell (1983). *Flora of Connemara and the Burren*. Cambridge: Royal Dublin Society and Cambridge University Press.

White, James Walter (1912). *The Bristol Flora*. Bristol: John Wright; London: Simpkin, Marshall.

Whitehouse, Sir Beckwith (1941). Fragarine: an inhibitor of uterine action, *British Medical Journal*, 13: 370–1.

Whitlock, Ralph (1976). *The Folklore of Wiltshire*. London: Batsford.

Whitlock, Ralph (1992). *Wiltshire Folklore and Legends*. London: Robert Hale.

Wigby, Frederick C. (1976). *Just a Country Boy*. Wymondham: Geo. R. Reeve.

Wilde, Lady [Jane] (1898). *Ancient Cures, Charms, and Usages of Ireland*. London: Ward and Downey.

Williams, Alfred (1922). *Round About the Upper Thames*. London: Duckworth.

Williams ab Ithel, John, ed. (1861). *The Physicians of Myddvai*. Llanodovery: D. J. Roderic; London: Longman.

Wilson, T. G. (1943). Some Irish folklore remedies for diseases of the ear, nose and throat, *Irish Journal of Medical Science*, 180–4.

Wise, John R. (1863). *The New Forest: Its History and Its Scenery.* London: Smith, Elder.

Withering, William (1785). *An Account of the Foxglove and Some of its Medical Uses* . . . . London: G. G. J. and J. Robinson.

Withering, William (1787–92). *A Botanical Arrangement of British Plants.* Ed. 2. 4 vols in 3. Birmingham: M. Swinney.

Withering, William (1796). *An Arrangement of British Plants.* Ed. 3. Birmingham: M. Swinney.

Withering, William, Jr, ed. (1830). *An Arrangement of British Plants.* Ed. 7. London: Longman.

Wood-Martin, W. G. (1902). *Traces of the Elder Faiths of Ireland: a Folklore Sketch.* Vol. 2. London: Longman.

Woodruffe-Peacock, E. Adrian (1894–7). Lincolnshire folk names for plants, *Lincolnshire Notes and Queries*, 4: suppl. 1–16; 5: suppl. 17–30.

Woodward, Donald, ed. (1982). *The Farming and Memorandum Books of Henry Best of Elmswell, 1642.* London: Oxford University Press.

Wright, Elizabeth Mary (1913). *Rustic Speech and Folk-lore.* London: Oxford University Press.

Yonge, Charlotte M. (1898). *John Keble's Parish: a History of Hursley and Otterbourne.* London: Macmillan.

Unpublished Sources

CECTL MSS—Centre for English Cultural Tradition and Language, University of Sheffield—undergraduate theses (Elizabeth Thompson, 1977; Henry Houston, 1982; Katharine Hamilton, 1988).

Cullum MS—Copy of William Hudson's *Flora Anglica* (ed. 1, 1762) annotated by Sir William Cullum—West Suffolk Record Office.

de Castre, William (1920). *Norfolk Beliefs*: manuscript notes in the Local Studies Department, Norwich Central Library.

EFS—English Folklore Survey. Manuscript notes held at University College London, from work done by the English Literature Department in the 1960s.

Farrelly MS—Undergraduate essay, 1979, 'The folk medicine of north Co. Meath' by Caroline Farrelly—Department of Irish Folklore, University College Dublin.

Garrad MS—Unpublished information communicated to one of the authors (D.E.A.) by Dr Larch S. Garrad.

Hatfield MS—Unpublished data on East Anglian herbal medicines collected by Dr Gabrielle Hatfield—in her personal possession.

IFC S—Irish Folklore Collection, University College Dublin—Schools' Manuscript Collection. This comprises the returns from the Irish Folklore Commission's Schools' Scheme, 1937–8, under which children in 5000 primary schools in all the 26 counties of the Republic of Ireland collected local folklore under the commission's direction and guidance. The herbal medicine material for Co. Cavan was extracted and published by Maloney (1972), and that for the Aran Islands and Co. Wicklow form the subject of postgraduate theses by Ó hEithir (1983) and McClafferty (1979), respectively, held in the college's Department of Irish Folklore. Ó Súilleabháin (1942) and Vickery (1995) also published a scatter of items selected from the collection as a whole at random, and Lucas (1960) drew on it for his monograph on the uses of gorse. For the purposes of the present study, Mrs Sylvia Reynolds in 1991–2 searched 148 out of the total of 1124 volumes, extracting herbal medicine data for every county but in different proportions: the larger counties were covered more fully and Co. Limerick most fully of all. A list of the volumes searched can be provided by the authors on request. Arising out of that work, a guide to the plant names and their attendant ambiguities was also produced (Reynolds 1993) for the benefit of other researchers.

Kermode MS—'Flora Monensis' by P. M. C. Kermode, c. 1900—Manx Museum, Douglas, Isle of Man.

Macpherson MS—Card index of folk remedies compiled in the 1950s by J. Harvey Macpherson—Folklore Society Archives.

Moore MS—Unpublished report, 'Botany of the County of Londonderry 1834–5', produced by David Moore for the Irish Ordnance Survey—herbarium library, National Botanic Gardens, Dublin.

Ó hEithir MS—Undergraduate essay, 1980, 'The folklore of whooping cough in Ireland'—Department of Irish Folklore, University College Dublin.

Parson MS—'Horseheath; some recollections of a Cambridgeshire village' by Catherine E. Parson (1952)—Cambridge County Record Office.

Paton MS—Notes by C. I. Paton in interleaved copy of S. A. P. Kermode's *List of Flowering Plants of the Isle of Man* (1900)—British Herbarium, Department of Botany, Natural History Museum, London.

Taylor MS—'Magic, witchcraft, charm-cures and customs in East Anglia' by Dr Mark R. Taylor (data for a never-published book, collected largely by correspondence, while Regional Medical Officer in Norwich 1920–7)—Norfolk Record Office, MS 4322, 57x1.

Vickery MSS—Folklore data collected by Roy Vickery, partly by correspondence—in his personal possession.

Williams MS—Data collected in the survey 'Folk Medicine in Living Memory in Wales, 1977–89', carried out by Dr Anne E. Williams for the Welsh Folk Museum, Cardiff—in her personal possession (to be drawn on for a book to be published by the University of Wales Press).

Index of Folk Uses

Sambucus nigra, 271
bites, of other animals
  Pinguicula vulgaris, 354
blackhead
  Lamium purpureum, 353
  Urtica spp., 358
black-leg
  Allium ursinum, 350
  Angelica sylvestris, 350
  Euphorbia spp., 352
  Ranunculus spp., 355
  Senecio vulgaris, 356
  Stellaria media, 357
  Taraxacum officinale, 357
bladder stones
  Anthriscus sylvestris? 182
  Palmaria palmata, 45
blasts (facial swellings)
  Bellis perennis, 295
  Senecio aquaticus, 356
  Senecio jacobaea, 356
bleeding, to staunch (see also nosebleeds)
  Achillea millefolium, 95, 301
  Antennaria dioica, 291
  Capsella bursa-pastoris, 120
  Centaurium erythraea, 195
  Cirsium spp., 351
  Equisetum spp., 55, 341
  Fontinalis antipyretica, 40
  Geranium robertianum, 176, 347
  Hedera helix, 180
  Heracleum sphondylium, 190
  Hypericum spp., 104
  Hypericum tetrapterum, 106
  Lamium album, 215
  Larix decidua, 65
  Linaria vulgaris, 253–4
  Lycoperdaceae, 50
  Malvaceae, 108
  Myosurus minimus, 75
  Nuphar luteum, 70
  Osmunda regalis, 58
  Persicaria lapathifolia, 95
  Persicaria maculosa, 95
  Pinus sylvestris, 65
  Piptoporus betulinus, 49
  Plantago spp., 245
  Poaceae: 'grass', 323
  Polygonatum multiflorum, 327

Potentilla anserina, 144
Prunella vulgaris, 222, 223
Ranunculus spp., 71–2
Rumex acetosa, 96
Rumex obtusifolius, 98, 99
Salix spp., 116
Sanicula europaea, 181
Sempervivum tectorum, 135
Sphagnum spp.? 40
Succisa pratensis, 276
Symphytum officinale, 208
Ulmus glabra, 84
Urtica spp., 86
Valeriana officinalis, 274
bleeding, uterine
  Achillea millefolium, 301
blindness
  Teucrium scorodonia, 357
blistering, to induce
  Anemone nemorosa, 71
  Ranunculus spp., 72
  Solanum dulcamara, 199
blisters
  Glechoma hederacea, 221
  linarich, 46
blood, cooling the
  Prunella vulgaris, 223
  Rorippa nasturtium-aquaticum, 118
  Tanacetum vulgare, 223
blood, to purify (see also cleansing of
    system)
  Allium ursinum, 329
  Apium graveolens, 188
  Arctium spp., 96
  Centaurium erythraea, 194
  Conopodium majus, 184
  Laminaria spp., 48
  Menyanthes trifoliata, 203
  Palmaria palmata, 45
  Persicaria bistorta, 94
  Rumex acetosa, 96
  Rumex hydrolapathum, 97
  Rumex obtusifolius, 99
  Scrophularia nodosa, 252
  Senecio vulgaris, 309
  Sorbus aucuparia, 155
  Stachys officinalis, 213
  Taraxacum officinale, 287
  Tussilago farfara, 310

Index of Scientific Names

Index of Vernacular Names

www.ingramcontent.com/pod-product-compliance
Ingram Content Group UK Ltd.
Pitfield, Milton Keynes, MK11 3LW, UK
UKHW021836270225
455667UK00014B/266